P9-DYP-758

649.122 Can 2011

Canadian Medical
Association complete book
of mother & baby

PRICE: $30.00 (3559/he   )

ASSOCIATION
MÉDICALE
CANADIENNE

CANADIAN
MEDICAL
ASSOCIATION

CANADIAN MEDICAL ASSOCIATION
Complete Book of
mother &
baby care

ASSOCIATION MÉDICALE CANADIENNE — CANADIAN MEDICAL ASSOCIATION

Canadian Medical Association
Complete Book of
mother &
baby care

Medical Editor ANNE BIRINGER MD, CCFP, FCFP

3RD EDITION, REVISED AND UPDATED

3RD EDITION

Dorling Kindersley
Senior Art Editor Sarah Ponder
Project Editor Suhel Ahmed
Publishing Manager Anna Davidson
Managing Editor Penny Warren
Managing Art Editor Glenda Fisher
Canadian Editor Barbara Campbell
Canadian Medical Editor Anne Biringer MD,
CCFP, FCFP
Canadian Medical Consultants Morton Goldbach
MD, FRCP(C); Lisa Vesik MEd, RD
UK Medical Consultants Ann Peters RN, HV;
Elizabeth Owen MD, FRCOG, MHPEd; Dr Su
Laurent FRCPCH
Senior Production Editor Jennifer Murray
Senior Production Controller Alice Sykes
DTP Miriam Dangerfield
Category Publisher Peggy Vance

Original Edition Consultants
Catherine Younger-Lewis MD, MJ; M. Shirley Gross
MDCM, CCFP; Sidney Kardash MD, FRCPC;
Mary Krywulak DMD, MS; Charmaine Roye
MDCM, FRCSC

DK India
Editorial Manager Suchismita Banerjee
Senior Editors Saloni Talwar, Neha Gupta
Design Managers Arunesh Talapatra, Ashita Murgai
Senior Designer Navidita Thapa
Designers Neerja Rawat, Akanksha Gupta, Pallavi
Narain, Anchal Kaushal, Rajnish Kashyap
DTP Co-ordinator Balwant Singh, Pankaj Sharma
DTP Designers Tarun Sharma, Jaipal Singh Chauhan,
Nand Kishore, Mohd. Usman, Chetan Singh

The CMA acknowledges the valuable contribution of Health Canada (Consumer Product Safety), the City of
Ottawa Public Health, and St. John Ambulance.

Copyright © 1990, 1995, 2001, 2005, 2011 Dorling Kindersley Limited
Text copyright © 1990, 1995, 2001, 2005, 2011 Elizabeth Fenwick
This Canadian edition Copyright © 2002, 2007, 2011 Dorling Kindersley Limited

Dorling Kindersley is represented in Canada by
Tourmaline Editions Inc.
662 King Street West, Suite 304
Toronto ON M5V 1M7

Publisher's note
Throughout this book, the pronouns "he" and "she" refer to both sexes,
except where a topic applies specifically to a boy or a girl.
The *Canadian Medical Association Complete Book of Mother & Baby Care* provides general information on
a wide range of pregnancy and baby care topics. The book is not a substitute for medical diagnosis, and you
are advised always to consult your doctor for specific information on personal health matters. The naming of
any organization, product, or alternative therapy in this book does not imply endorsement by the CMA or by
the publisher; the omission of any such name does not imply disapproval by the CMA or by the publisher.
Neither the publisher nor the CMA assumes any responsibility for liability arising from any error in or
omission from the book, or from the use of any information contained in it.

All rights reserved. No part of this publication may be reproduced, stored in a retrieval system, or transmitted
in any form or by any means, electronic, mechanical, photocopying, recording, or otherwise, without the prior
written permission of the copyright owner.

Library and Archives Canada Cataloguing in Publication
Canadian Medical Association complete book of mother & baby care /
Anne Biringer, medical editor. -- 3rd Canadian ed., rev. & updated.
Includes index.
ISBN 978-1-55363-154-5
1. Infants--Care. 2. Child care. 3. Pregnancy. I. Biringer, Anne
II. Canadian Medical Association III. Title: Complete book of mother & baby care.
RG525.C34 2011   649'.122   C2010-906172-1

Printed and bound in Toppan, China
See our complete catalogue at
www.dk.com

Introduction

Every year close to 400,000 babies are born in Canada, and if you are reading this book odds are that you were or will be involved in one of those births. Your new baby is lucky. Thanks to advances in health care and in the social programs now available for children, the lives of Canadian babies born today are more than one-third longer than they were just 80 years ago.

However, regardless of the advances we've made, parenting is not an easy job. There's a lot to learn, and many unforeseen events lie ahead of you. Although parents may handle these challenges in different ways, there's often an "easiest" or "best" way available. *Complete Book of Mother & Baby Care* was written to provide you with that "best way."

It offers sensible, user-friendly tips on nutrition, exercise, self-care and baby care, and on getting the most out of medical and obstetric care (including important questions to ask your physician). Best of all, this edition has been completely revised to reflect changes in health and wellness care in early childhood and includes new online resources and updated information in areas such as immunization and prenatal tests. It also features hundreds of beautiful illustrations and clearly written text covering the period from conception to early childhood.

This book is more than a self-help or "how-to" book: it was written and reviewed by health professionals who are experts in the field, and it has the Canadian Medical Association's name – and stamp of approval – on it. It tells parents what they need to know about the way physicians are currently practising obstetrics and pediatrics, about when to call the doctor, and about what to do during an emergency while awaiting medical help.

I hope this practical book helps you at every stage of your pregnancy and delivery, and in providing care for your young child.

Jeffrey Turnbull, MD, FRCPC
President, Canadian Medical Association

Contents

Pregnancy and birth 8–73

Caring for your baby 74–177

Your child's health   178–253

pregnancy
and birth

An illustrated guide to a healthy and happy pregnancy, incorporating practical self-help advice for labour and birth.

Thinking about pregnancy

There are a number of steps you can take to increase your chances of conceiving and giving birth to a normal, healthy baby. Ideally, you and your partner should plan for pregnancy at least three months before you conceive as it is in the first few weeks, when you may not even know you are pregnant, that a baby's development can be most easily affected. Planning for pregnancy gives you the time you need to consider any risks, and, if necessary, to do something positive about them.

Checklist for pregnancy

Use these questions as a checklist if you want to have a baby or you find that you are pregnant. A few may not apply to you, but it's important to ask yourself all of them. Talk to your partner, too, as some of the questions relate directly to him. If you feel worried by any of the points, see your doctor.

Are you immune to rubella?

Rubella, or German measles, can cause serious defects in the baby if you develop it in pregnancy, especially during early pregnancy. At least three months before you start trying to become pregnant, ask your doctor for a blood test to make sure that you are immune. If you are not, he can give you a vaccination.

Have you or your partner a family history of inherited disease?

If either you or your partner has a close relative with an inherited disease there is a chance that it might be passed on to your baby. See your doctor before trying to become pregnant, and if necessary he can refer you to a genetic counsellor who can assess the level of risk that you will be taking. It's reassuring to know that, in many cases, only if both partners carry the gene that causes the disease does the child run a real risk of inheriting it.

Do you have a long-standing medical condition?

If you have a medical disorder, such as diabetes or epilepsy, you should talk to your doctor before trying to become pregnant. Your doctor may want to change your drug treatment, either because the drugs you are on might

affect the baby, or because they might make it more difficult for you to conceive.

If you are on the pill, when should you stop taking it?

It is best to stop taking the pill well before trying to conceive to allow your body time to return to its normal cycle. Wait until you have had three menstrual periods before trying to become pregnant

"At what age are you in the best physical condition to have a baby?"

Q&A

This is probably in your twenties, although more women are deciding to start a family at a later date, when they feel emotionally and financially ready for a baby. Risks of a difficult pregnancy do increase if you are over 35 years old, but this reduces if you lead a healthy lifestyle. The risk of having a Down syndrome baby increases with age. Women under 18 run a greater risk of having a stillbirth or low-birthweight baby, but regular prenatal care and keeping healthy minimize this.

as conceiving during this stage will make it more difficult to predict your baby's due date (find an alternative means of birth control during this time).

Might you be at risk from sexually transmitted infections (STIs)?

Although you will be routinely screened for some sexually transmitted infections once pregnant, such as HIV (see page 36), the most common STI in young women is chlamydia. Although it can be easily treated with antibiotics, unfortunately in about 75 percent of people there are no symptoms. If undetected, it can be transmitted to your baby and lead to possible pregnancy complications, so make sure you ask for a screening test if you think you might be at risk. If you are under 25 and sexually active, you have a one in 10 chance of having chlamydia. If you have had two partners within a year, or recently changed partners, your risk is also increased.

Does your work bring you into contact with any risks?

Your employer has a responsibility to make sure that you are not exposed to any risks in your work that might affect your chances of conception or put your baby at risk. Talk to your employer about carrying

out a specific risk assessment once you notify them that you are pregnant. This should take into account any advice provided by your health professional.

How much do you weigh?
Ideally, your weight should be normal for your height for at least six months before conceiving, so if you are seriously overweight or underweight see your doctor for advice on attaining the right weight. Unless you have a serious weight problem, never diet in pregnancy.

Are you eating healthily?
Your chances of conceiving, and of having a healthy baby, increase if you eat a healthy balanced diet.

Do you smoke or drink?
You and your partner should both stop smoking and drinking as soon as you want to become pregnant – tobacco and alcohol affect fertility and can harm the growing baby before and after birth.

Are you exercising regularly?
To keep fit, aim for at least 20 minutes of exercise each day. Walking and swimming are great before and during pregnancy. If you have concerns about a particular exercise program, speak to your doctor.

Folic acid

From the time you stop using contraception until the 12th week of pregnancy you should take a folic acid supplement. Folic acid, also called folate or folacin, is one of the B vitamins. It is one of the few nutrients that is known to prevent neural tube defects (NTDs) such as spina bifida or anencephaly. The neural tube, which goes on to form the baby's spine, develops very soon after conception, probably even before you realize that you are pregnant. Without sufficient folic acid, the neural tube may fail to fuse completely along its length, exposing the spinal cord and resulting in the condition known as spina bifida. Infants with anencephaly die shortly after birth because a large part of the brain is absent.

Sources of folic acid
Research has shown that an increased intake of folic acid can prevent up to 70 percent of cases of spina bifida.

Good natural food sources of folic acid include dark green leafy vegetables (spinach and broccoli), citrus fruits, legumes (kidney beans, chick peas), wheatgerm, yeast, and egg yolk. Try to eat vegetables lightly steamed or raw. Some foods have also been fortified with folic acid. These include grain products such as bread, rice, pasta, and breakfast cereals.

However, you should not depend on food sources alone. To be on the safe side you should start to take a folic acid supplement as soon as you decide to stop using contraception. Multivitamin tablets often contain some folic acid, but not enough to protect your baby. To reduce the risk of spina bifida, you need to take 0.4 to 1mg of folic acid daily before conception and throughout pregnancy. Tablets can be bought over the counter without a prescription from any pharmacy. If you have had a child with a neural tube defect, or if you have diabetes, epilepsy, or take certain medications, you have a higher risk of having a child with spina bifida. In this instance, your doctor will advise you to take a higher dose (5mg) of folic acid each day.

The developing embryo
Your unborn baby will stand a better chance of developing normally if you take a folic acid supplement. This should be taken before conception and throughout your entire pregnancy.

A pregnancy calendar

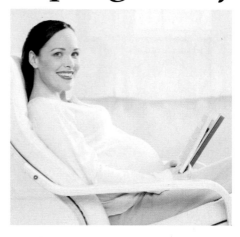

This month-by-month calendar charts the progress of one woman's pregnancy. There is advice on what to do at each stage, as well as reassuring answers to questions and worries you might have. Every pregnancy varies, so don't be surprised if some of the changes described don't happen to you at exactly the same time. The calendar counts day one of pregnancy as the first day of your last menstrual period. So two weeks after conception, you are four weeks pregnant.

Becoming pregnant

If you are thinking of becoming pregnant, check that your lifestyle involves nothing that might harm the baby. All the major organs of his body are formed during the first three months of pregnancy and it is now that his health can be harmed most easily. Once you have conceived you will experience a number of changes, such as heavy breasts or feeling sick. Most of these changes are set off by the increase in hormone levels during the early weeks as your body prepares to nurture and accommodate your baby.

Early signs of pregnancy

One or more of these changes can signify that you are pregnant. You may not notice any of them at first, but still instinctively know you are pregnant because you "feel" different.

● A missed period (amenorrhoea). This is usually one of the first signs of pregnancy, but if your periods are irregular, or you are anxious, busy, or ill, or are underweight, this may not be a reliable guide. It is also possible to have slight bleeding around the time you would normally expect your period, after you have conceived.

● Breasts are enlarged and tender, and perhaps tingle a little. The veins over the surface of the breasts may become more prominent.

● A feeling of deep tiredness, not just in the evening, but also during the day.

● Feeling faint, and perhaps dizzy.

● An increase in normal vaginal discharge.

● Nausea and perhaps vomiting; this can happen at any time of day. Certain odours may make you feel nauseous, particularly cooking smells.

● Some foods taste different from normal, and you may develop a strong dislike of some things, such as alcohol, coffee, and cigarette smoke, and a craving for others.

● Feeling unusually emotional, due primarily to hormone changes.

● A frequent need to urinate, although this may be only in very small quantities.

● A strange metallic taste in the mouth.

Confirming the pregnancy

Two weeks after conception a pregnancy hormone, HCG (human chorionic gonadotrophin), appears in your urine. At this stage, a test of the urine will confirm whether or not you are pregnant. Your doctor or a family planning clinic can test for this hormone in a urine or blood sample. Alternatively, you can buy a home pregnancy testing kit from a drugstore and do the test yourself. Follow the instructions carefully as each test may work slightly differently. Many suggest that you do the test with the first urine you pass in the morning as it contains the highest concentration of hormones.

Calculating your delivery date

Pregnancy lasts about 266 days from conception to birth. The most likely time of conception is when you ovulate. In a normal 28-day cycle this happens about 14 days before the next period is due, so to calculate your approximate delivery date count 280 days (266 plus 14) from the first day of your last period. Remember, this is only a guide. Although the average pregnancy is 40 weeks, a normal pregnancy can last for up to 42 weeks.

Weight gain goals

Optimal weight gain is determined by your pre-pregnancy weight. If you are at a healthy weight (BMI between 18.5 and 24.9), you should aim to gain between 11.5 and 16kg (25–35lb). However, if you are underweight (BMI under 18.5), you should gain more (approximately 12.5–18kg/27½–39½lb) to increase your

A healthy pregnancy
From conception onwards, it is important to avoid ingesting any substance that could harm your unborn baby.

chances of a healthy pregnancy. Likewise, if you are overweight, your weight gain should be limited to between 7 and 11kg (15½–24lb). If your BMI is over 30, you should aim to gain only 7kg (15½lb).

What to avoid

Avoid smoking, alcohol, and any form of medication (unless the medication is confirmed as safe by your doctor) throughout pregnancy, but especially in the first three months when the baby's organs are forming.

Smoking

This deprives the baby of oxygen. Babies of mothers who smoke are more likely to be premature and have a low birthweight. Smoking also increases the chances of having a miscarriage, a stillbirth, a malformed baby, or a baby that dies after birth, so stop smoking completely. If you are having trouble quitting or cutting down, ask your health care provider for help. Passive smoking poses similar risks to your baby's health and could be a factor in causing crib death, so avoid smoky atmospheres when pregnant. If your partner smokes, encourage him to give it up.

Alcohol

There is no known safe level of alcohol consumption in pregnancy. For this reason, it is recommended not to drink at all while pregnant or when planning a pregnancy. Regular excessive alcohol consumption can cause serious harm to the baby and "binge drinking" is particularly dangerous.

Medication

Many drugs can have harmful or unknown effects on your unborn baby, so avoid taking medication in pregnancy unless it is prescribed by a doctor who knows that you are pregnant. This includes many of the remedies you would normally take for minor complaints, such as aspirin. Herbal remedies are sometimes perceived as being safer than pharmaceutical drugs, but many contain powerful active ingredients and all should be avoided without the advice of a qualified medical herbalist. If you need medication to control an existing condition such as diabetes, your doctor may have to alter your dose.

Other risks

Cat and dog feces, and raw or undercooked meat, may contain a parasite called toxoplasma, which can seriously harm the unborn baby. Avoid emptying pet litter trays (if you must, wear rubber gloves and then wash your hands). Wear gloves for all gardening jobs and thoroughly wash all fruit and vegetables before eating to remove any soil. To avoid the risk of listeriosis and salmonella, wash your hands after handling raw meat, and don't eat undercooked meat or fish, raw/lightly cooked egg, soft and blue-veined cheeses, or pâté. Avoid eating shellfish, shark, swordfish, and marlin, which may carry the risk of food poisoning. Refer to page 53 for more on foods to avoid.

The start of life

During the first eight weeks of pregnancy the baby develops from a single cell at conception to a fetus approximately 2.5cm (1in) long, and begins to look human.

Conception to week four

1 Ovulation
Around day 14 of your menstrual cycle, a ripe egg is released from one of your ovaries, and fertilization becomes possible. The egg is caught by the fingers at the end of the Fallopian tube, and drawn into it. The egg can survive for up to 24 hours as it waits to be fertilized. If it isn't fertilized, it passes out of the vagina with the lining of the womb in your next monthly period.

3 The cell divides
The cell starts to divide and carries on dividing into more cells as it travels down the Fallopian tube.

4 Reaching the womb
On about the fourth day after fertilization, the cells reach the womb. They form a ball of about 100 cells with a fluid-filled centre, which produces HCG hormone, and floats about in the cavity for the next few days.

The swim of the sperm

During orgasm, a man may ejaculate between 200 and 400 million sperm into a woman's vagina. Most will perish, but some swim through the mucus secreted by the cervix (the neck of the womb), and cross the womb into the Fallopian tube. If an egg hasn't been released, the sperm can survive in the tube for up to 48 hours.

Position of the womb

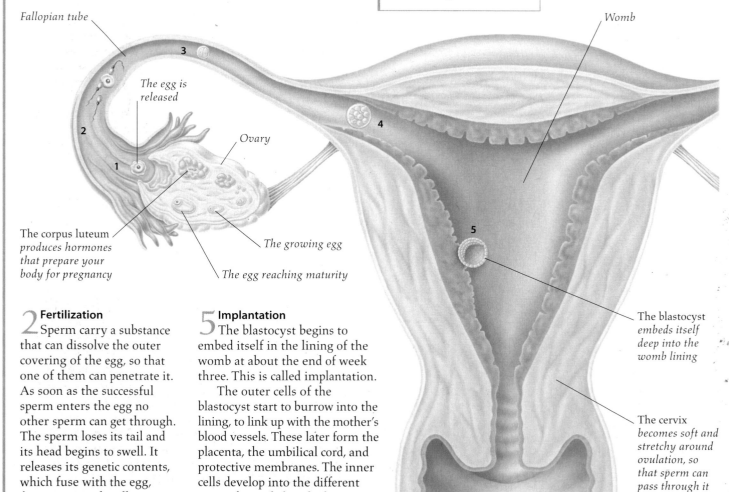

Fallopian tube

The egg is released

Ovary

The corpus luteum produces hormones that prepare your body for pregnancy

The growing egg

The egg reaching maturity

Womb

The blastocyst embeds itself deep into the womb lining

The cervix becomes soft and stretchy around ovulation, so that sperm can pass through it more easily

2 Fertilization
Sperm carry a substance that can dissolve the outer covering of the egg, so that one of them can penetrate it. As soon as the successful sperm enters the egg no other sperm can get through. The sperm loses its tail and its head begins to swell. It releases its genetic contents, which fuse with the egg, forming a single cell.

5 Implantation
The blastocyst begins to embed itself in the lining of the womb at about the end of week three. This is called implantation.
   The outer cells of the blastocyst start to burrow into the lining, to link up with the mother's blood vessels. These later form the placenta, the umbilical cord, and protective membranes. The inner cells develop into the different parts of your baby's body.

About week six

About week seven

About week eight

Weeks five to six

● The embryo is floating in a fluid-filled sac.
● It has a simple brain, spine, and central nervous system.
● Four shallow pits have appeared on the head, which will later become the baby's eyes and ears.
● The embryo has the beginnings of a digestive system, a mouth, and a jaw.
● The stomach and chest are developing. The heart can be seen as a large bulge at the front of the chest; by the end of the week it will start beating.
● A system of blood vessels is forming.
● Protruding buds mark the beginning of the baby's arms and legs.

Length: The embryo is now 6mm (¼in), about the size of an apple seed.

Week seven

● The head looks large and is bent onto the chest. A face is forming, though the eyes are on the sides of the head and still sealed. Black pigment can be seen under the skin overlying the eyes.
● The arms and legs are clearly visible, with clefts at the end, which become fingers and toes.
● The heart starts to circulate blood around the embryo's body.
● The outline of the baby's nervous system is already nearly complete.
● Bone cells are beginning to develop.
● The embryo has lungs, an intestine, a liver, kidneys, and internal sex organs, but none are yet fully formed.

Length: The embryo is now 1.3cm (½in), about the size of a small grape.

Week eight

● The embryo can now be called a fetus, which means "young one."
● All the major internal organs have developed, although they are still in a simple form.
● A face is recognizable: the nose seems to have a tip, the nostrils have formed, and the two sides of the jaw have joined to make a mouth. There is already a tongue.

● The inner parts of the ears, responsible for balance and hearing, are forming.
● The fingers and toes are becoming more distinct.
● The arms and legs have grown longer, and shoulders, elbows, hips, and knees are detectable.
● Nerve cells in the brain are branching to connect with one another to form a primitive neural pathway.
● The baby moves around quite a lot, though you can't feel him yet.

Length: The fetus is now 2.5cm (1in), about the size of an average strawberry.

Twins

Currently, about one in 32 pregnancies results in twins. This figure has increased dramatically since 1974, and it's mainly due to fertility treatments. About 80 to 90 percent of twins will be fraternal, and 10 to 20 percent will be identical.
Fraternal twins occur when two separate eggs are fertilized by two separate sperm. The twins each have their own placenta, may or may not be the same sex, and are no more alike than any other brothers or sisters.
Identical twins are produced when the egg is fertilized and divides into two separate halves, each of which develops into an identical baby. The twins usually share a placenta, are always of the same sex, and have the same physical characteristics and genetic makeup.

"Can I do anything to influence the baby's sex?" **Q&A**

The baby's sex is determined by the man's sperm, which can be either male or female. Research suggests that male sperm do not survive as long as female sperm, so you may increase your chances of having a boy if you make love when you are most fertile (about 14 days before your period is due); and of having a girl if you have intercourse up to three days before you expect to be fertile. It might, therefore, be a good idea to keep a chart of your cycle before you try to get pregnant. None of these techniques have been proven, however.

week 12

The baby looks much more human although his head is still large in proportion to his body, and his limbs, although fully formed, are small. You should find that the discomforts of early pregnancy are beginning to wear off. Make sure you have your first visit with your doctor or midwife and your first ultrasound around now.

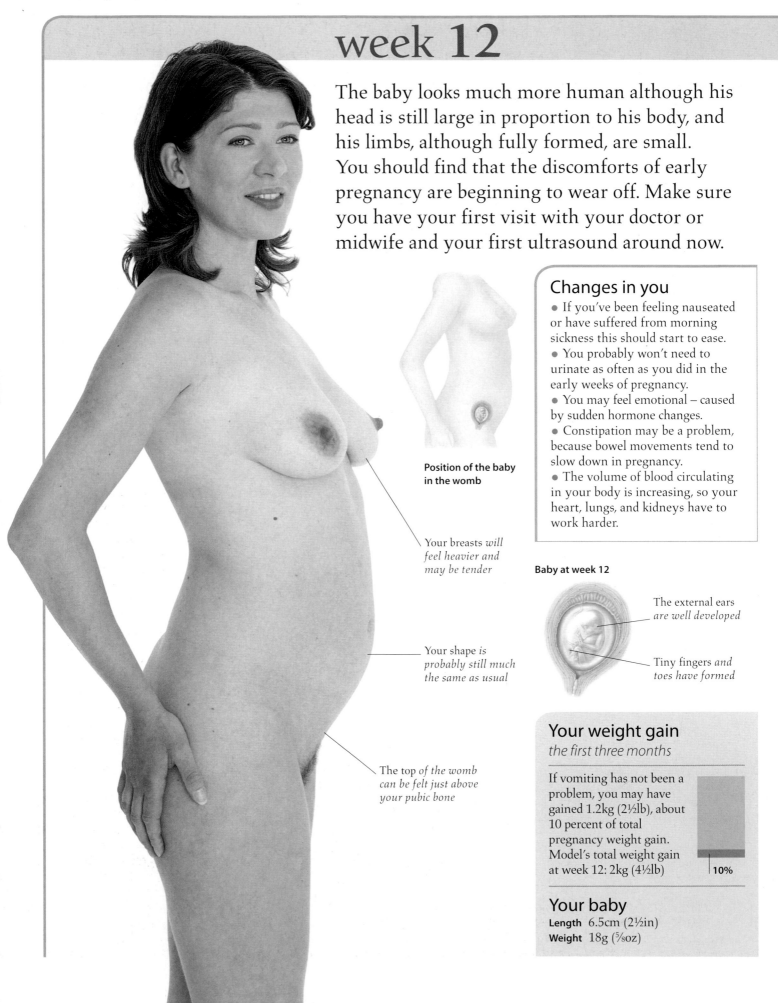

Position of the baby in the womb

Changes in you

- If you've been feeling nauseated or have suffered from morning sickness this should start to ease.
- You probably won't need to urinate as often as you did in the early weeks of pregnancy.
- You may feel emotional – caused by sudden hormone changes.
- Constipation may be a problem, because bowel movements tend to slow down in pregnancy.
- The volume of blood circulating in your body is increasing, so your heart, lungs, and kidneys have to work harder.

Baby at week 12

The external ears *are well developed*

Tiny fingers *and toes have formed*

Your breasts *will feel heavier and may be tender*

Your shape *is probably still much the same as usual*

The top *of the womb can be felt just above your pubic bone*

Your weight gain
the first three months

If vomiting has not been a problem, you may have gained 1.2kg (2½lb), about 10 percent of total pregnancy weight gain. Model's total weight gain at week 12: 2kg (4½lb)

10%

Your baby
Length 6.5cm (2½in)
Weight 18g (⅝oz)

What to do

- Buy a bra that will support your breasts well.
- Check that you are eating a varied diet of fresh foods.
- Guard against constipation by drinking a lot of water and including high-fibre foods in your diet.
- Tell your employer that you are pregnant, so that you can adjust your work schedule.
- Visit the doctor or midwife for your first prenatal check-up.
- You may be offered your first ultrasound scan for dating and screening.
- Find out about insurance benefits and parental leave policies.
- Make an appointment with your dentist for a check-up.
- Find out about prenatal classes in your area.
- Practise prenatal exercises regularly. Go swimming.

Your growing baby

- All of the internal organs are formed, and most are working, so the baby is less likely to be harmed by infections or drugs.
- The eyelids have developed, and are closed over the eyes.
- The baby has earlobes.
- The limbs are formed. Miniature fingernails and toenails are growing.
- Muscles are developing, so the baby moves much more. He can curl and fan his toes. He can make a fist with his tiny fingers.
- He can move the muscles of his mouth to frown, purse his lips, and open and close his mouth.
- He can suck. He swallows the fluid that surrounds him. He passes urine

Prenatal classes

Start thinking about the type of class that will best suit you and your partner. Often you can go to introductory classes now – on ways to keep healthy in pregnancy, for example – and the prenatal classes themselves start eight to 10 weeks before the baby is due. Prenatal exercise classes may continue throughout pregnancy.

Choosing a class

Prepared childbirth classes are run by hospitals, individual instructors, as well as various organizations and local groups such as the YWCA, the community health centre, or (in Quebec) the CLSC. To find one, start by checking the professional advertising section of community newspapers and bulletin boards. Ask your doctor or friends for recommendations. Make sure that you reserve a spot early, even if classes won't begin until you are 28 to 32 weeks pregnant. Most feature a weekly two-hour session, scheduled over a six- to eight-week period. To find the one

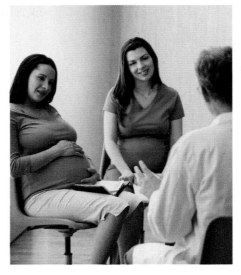

Prenatal class
You will meet trained teachers and other prospective mothers in these classes.

that suits your feelings about pregnancy, labour, and delivery best, you might want to observe a session before you sign up.

What you will learn

Though the course content may vary according to the philosophy of the instructor, all childbirth classes teach couples basic information about pregnancy, the stages and pain of labour and delivery, relaxation techniques, physical exercises, medication and anaesthesia, and everything you might need to know about different hospital procedures and policies. A tour of the hospital is often included. Classes can be invaluable for first-time mothers and fathers, and even in a second or third pregnancy the review is almost always worthwhile. Most emphasize the close working relationship a woman will want to have with the person she chooses to have by her side during the birth, her labour partner. If your baby's father isn't going to be there, a relative or close friend can join in the preparation. Some classes cover the postnatal period and include tips on caring for a newborn, breastfeeding, postpartum depression, and exercises for getting back into shape after the birth.

Tips for labour
Massage is one of the techniques you and your partner may be taught at a prenatal class to help you cope with labour.

week 16

You are now into the second three months of pregnancy and you will definitely begin to look pregnant and start feeling energized. Your baby is fully formed, and has been nourished by the placenta since week 14. Over the remaining weeks he grows and matures so that he is capable of independent life.

Position of the baby in the womb

Changes in you
- You should feel much better.
- There will be a growing feeling of excitement and pleasure.
- Changes in skin pigmentation may occur: your nipples and the surrounding skin may darken, and a dark line (the linea nigra) may appear down the centre of your stomach. This fades soon after birth.
- Your appetite will be increasing as the baby grows.
- Your ordinary clothes will probably be tight, but you may not be quite ready for maternity clothes.

Baby at week 16

His head *looks too large for his body*

His fingers *have their own unique fingerprint pattern*

Your breasts *may still be about their normal size; you will notice them enlarging over the next weeks*

Your bump *starts to show as a gentle rounding of the stomach. You will be starting to lose your waistline*

Moles and freckles *may become darker with the increase in skin pigmentation*

Your weight gain
the second three months

During the next three months you can expect to gain about 5–7kg (11–15½lb), 50 to 60 percent of total pregnancy weight gain. Model's total weight gain at week 16: 2.5kg (5½lb).

60%

Your baby
Length 16cm (6in)
Weight 135g (4¾oz)

What to do

- Give up smoking if you have not already done so and encourage your partner to do the same. Make the living area a smoke-free zone.
- Don't indulge in overeating; eat healthily and watch your weight gain.
- Continue to take iron supplements as prescribed by your doctor. Take supplements on a full stomach.
- Prenatal visits are scheduled once a month now. You may be offered blood tests to screen for genetic abnormalties. Amniocentesis (see page 36–7) can be done now if you are at higher risk of having a baby with abnormalities.

Your growing baby

- The eyebrows and eyelashes are growing, and the baby has fine downy hair on his face and body. This is called lanugo.
- His skin is so thin that it is transparent; networks of blood vessels can be seen underneath.
- Joints have formed in his arms and legs, and hard bones are beginning to develop.
- His sex organs are sufficiently mature for his sex to be evident, but this is not always detectable by an ultrasound scan.
- The baby makes breathing movements with his chest.
- He moves around vigorously, but you probably won't be able to feel his movements yet.
- His heart is beating about twice as fast as your own; the doctor or midwife can hear it with a fetal doppler (a special listening device) after approximately week 14.

See also:

Amniocentesis *pages 36–7*
Eating healthily *pages 50–3*
Relaxation and breathing *pages 48–9*
Skin colour *page 21*
Smoking *page 13*
Supplements *page 52*
Ultrasound *page 36*

Mixed feelings

You and your partner are bound to have mixed emotions about the pregnancy, so don't be surprised if as well as feeling elated and excited, you sometimes feel low. Try to tolerate and understand any negative feelings – they are normal emotions during pregnancy.

Common worries

The best way to dispel any worries you may have about your baby or parenthood is to talk about them frankly with your partner. It also helps to find out as much as you can about pregnancy, so you understand the changes taking place.

You

It's only natural for your feelings of excitement and anticipation to be clouded sometimes by more negative thoughts. You may worry about loving the baby, but once he's born and you get to know each other, love will grow. You may also feel depressed about your changing shape, and even resent the baby for putting your body through such strains. But most major bodily changes disappear after birth, and with some gentle exercising your shape will return.

Your partner

Up to now your partner may have felt left out, and perhaps jealous of all the attention the baby is receiving. However, he or she should now start to feel positive and excited as your baby becomes a reality. If you are worried about money and having enough to support your new family, try to plan and budget.

Non-traditional families

There are many ways to make a family, not all of which involve a man and a woman. The new baby may have two mothers or two fathers. Some women parent alone, either by circumstance or by choice. Regardless of your social situation, you should surround yourself with friends and family, who will act as your support network. You can even get in touch with organizations for similar families that offer support and advice throughout pregnancy and after the birth.

"How can I be sure the baby will be all right?" Q&A

The chances of the baby being abnormal are very small. Most abnormalities occur in the first few weeks, and usually end in an early miscarriage. By week 13, the baby is fully formed and from then on very little can go wrong. If you check that your lifestyle involves nothing that could harm him, you can reduce the risk still further.

week 20

You will probably have a strong sense of well-being and may look and feel radiant during the middle months of pregnancy. If you're feeling well, it's often a good idea to take a holiday. By now you will be able to feel the baby move, and a second ultrasound scan will check that he is growing normally.

Your nipples become darker during pregnancy

Position of the baby in the womb

Changes in you

● Skin pigmentation may be more noticeable, but will fade after birth.
● Your breasts may produce colostrum, a thin cloudy substance that provides all your baby needs in the first days after birth.
● You may be suffering from some of the common problems of pregnancy, such as bleeding gums and an increase in vaginal discharge. The joints and ligaments of your body have relaxed, so you are more likely to suffer from back trouble and other aches and pains.

Your breasts will have probably increased dramatically in size by now

Baby at week 20

His legs are in proportion to the rest of his body

The baby can grip firmly with his hands

The top of the womb is level with your navel

You will first feel your baby's movements as a faint fluttering inside your abdomen, like bubbles rising

Your weight gain
at around week 20 of pregnancy

During this month you should gain about 0.5kg (1lb) a week. Take extra care to eat healthily now: the next few weeks is the period of maximum growth for the baby. Model's weight gain to date: 3kg (6½lb)

Your baby
Length 25cm (10in)
Weight 340g (12oz)

What to do

- Make sure you are holding yourself well, and that you avoid overstretching or straining your back. Wear low-heeled shoes.
- Take the practical steps suggested on pages 40–2 to relieve any other discomforts that you may have.
- Start to think about essential clothes and equipment for the baby.

"Is a long journey advisable?" Q&A

There's usually no reason why you shouldn't travel in pregnancy, but preferably not on your own, especially on a long car journey. Wear loose, comfortable clothes, and break the journey up by walking around for a few minutes at least every two hours, to help your circulation. Stay hydrated and carry healthy snacks to maintain blood sugar levels. Always remember to take your pregnancy record with you.

Your growing baby

- Hair appears on the baby's head.
- Teeth are developing.
- Vernix, the white and greasy substance that protects the baby's skin in the womb, forms.
- The baby's arms and legs are well developed.
- Your own antibodies will be transferred to the baby through your blood to help him resist disease in the first weeks after birth.
- The baby is very active; you should have felt his movements for the first time as a faint fluttering. He may even react to noises outside the womb, but don't worry if he doesn't move around much – it's fairly common for babies to have a quiet period now.

See also:
Common complaints *pages 40–2*
Eating healthily *pages 50–3*
Essentials for the baby *page 27*
Protecting your back *page 44*

Looking good

You may look and feel your best during the middle months of pregnancy, with lustrous hair, rosy cheeks, and healthy skin, but not everyone blooms; the high hormone levels can have less flattering effects on your skin, nails, and hair, though any adverse changes usually disappear after giving birth.

Your hair
Your hair may seem thicker during pregnancy. This is due to higher hormone levels causing the hair to stay in its active growing phase for longer.

Hair

Thick, shiny hair is often a bonus of pregnancy. However, not all hair improves, and greasy hair may become more oily, and dry hair, drier and more brittle, so that you may seem to lose more hair than usual. Facial and body hair also tends to darken.

What to do
If your hair is dry and splits easily, use a mild shampoo and conditioner, and don't brush it too often or too vigorously. Wash greasy hair frequently to keep it shiny. As hair texture is so unpredictable during pregnancy, avoid having your hair coloured too often – colouring it occasionally throughout your pregnancy should be fine. However, if you have any concerns about the chemicals, it is best to check with your health professional first.

Skin texture

Your skin will probably improve in pregnancy: the blemishes disappear, and skin texture becomes smooth and silky. However, you may find that your skin becomes very dry, or greasy, and perhaps spotty.

What to do
Cleanse your skin thoroughly. If it is dry, gently rub moisturizer over the dry areas, and add bath oil to your bath water. Use as little soap as possible.

Skin colour

An increase in skin pigmentation is normal during pregnancy. Moles, birthmarks, scars, and especially freckles usually darken and grow in size, and a brown line often appears on the stomach. You may also notice a brownish patch, or "butterfly mask," across your face and neck. Don't worry, as this disappears soon after the birth.

What to do
Avoid strong sunlight as this makes pigmentation worse, but if you have to go out in the sun, use sun cream with a strong UV filter, cover up exposed skin, and wear a hat. Don't bleach the "butterfly" mask; if you want to disguise it, use a skin-blemish covering stick.

Nails

You may notice that your nails split and break more easily than usual.

What to do
Wear protective gloves for household chores and gardening.

week 24

This is often the best month of pregnancy. You will probably look well and feel happy and contented. If you have not been gaining weight very rapidly so far, you may put on a lot this month. You will start to appear visibly pregnant.

Your face *may look rather puffy because your body holds extra water*

Your areolas, *the dark areas around your nipples, may become more prominent*

Your bump *is enlarging rapidly*

Extra weight *on your thighs and upper body may be the result of your body retaining water, so it won't be permanent*

Position of the baby in the womb

Changes in you

● It's quite common to experience sudden gain in weight around this month or the following one.
● You may find that loose-fitting, unrestricting clothes are more comfortable from now until the end of your pregnancy.
● Sweating may be a problem because you tend to feel the heat more. Make sure you drink plenty of water, and try to avoid wearing any synthetic materials.

Baby at week 24

His eyes *appear to bulge because his face is thin*

His skin *is becoming thicker*

Your weight gain
at around week 24 of pregnancy

You will probably gain weight at the rate of about 0.5kg (1lb) a week; if you were underweight when your pregnancy began you might gain at a faster rate than this. Model's weight gain to date: 4.5kg (10lbs)

Your baby
Length 33cm (13in)
Weight 570g (1¼lb)

What to do

- If you have flat or inverted nipples and you want to breastfeed, you should be able to do so; talk to your doctor or midwife.
- Rest as much as possible during the day.
- Continue to exercise gently, but regularly. Practise relaxation and breathing exercises.
- As your uterus gets bigger, you may feel dizzy lying on your back. Roll onto your side and position yourself with pillows for comfort.
- By now you will have seen an image of your baby on the anatomy ultrasound scan.

"What is the best kind of bra?" **Q&A**

To give your breasts the support they need in pregnancy, choose a bra (preferably cotton) with a deep band under the cups, broad shoulder straps, and an adjustable back that gives you support all the way round. Check your size regularly, as your breasts will continue to swell throughout pregnancy. By full term, you may need a cup two sizes larger than usual. If your breasts become very heavy, wear a lightweight bra at night.

Your growing baby

- No fat has been laid down yet, so the baby is still lean.
- The sweat glands are forming.
- Arm and leg muscles are well developed, and the baby tries them out regularly. He has periods of frenzied activity, when you feel him moving around, alternating with periods of calm.
- The baby can cough and hiccup; you may feel the hiccups as a knocking movement.

See also:
Prenatal exercises *pages 45–7*
Pregnancy clothes *page 25*
Relaxation and breathing *pages 48–9*

The baby in the womb

While your baby is developing physically, he is also becoming an aware, responsive person with feelings. He lies tightly curled up in the womb, cushioned by the amniotic fluid that surrounds him. He is entirely reliant on your placenta for food and oxygen, and for the disposal of his waste products. However, he looks and behaves much the same as a baby at birth.

Sight
His eyelids are still sealed, but by week 28 they become unsealed, and he may see, and open and close his eyes.

Hearing
He can hear your voice, and if he's asleep can be woken by loud music. He may prefer some types of music, and show this by his movements. He jumps at sudden noises.

Facial expressions
He frowns, squints, purses his lips, and opens and closes his mouth. He smiles, too.

Life-support system
The baby is nourished by the placenta and protected by warm amniotic fluid, which can change every four hours. It regulates the baby's temperature, and protects against infection and sudden bumps.

Movements
He kicks and punches, and sometimes turns somersaults.

Sleeping patterns
He sleeps and wakes randomly, and will probably be most active when you are trying to sleep.

Personality
The part of the brain concerned with personality and intelligence becomes far more complex during the seventh month, so your baby's personality may soon be developing.

Sucking, swallowing, and breathing
He sucks his thumb, and swallows the warm water (the amniotic fluid) that surrounds him, passing it out of his body as urine. Sometimes he drinks too much of the fluid and hiccups. He makes breathing movements with his chest, practising for life outside the womb.

Taste
His taste buds are forming, and by week 28, he can respond to sweet, sour, and bitter tastes.

The placenta supplies all the nutrients the baby needs; almost anything entering your body, good or bad, is filtered through to him.

The umbilical cord, a rope of three blood vessels, links the placenta to the baby.

week 28

With only three months of pregnancy left to go, you may be starting to feel large and clumsy, and perhaps forgetful. During the last months your baby lays down fat stores. He is very active, and you may even be able to see him moving around.

Stand tall and avoid arching your back as you grow larger

Position of the baby in the womb

Changes in you

● You may be troubled by heartburn, indigestion, and cramps.
● You may notice red stretchmarks on your stomach.
● You may sometimes feel faint Braxton Hicks, or false, contractions.
● You may be having vivid dreams about the birth and the baby. This is quite normal. These dreams do not indicate that there is anything wrong with the baby.

Baby at week 28

The veins on your breasts will probably become more noticeable during pregnancy

His face and body are covered with vernix, which waterproofs the skin

His eyes have become unsealed

Hearing is well developed

The top of the womb is about halfway between your navel and breastbone

Your weight gain
the third three months

During the final months you will probably gain about 4kg (9lbs), 30 percent of total pregnancy weight gain. Model's total weight gain at week 28: 9kg (19lbs)

30%

Your baby
Length 37cm (14½in)
Weight 900g–1kg (2–2¼lb)

Weight gain can be on your buttocks and thighs, as well as your stomach

What to do

- Make sure you are getting enough rest during the day and at night.
- Be aware of baby's movements. Ask your care provider how they recommend monitoring fetal movements.
- If you are still working full-time, meet with the human resources department to discuss your plans. Some women continue to work until labour, while others need time to prepare and rest at home before the birth. Inform your employer in writing when you intend to stop work, and if you're planning to go back after the baby is born.
- Prenatal visits are every two weeks from now until week 36. At this visit you may have blood tests for anemia, gestational diabetes, and antibodies.
- If you're planning a trip involving air travel, check with your doctor, the airline, and your insurance company.

Your growing baby

- His skin is red and wrinkled, but fat starts to accumulate beneath it.
- There have been dramatic developments in the thinking part of the brain, which becomes bigger and more complex. A seven-month-old baby can feel pain, and responds in much the same way as a full-term baby.
- The baby has far more taste buds than he will have at birth, so his sense of taste is acute.
- His lungs are still not mature, and need to develop a substance called surfactant, which stops them collapsing between each breath.
- The baby's heartbeat can be heard distinctly, using either a fetal stethoscope or a Doppler ultrasound device.
- A baby born now could survive, given special care.

See also:
Common complaints *pages 40–2*
Protecting your back *page 44*
Stretchmarks *page 42*

Your pregnancy wardrobe

Up to five or even six months of your pregnancy, many of your normal clothes may be wearable if they fit loosely or you use a little creativity. However, a few new outfits may greatly improve your morale and you don't have to buy special maternity wear. Look for clothes that are attractive, comfortable, and easy to care for.

Comfortable tops
Go for stretchy fabrics in soft natural fibres.

Choose a style with plenty of room across the chest to accommodate your growing breasts

Loose-fitting bottoms
Pants with special stretch panels or thick elastic waistbands are comfortable and unrestricting; they are convenient because they expand as your bump grows.

Dressing up
A simple dress can look casual, but is also easy to dress up. Check that there's enough length in the hem so the dress hangs evenly as you grow larger. Maternity dresses are usually 2.5cm (1in) longer at the front to allow for this.

What to choose

You tend to feel the heat more during pregnancy, so look for lightweight, loose-fitting clothes, made of cotton or other natural fibres. If it's cold, put on several layers. Avoid anything that is tight around the waist or that restricts blood flow in your legs, such as tight knee-high socks.

Comfortable, low-heeled shoes are essential. You probably won't be able to wear lace-ups soon, as you will have difficulty bending down to tie them. Your shoe size may even change.

A versatile fabric will stretch to fit your changing shape

week 32

You need all the rest you can get, so try to lie down in the middle of the day. You will probably be feeling weary of your pregnant state. Now is the time to start going to childbirth classes, which will run until the end of your pregnancy.

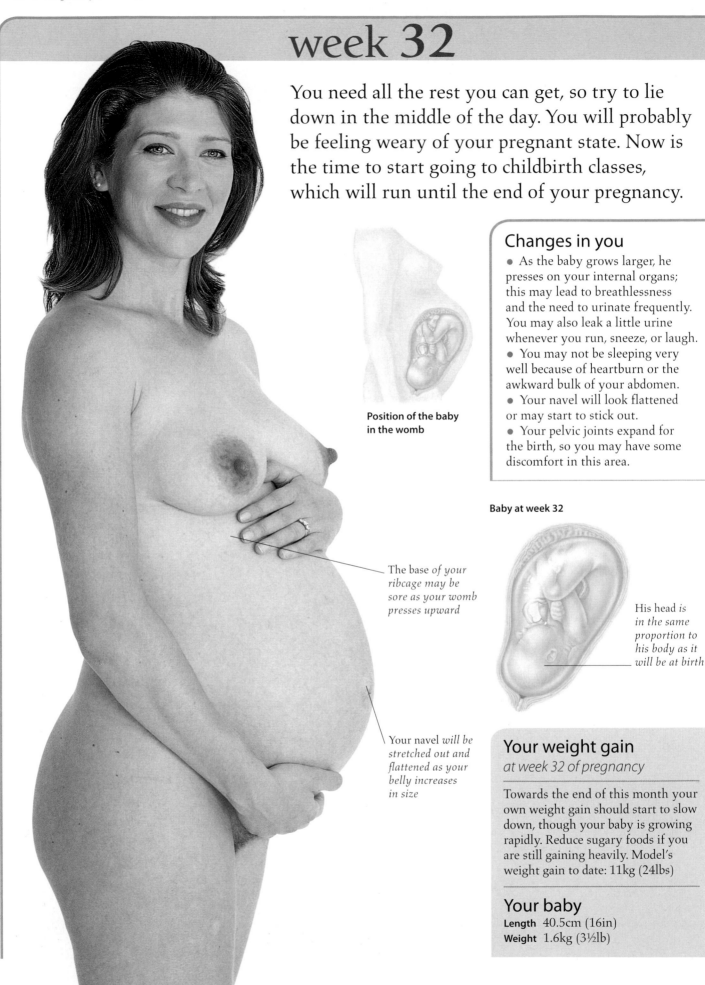

Position of the baby in the womb

Changes in you

● As the baby grows larger, he presses on your internal organs; this may lead to breathlessness and the need to urinate frequently. You may also leak a little urine whenever you run, sneeze, or laugh.
● You may not be sleeping very well because of heartburn or the awkward bulk of your abdomen.
● Your navel will look flattened or may start to stick out.
● Your pelvic joints expand for the birth, so you may have some discomfort in this area.

Baby at week 32

The base *of your ribcage may be sore as your womb presses upward*

His head is in the same proportion to his body as it will be at birth

Your navel *will be stretched out and flattened as your belly increases in size*

Your weight gain
at week 32 of pregnancy

Towards the end of this month your own weight gain should start to slow down, though your baby is growing rapidly. Reduce sugary foods if you are still gaining heavily. Model's weight gain to date: 11kg (24lbs)

Your baby
Length 40.5cm (16in)
Weight 1.6kg (3½lb)

What to do
- Break up the day by putting your feet up for an hour or two, if possible.
- If you have difficulty sleeping, practise relaxation techniques before going to bed, and try sleeping on your side, with one leg bent and supported on a pillow. Try not to worry if you still can't sleep; it's very normal to be wide awake at night during this stage of pregnancy.
- Keep up with your pelvic floor exercises; especially if you are suffering from leaking urine.
- Start attending prenatal classes if they haven't begun already.
- Your prenatal visit will include a thorough review of screening tests performed at 28 weeks.

Q&A
"I'm worried about harming the baby during intercourse. Is there any danger of this?"
This is a common worry but an unnecessary one if your pregnancy is normal. The baby is cushioned by the bag of fluid surrounding him, so he cannot be harmed when you make love. The doctor or midwife will tell you if there is any danger, such as a low-lying placenta.

Your growing baby
- The baby looks much the same as he will at birth, but his body still needs to fill out more.
- He can now sense the difference between light and dark.
- Because there is less room in the womb, he will probably have turned into a head-down position by now, ready for birth.

See also:
Prenatal classes *page 17*
Breathlessness *page 40*
Frequent urination *page 41*
Pelvic floor *page 45*
Relaxation techniques *pages 48–9*

Essentials for your baby

Buy the following basic equipment and clothing for your new baby, then add anything else you need when he's born.

Equipment
Buy new equipment if you can. Check second-hand items carefully to ensure they are safe. You will need:
- a crib or bassinet
- appropriate bedding
- a soft blanket
- an infant car seat, if you have a car
- a baby bath
- two soft towels
- changing mat or table
- diapers and changing equipment
- bottle-feeding equipment (if you are going to bottle-feed and as a back-up if you are breastfeeding).

Clothes
Buy a minimum number of "newborn" clothes – your baby will grow fast. You will need:
- undershirts
- stretchsuits
- sweaters
- infant sleeping or drawstring gowns
- soft socks or booties
- sun hat or warm hat.

Enjoying sex

Making love is often particularly enjoyable during pregnancy because you become aroused more easily as a result of the increase in hormone levels, and there are no worries about contraception.

Other ways of loving
There may be times when you lose interest in sex, especially in the first and last weeks. This doesn't mean that you have to stop showing your loving feelings for each other. Even if you feel too tired or heavy to make love, you can find other ways of showing your affection, such as kissing, cuddling, stroking, and touching.

A change of position
In the last weeks of pregnancy, you may find the traditional man-on-top position rather uncomfortable. Experiment with other positions; perhaps sitting on your partner's lap, kneeling with him behind, or both lying side by side.

week 36

By now you may have stopped work. You may be longing for the pregnancy to be over, yet feel apprehensive about the birth and becoming a parent. The baby takes up all the space in the womb, so he kicks and punches rather than shifts his whole body.

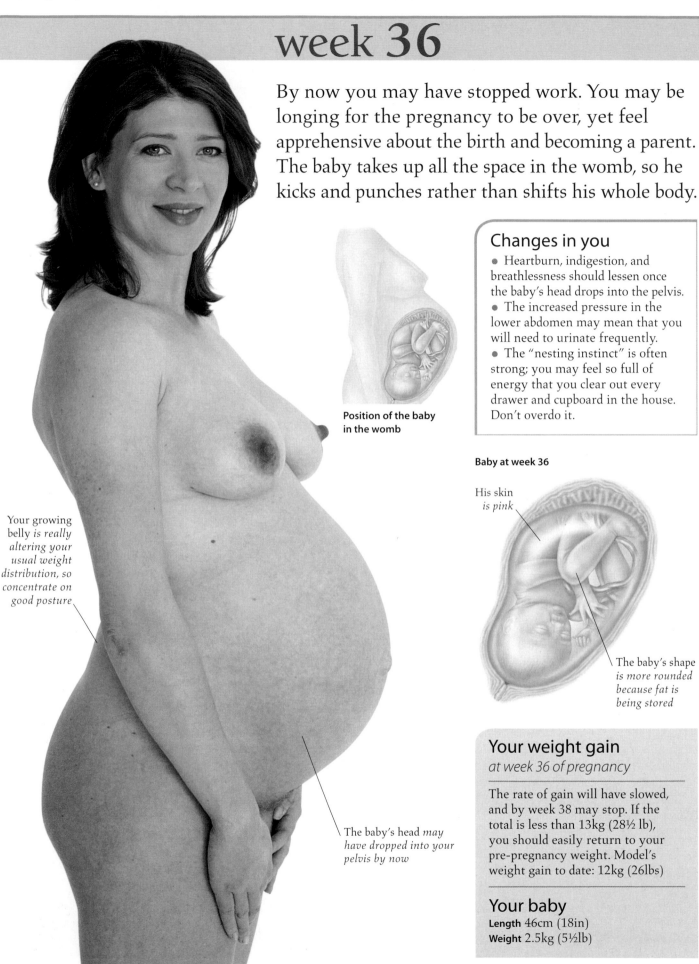

Position of the baby in the womb

Changes in you

- Heartburn, indigestion, and breathlessness should lessen once the baby's head drops into the pelvis.
- The increased pressure in the lower abdomen may mean that you will need to urinate frequently.
- The "nesting instinct" is often strong; you may feel so full of energy that you clear out every drawer and cupboard in the house. Don't overdo it.

Baby at week 36

His skin *is pink*

The baby's shape *is more rounded because fat is being stored*

Your growing belly *is really altering your usual weight distribution, so concentrate on good posture*

The baby's head *may have dropped into your pelvis by now*

Your weight gain
at week 36 of pregnancy

The rate of gain will have slowed, and by week 38 may stop. If the total is less than 13kg (28½ lb), you should easily return to your pre-pregnancy weight. Model's weight gain to date: 12kg (26lbs)

Your baby
Length 46cm (18in)
Weight 2.5kg (5½lb)

What to do

- Put your feet up whenever you can to guard against swollen ankles and varicose veins.
- Prenatal visits are weekly now.
- If you are having your baby in hospital, take a tour of the delivery room and maternity area.
- Buy your nursing bras.
- Stock the food cupboards for when you return from the hospital. If you have a freezer, take this opportunity to make nutritious, freezable meals that you can have after the baby is born.
- Pack your suitcase for hospital; if you are having a home birth, assemble all the things you need.

Q&A

"Should I have my partner with me during labour?"

Labour can be a long process, and a rather lonely one unless you have someone to share it with, and a natural choice is your partner, whose presence can be beneficial for both. But if this isn't possible, having a relative or a friend as a companion can be very reassuring.

Your growing baby

- If this is your first baby, his head will probably have descended into the pelvis ready for birth.
- Soft nails have grown to the tips of his fingers and toes.
- In a boy, the testicles should have descended.
- The baby will gain about 28g (1oz) every day from now onwards

See also:
Plan for baby's arrival *page 27*
Frequent urination *page 41*
Preparing for the birth *pages 54–5*
Protecting your back *page 44*
Relaxation techniques *pages 48–9*
Swollen ankles *page 42*
Varicose veins *page 42*

Resting in later pregnancy

During the last weeks, you will probably get tired very easily. You may not be sleeping as well as usual, and you will also feel exhausted by the extra weight you are carrying around.

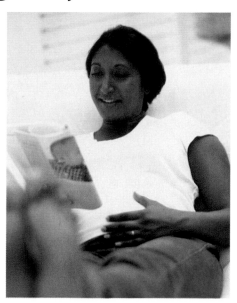

Avoid tiring yourself

Put your feet up whenever you need to during the day. Think of quiet things to do when you rest: practise relaxation exercises, listen to soothing music, read a book, or perhaps knit something for the baby. It also helps if you try to do things at a slower pace than usual, so that you don't overexert yourself.

Your nursing bra

If you want to breastfeed, you will need at least two plain cotton nursing bras with firm support straps. To make sure these are the right size, it's best to buy them no earlier than week 36.

What to look for

There are two main types of bra: one has flaps, which open to expose the nipple and some of the surrounding breast; the other fastens at the front, so you can expose the whole breast. The front-opening kind is best, as it allows the baby to feel and fondle the breast while he's sucking. It also allows the milk to flow freely.

Measuring up

Take the measurements while wearing one of your ordinary pregnancy bras.

1 Measure around your body below your breasts. Add 12cm (5in) to get your final chest measurement.

2 Measure around the fullest part of your breasts. If this equals your chest measurement, you need an A cup. If it is 2.5cm (1in) more, you need a B cup. If it is 5cm (2in) more, you need a C cup. Alternatively, you can opt to get fitted in a store specializing in maternity bras. In fact, professional fitting is often the best option.

week 40

By this stage, you will feel very ungainly and will be bumping into objects because of your size. You will be impatient to give birth, but also excited and relieved that you are nearly there. Rest as much as possible, and enjoy these last baby-free days.

Changes in you

- You will have a feeling of heaviness in your lower abdomen.
- Your cervix will be softening in preparation for labour.
- Braxton Hicks contractions may be so noticeable that you think you are in labour, but they won't be regular.

Your weight gain
at week 40 of pregnancy

In the final two weeks, you may actually lose a little weight. This is a sign that your baby is fully mature, and you can expect labour to start within 10 days. Model's weight gain is negligible from week 36 onwards.

Your baby
Length 51cm (20in)
Weight 3.4kg (7½lb)

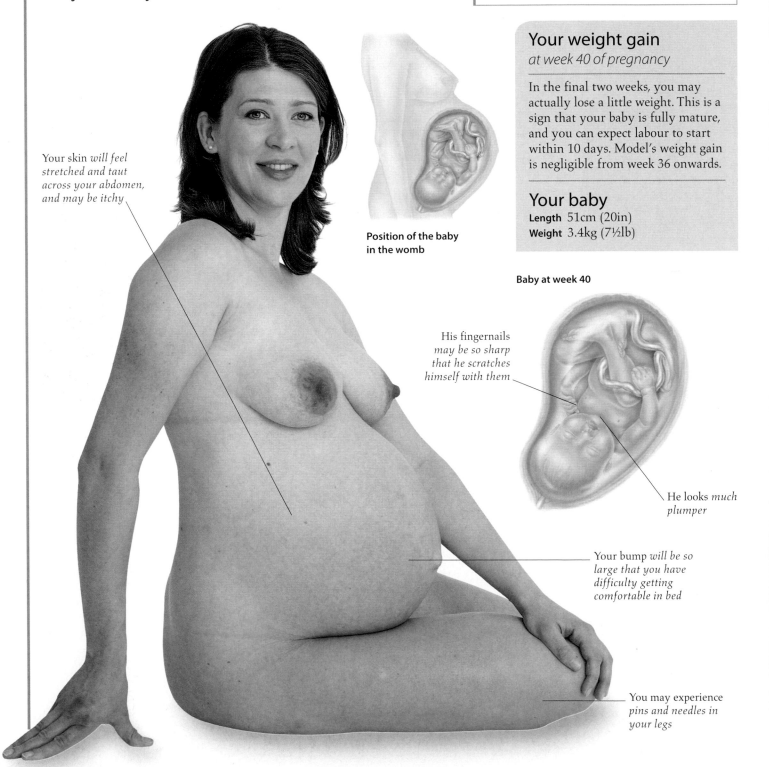

Your skin *will feel stretched and taut across your abdomen, and may be itchy*

Position of the baby in the womb

Baby at week 40

His fingernails *may be so sharp that he scratches himself with them*

He looks *much plumper*

Your bump *will be so large that you have difficulty getting comfortable in bed*

You may experience *pins and needles in your legs*

What to do

- Continue to monitor baby's movements. If you don't feel at least six movements within two hours, call your doctor or midwife immediately.
- If the Braxton Hicks contractions are stronger and more frequent, practise your breathing.
- Don't worry if your baby doesn't arrive on time – it's perfectly normal for a baby to be born up to two weeks either side of the expected delivery date.

Total weight gain

The average amount of weight gain during pregnancy varies between 10 to 12kg (22–27lbs), but you may put on more or less weight. The total weight gain is made up as follows:

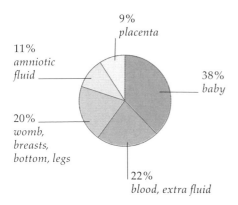

9%
placenta

11%
amniotic fluid

38%
baby

20%
womb, breasts, bottom, legs

22%
blood, extra fluid

Your growing baby

- Most of the lanugo hair (soft prenatal hair) has disappeared, though there may still be a little over his shoulders, arms, and legs.
- He may be covered in vernix, or just have traces in skin folds.
- A dark substance called meconium gathers in the baby's intestines; this will be passed in his first bowel movement after birth.
- If this is your second or later baby, his head may engage now.

See also:
Braxton Hicks contractions *page 56*
Breathing techniques *page 49*

Becoming a mother

After all the weeks of preparation and planning, you are fully ready to give birth. Afterwards, you can hold your baby in your arms. You will probably feel overwhelmingly protective towards this tiny person, who is dependent on you for everything.

The first weeks

Life in the early weeks following the arrival of your baby revolves around him and his needs, whether he needs feeding, diaper changing, or comforting. But once you get to know each other, and you become more adept at handling your baby and understanding what he requires, both of you will become more settled and life will fall into some sort of routine once again.

Prenatal care

Having a baby nowadays is very safe. This is largely because of the availability of prenatal care, a system of checks and tests at regular intervals throughout pregnancy designed to confirm that all is well with you and your baby. It is important for prenatal care to start early in pregnancy, as the first set of checks provides a baseline for assessing any changes later on. Ask your doctor about the available choices after the pregnancy is confirmed, and he can make the arrangements.

Where to have your baby

Providing you have a normal pregnancy, an important decision you will need to make is where to have your baby. Most babies today are born in a hospital, with medical staff available round the clock. In some areas you may be able to choose to have your baby in a birthing centre. It may also be possible to have your baby at home. Your doctor or midwife will make arrangements for your prenatal care according to your choice of where you want to have your baby.

Who will deliver the baby?

You can choose a family doctor, an obstetrician, or in most provinces, a midwife to deliver your baby. Family doctors and midwives generally care for uncomplicated pregnancies, whereas obstetricians have specialized training enabling them to care for complicated pregnancies and perform Caesarean sections. Family doctors and midwives both provide care for the newborn baby; however, if you choose an obstetrician, you will need to find another doctor for the baby

Most doctors and midwives work in groups. Although some care providers will attend your birth at any time, others will only attend on the days that they are "on call" in order to ensure personal time off and well rested caregivers. However, even if your primary doctor or midwife does not attend the birth, the groups usually have good communication and consistent philosophies of care between members of the group.

Hospital birth

The majority of Canadian babies are born in the hospital. A hospital has all the equipment and expertise needed for pain relief, for monitoring the baby's progress, for intervening in the birth to help you and the baby if necessary, and for providing emergency care for you both. After the birth, the duration of your stay in hospital varies, but it may be possible for you to go home the same day. The average stay is one to two days. Obstetricians, family doctors, and midwives all care for women planning hospital births.

Facilities vary among hospitals, so it's worth seeing what your local hospital has to offer before you decide. Some offer home-like birthing suites, and some have large tubs that may make labour more comfortable. If you attend prenatal classes (see page 17), you will be encouraged to look around the delivery room and maternity wards in advance to familiarize yourself with them.

Birth centres

Some jurisdictions offer women with uncomplicated pregnancies the possibility of giving birth in a birth centre. These units can be either attached to a hospital or "free standing" and offer a more home-like environment. They are designed to deal with normal pregnancies and deliveries in a low-tech and informal environment with the attendance of either midwives or family doctors. However, these small units do not have the full medical facilities of a hospital.

Home birth

Midwives are the only maternity care providers who offer the option of home birth. If you are healthy, have had a normal pregnancy, and feel you would be more comfortable in familiar surroundings, you may be able to have your baby at home. A home birth may be more suitable if you have had previous births that were uncomplicated. If you choose home birth, make sure that your midwife is fully licensed and experienced with home birth. Discuss contingency plans such as how to get to the hospital in case of an emergency, and remember that pain relief options at home are limited. Because of the possibility of unexpected emergencies, some medical organizations such as the CMA do not endorse home births.

Doulas

Doulas are private, non medical labour support coaches who provide emotional support and physical comfort measures. Some doulas provide postpartum and breastfeeding support.

Questions to ask

Hospital policies vary, so discuss any issues that are important to you with your doctor or midwife. It's natural to have pre-conceived ideas about labour and birth, but the reality is often quite different. However sure you are that you don't want pain relief, keep an open mind and ask for it if you need it. This list covers some questions you might like to ask.

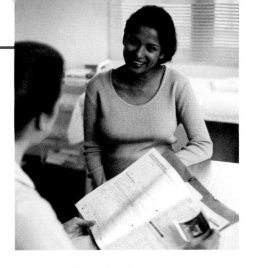

About labour

Can my partner and/or a friend stay with me throughout labour?

Will I be able to move around as I please during labour?

What is the hospital policy on pain relief, routine electronic monitoring, and induction (see pages 64, 65, and 66)?

What kind of pain relief (see pages 64 and 65) will I be offered?

About the birth

Can I give birth in any position I choose to? Are chairs, large cushions, birthing balls, and birth stools available?

Will I be able to use a birthing pool (see page 58)?

What is the hospital policy on episiotomies and Caesareans (see pages 63, 66, and 67)?

What types of birthing rooms are available?

About after the birth

How long will I stay in hospital after delivery?

Will I be able to have my baby with me all the time, including nights?

Is there open visiting for my partner?

Is there a special care baby unit in case my baby needs treatment?

Does the hospital's policy support (and give advice on) breastfeeding?

Your maternity records

Test results and other details about your pregnancy are kept in your medical files. Do not hesitate to ask for an explanation of any test for which you are scheduled. The following is a sampling of medical terminology and the abbreviations used, which you may see written down on your medical chart.

AFP	Alpha fetoprotein	**IPS**	Integrated prenatal screen
Alb	Albumin (a protein) found in urine	**LFTS**	Liver function tests
		LMP	Last menstrual period
BP	Blood pressure	**LSCS**	Lower segment caesarean section
Br	The baby is bottom down (Breech)	**MSS**	Maternal serum screen
C/Ceph or Vx	The baby is in the normal (head down – Vertex) position	**MSU**	Mid-stream urine sample
CS	Caesarean section	**NAD**	Nothing abnormal discovered
E/Eng	The baby's head has engaged	**Para O**	A woman who has had no other children
EDD/EDC	Estimated date of delivery/confinement	**Presentation**	Which way up the baby is
Edema	Swelling present	**Primigravida**	First pregnancy
Fe	Iron supplements	**Rh+**	Rhesus blood group positive
FH	Fetal heart		
FHH or FH√	Fetal heart heard	**Rh-**	Rhesus blood group negative
FHNH	Fetal heart not heard		
FMF	Fetal movements felt	**RTC**	Return to clinic
Fundus	Top of the womb	**SGA**	Small for dates
GBS	Group B strep	**TBA**	To come into hospital; or, to be arranged
GCT	Glucose challenge test		
Hb or Hgb	Hemoglobin levels in the blood	**Tr**	A trace found
		U/S	Ultrasound
HBsAg	Hepatitis blood test	**VDRL**	Test for syphilis
HTN	High blood pressure	**VE**	Vaginal examination

Abbreviations are used to describe the way the baby is lying in the womb. These are some of the positions:

LOT: left occipito-transverse

ROT: right occipito-transverse

LOA: left occipito-anterior

ROA: right occipito-anterior

LOP: left occipito-posterior

ROP: right occipito-posterior

Your prenatal appointments

Your first prenatal check-up takes place at about 10 weeks, and you will be asked to go every four weeks until 28 weeks. Visits become more frequent after this: every two weeks until you are 36 weeks pregnant, and every week in the last month. Routine tests are carried out by the doctor or midwife at every visit to check that the pregnancy is progressing normally. Write down questions you have beforehand.

Blood tests
first visit
Some blood will be taken from your arm to check:
• your blood group and rhesus (Rh) factor (see page 38)
• that you are not anemic (see page 38); your blood will be tested for this again at about 28 weeks
• that you are immune to rubella (see page 10)
• that you do not have a sexually transmitted disease, such as syphilis, which must be treated before week 20 if it is not to harm the baby
• for sickle cell trait, if you and your partner are of West Indian or African descent, and thalassemia, if your families come from the Mediterranean, South Asia, or the Middle and Far East. These forms of anemia are inherited, and thus can be passed on to the baby.
• for viruses that cause hepatitis and HIV.

General examination
first visit
The doctor or midwife will examine you physically to rule out any medical problems. This is a complete examination with particular focus on your blood pressure, heart and lungs, abdomen, breasts, and an internal examination.

You may also have a Pap smear and test for infections such as chlamydia and gonorrhea at this time. You will probably be asked about your dental health and encouraged to go for a check-up.

Weight
first visit
You will be weighed at your first visit, as part of the general examination. Don't worry if you lose weight during the first three months because of morning sickness, as this is quite common. If you gain weight suddenly in late pregnancy, this can be a sign of pre-eclampsia (see page 38).

Urine sample
every visit
Most clinics test a sample of urine at every visit for:
• traces of protein, which may indicate the possibility of pre-eclampsia (see page 38) in later pregnancy.

In early pregnancy and again at 28 weeks, your urine may be checked for:
• bacteria (germs), in case you have an asymptomatic urine infection. This can cause problems in later pregnancy. It can be easily treated with antibiotics.

Initial appointment
At the first visit, the doctor or midwife will ask some questions about you and your partner to find out whether there is anything that could affect the pregnancy or your baby. Prenatal procedures may vary from place to place, but you can expect to be asked about:
• personal details, such as your date of birth, and what work you and your partner do, and your address
• your religious or ethnic background, as some conditions such as thalassemia are inherited and affect only certain ethnic groups (see above)
• your health: any serious illnesses or operations you may have had in the past, whether you are currently being treated for any disease, and whether you have any allergies, or are taking any medications
• whether you smoke, or consume alcohol or recreational drugs, all of which could affect your pregnancy and your developing baby
• your family's medical history: whether there are twins or any inherited illnesses in you or your partner's family
• the type of contraceptives you used before you became pregnant, and when you stopped using it
• your periods: when they began, whether they are regular, when the first day of your last period was, and how long your cycle is
• any previous pregnancies, including miscarriages and terminations.

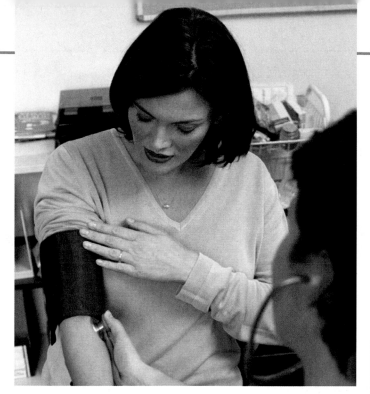

collect more water in their bodies than they would otherwise, but excessive swelling may be a sign of pre-eclampsia (see page 38). Your legs will also be checked for varicose veins (see page 42).

Feeling the abdomen
every visit
The doctor or midwife will gently feel your abdomen to check the position of the top of the womb, which gives her a good idea of the rate of the baby's growth. Later in your pregnancy, checks will be made to ensure that your baby has turned the right way round (head first), and, in the final weeks, that the head is dropping into your pelvis (engaging).

Blood pressure
every visit
Blood pressure may be slightly lower in pregnancy, and it is measured regularly to detect any sudden rises and keep it under control. Normal blood pressure is about 120/70, and there will be cause for concern if your blood pressure rises above 140/90. Raised blood pressure can be a sign of a number of problems, including pre-eclampsia (see page 38).

Legs, ankles, and hands
every visit
The doctor or midwife will look at your lower legs, ankles, and hands, and feel them to check there is no swelling or puffiness. A little swelling in the last weeks of pregnancy is normal, especially at the end of the day, since during pregnancy women normally

Listening to the baby's heartbeat
every visit (after week 14)
From early in pregnancy, this may be done with a fetal doppler (see above), which amplifies the baby's heartbeat so you can hear it too.

Screening and diagnostic tests in pregnancy

During your pregnancy you will probably be offered tests to look for conditions that might cause your baby to have a disability. Some of these tests are offered as a routine part of prenatal care and others when it is thought that there is a chance of an abnormality. The object of the tests is to detect any serious problem as early as possible so that the pregnancy can, if you wish, be safely terminated. The most likely outcome is that they will give you the reassurance that your baby is normal.

Your choice
You don't have to have any of these tests if you don't want to, and indeed you may prefer not to if you are certain that, whatever the outcome, you would never consider terminating the pregnancy. Even so, you might want to be prepared for a baby with a disability before the birth and, if the condition is treatable, to discuss and plan the treatment in advance.

Types of tests that you may be offered
Screening tests
A screening test will not detect any abnormality. It will only show whether you are more likely to have a baby with a particular disability. If the results show you are in a "high risk" group ("screen positive"), you will be offered a diagnostic test, but this does not mean there is anything wrong with your baby.

Diagnostic tests
If a screening test shows you are "high risk," you may be offered a diagnostic test that will give you a firm answer and show whether or not your baby has a particular abnormality. All diagnostic tests, except an "anatomy" ultrasound scan, involve taking samples from inside your uterus, and they carry an increased risk of miscarriage. If you are unsure whether to agree to a test or want to discuss it further, ask.

Ultrasound scan

An ultrasound scan is a test offered routinely at some stage of your pregnancy. A thin layer of gel is rubbed over your stomach and a hand-held instrument, a transducer, is passed gently over it. This beams and receives sound waves that are built into an image of your baby on the screen.

The scan is painless and takes about 15–45 minutes. Ultrasound does not use radiation, and there is no evidence that it causes harm to the developing fetus. Nevertheless, ultrasound should only be used when there is a medical indication for the test.

Early scan

If you have a history of miscarriage, or have had any pain or bleeding, you may be offered a very early scan, at 6–11 weeks. This will confirm that the pregnancy is safely established, and may also detect an ectopic pregnancy. If you have an early scan, the transducer may be placed in your vagina, but there is no risk that this will cause a miscarriage.

11–14 week scan (for dating pregnancy and nuchal translucency)

You may be given a scan when you are between 11 and 14 weeks pregnant, to help date your pregnancy accurately. In some areas, this scan is also used to help calculate the risk of Down syndrome by measuring fluid accumulation at the back of the baby's neck. All babies have some fluid there between 11 and 13 weeks, but most babies with Down syndrome have an increased amount. This test result, combined with selected blood tests, is used to help calculate the risk of Down syndrome and help you to decide whether you wish to have further diagnostic testing.

18–20 week anatomy scan

This scan is offered routinely to confirm the date of the pregnancy, to make sure the baby's growth is normal, and that his heart, brain, other organs, spine, and limbs are all developing normally. It will also show any condition that might complicate the delivery.

Further scans

You may be offered additional scans later in pregnancy if you are expecting twins, or if your doctor thinks that your baby is not growing properly. A scan within the last six weeks of pregnancy may be offered to check on the "lie" of the baby and the position of the placenta.

Biophysical profile scan (BPP) (as necessary)

This scan is used later in pregnancy when there is concern about baby's growth and health. It evaluates the placenta and other indicators such as movement, breathing, and the amount of amniotic fluid.

Prenatal screening tests for Down syndrome, trisomy 18, and neural tube defects

You will be offered testing to assess your risk of having a baby with Down syndrome and other abnormalities. These are blood tests, sometimes with an ultrasound (for nuchal translucency), which are done starting at 11 weeks. These tests do not make the diagnosis, they simply tell you whether you are at higher risk of having a baby affected by these conditions. If you are at higher risk, you will be offered further diagnostic tests.

The tests are optional, and it is your choice whether or not to have screening tests. Not all test are offered everywhere, and you may want to discuss the options with your health care provider. The chart opposite explains the different ways of testing for these conditions.

HIV testing (first appointment)

You will be offered a test for HIV (the Human Immunodeficiency Virus). The virus can be transmitted to your baby during pregnancy, at birth, or even during breastfeeding. However, if your doctor knows that you are HIV+ve, precautions can be taken to minimize the risk of the infection being passed to your baby during pregnancy and birth. It is worth having the test even if you do not think that you or your partner are at risk.

Hepatitis B testing (first appointment)

Mothers who carry the hepatitis B virus can pass it on to their baby. However, this can be prevented by giving antibodies and vaccine to the baby.

Other blood tests (first appointment)

Your blood will be checked for anemia (low blood count), antibodies to rubella (German measles, which can harm the unborn child if the mother contracts it during pregnancy), syphilis, blood group, and antibodies. Specific tests will be offered if your medical or family history suggests that you may be at risk of a certain disorder.

Amniocentesis (weeks 15–20, usually at week 16)

Amniocentesis can be used to detect some abnormalities in the baby, such

Ultrasound scan
It can be very exciting to see your baby on the ultrasound monitor, and it will reassure you that your baby's development is normal.

as Down syndrome. It is not offered routinely, as there is a risk of miscarriage in about one woman in 200 to 400. You may be offered the test if:

● you are over 35, when there is a higher risk of a Down syndrome baby
● you have a family history of an inherited disease
● your screening test was positive.

An ultrasound scan is done to check the position of the baby and the placenta. A hollow needle is inserted through the wall of the stomach into the womb, and a sample of the fluid that surrounds the baby, and which contains some of her cells, is taken. The cells are then tested for abnormality. The test results can take three weeks.

Chorionic villus sampling (CVS)
(11–13 weeks)

Some inherited disorders can be detected by examining a small piece of the tissue that forms part of the placenta. The sample can be obtained either through the vagina, or by inserting a needle directly into the uterus through the abdominal wall, guided by an ultrasound scan. The test carries a slightly greater risk of miscarriage than amniocentesis (roughly 1 in 100) but the results are available earlier in pregnancy.

Fetal blood sampling
(after 16 weeks)

Blood from the baby's hepatic vein can be used to diagnose a range of rare genetic and metabolic diseases including clarification of inconclusive amniocentesis and CVS. It can also diagnose and treat (by blood transfusion) fetal anemia while the baby is still in utero.

Non-invasive chromosomal screening tests

	First trimester screening (FTS)	Integrated prenatal screening (IPS)	Serum integrated prenatal screening (SIPS)	Quadruple screening
1st blood sample	11–14 weeks	11–14 weeks	11–14 weeks	None
Nuchal translucency scan *	11–14 weeks	11–14 weeks	None	None
2nd blood sample	None	15–20 weeks	15–20 weeks	15–20 weeks
Results available	12–15 weeks	16–21 weeks	16–21 weeks	16–21 weeks
Detection rate (accuracy)	80–85%	85–90%	80–90%	75–85%
False positive rate	3–9%	2–4%	2–7%	5–10%

* Nuchal translucency scans not available in all centres.
Detection rate: Of every 100 pregnancies with Down syndrome, this percentage will be detected by the test.
False positive rate: Of every 100 pregnancies, this percentage will test positive but NOT have Down syndrome.
Table adapted with permission from Carroll et al. Genetics Education Project, 2008.
www.mtsinai.on.ca/FamMedGen/

High risk pregnancies

Nearly all pregnancies are normal and straightforward, but there may be circumstances that make your doctor think there is greater risk of complications, and hence you need to be monitored closely during pregnancy. This could be because you have a general medical condition, or perhaps you are expecting twins. Sometimes symptoms develop that also warn the doctor that special care is needed.

Anemia

Many women are slightly anemic before pregnancy, and this is usually due to an iron deficiency. It's important to correct this in order to cope with the increased demands of pregnancy, and any bleeding during labour.
Treatment Try to prevent the problem by eating a varied diet, with plenty of iron-rich foods. However, you should avoid liver and liver products in pregnancy (see page 52). If blood tests at the clinic show that you are anemic, the doctor or midwife may prescribe iron supplements. Take iron tablets directly after a meal, with fluid, as otherwise they can cause constipation or nausea.

Diabetes

Diabetes must be carefully controlled before conception and during pregnancy. If this is done, there's no reason why the pregnancy shouldn't be straightforward. Some women develop gestational diabetes, a mild form of the disease which appears for the first time in pregnancy. This condition is usually controlled by diet and nearly always disappears soon after delivery.
Treatment It's imperative that your blood-sugar level remains stable, so the doctor may adjust your insulin intake for the pregnancy. You may need more frequent prenatal visits.

Incompetent cervix

In a normal pregnancy, the cervix (neck of the womb) stays closed until the beginning of labour. But if miscarriages frequently occur after the third month of pregnancy, it could be because the neck of the womb is weak and so it opens up, allowing the baby to pass through.
Treatment Your doctor may suggest a small operation to stitch the cervix firmly closed at the beginning of pregnancy. The stitch is then removed towards the end of pregnancy, or as labour starts.

Pre-eclampsia

This is one of the more common problems in late pregnancy. Warning signs are: raised blood pressure above 140/90; excessive weight gain; swollen ankles, feet, or hands; and protein in the urine. If you develop any of these symptoms, the doctor will monitor you very carefully.

If high blood pressure is untreated, it could progress to the extremely dangerous condition called eclampsia, where seizures occur.
Treatment At the moment there is no effective way to prevent pre-eclampsia. If the signs are severe, you will be admitted to hospital even though you might be feeling fine. If your blood pressure is high, you may be given a drug to lower it. Labour may be induced (see page 66), especially in late pregnancy.

Rhesus (Rh)-negative mothers

Your blood is tested at the first prenatal visit to see if it is Rh positive or negative. About 15 percent of people are Rh negative, and if you are one of these you will only have a problem in pregnancy if you give birth to a Rh-positive baby. Your blood groups will be incompatible, and although this won't harm a first baby, you could have problems with later pregnancies.
Treatment A protective injection of Rh immunoglobulin (RhIg) is given to all Rh-negative women at 28 weeks. It is also given after any bleeding and after the birth of a Rh-positive baby to prevent problems in future pregnancies.

"Small for dates" babies

A baby who doesn't grow properly in the womb and is small at birth is called a "small for dates" baby. This may happen because the expectant mother smokes or eats a poor diet, or because the placenta is inefficient (usually when

Anemia Eating foods that are a good source of iron, such as spinach, will help to guard against the problem.

Emergency signs
Call for emergency help immediately if you have:
- a severe headache that won't go away
- misty or blurred vision
- severe, prolonged stomach or back pains
- vaginal bleeding
- a leakage of fluid, which suggests your waters have broken early
- frequent, painful urination (drink plenty of water in the meantime).

Consult your doctor within 24 hours if you have:
- swollen hands, face, and ankles
- severe, frequent vomiting
- a temperature of 38.3°C (101°F)
- no movement or fewer than 10 kicks from your baby for 12 hours after week 28.

Miscarriage

A miscarriage is the ending of a pregnancy before 20 weeks, and may occur in up to one in five pregnancies. Most miscarriages occur in the first 12 weeks, often before the woman even knows she is pregnant, and usually because the baby is not developing normally. Bleeding from the vagina accompanied by lower backache and severe stomach cramps are usually the first signs. You should call your doctor immediately if this happens.

Threatened miscarriage

If the bleeding is mild and painless, and occurs around the time of a missed period, you may not necessarily miscarry. You may be given an ultrasound scan (see page 36), which will show whether all is well.

True miscarriage

If the bleeding is heavy and you are in pain, it probably means that a miscarriage is inevitable. You may fully miscarry on your own. However, some women require either medications or a D and C (cleaning of the womb) to complete the process.

Your feelings

Even if you lose the baby early in pregnancy, you will feel an intense sense of loss and will probably feel very emotional. Other people don't always understand that you need to mourn the loss of your baby. Worrying about whether you can ever have a normal, healthy baby is common. You may feel guilty, too, though you should not blame yourself – it really isn't your fault. You can try for another baby as soon as you like, although some doctors suggest waiting until one to three menstrual cycles have passed. Unless you have had several miscarriages, there is no reason why you shouldn't experience a successful pregnancy the next time.

pregnancy, call your doctor without delay. Before 24 weeks, it can be a sign of an impending miscarriage. After this time, it may mean that the placenta is bleeding. This can happen if the placenta has started to separate from the wall of the womb (placental abruption) or if the placenta is too low down in the womb and covers, or partially covers, the cervix (placenta previa).

Treatment The placenta is the baby's lifeline, so if the doctor thinks that there is a risk to it, you will probably be admitted to hospital immediately, where the position of the placenta can be checked. You may stay in hospital until after the birth. If you have lost a lot of blood, you may be given a blood transfusion, and the baby will probably be delivered as soon as possible, by induction or Caesarean section (see pages 66 and 67). But if bleeding is only slight and occurs several weeks before the baby is due, the doctor may decide to wait for you to start labour naturally, while keeping you under close observation.

---

the mother has a general medical condition, such as diabetes or high blood pressure).

Treatment If tests show your baby is small, you will be monitored closely throughout pregnancy to check his health, and whether the flow of blood to the placenta is adequate. If the baby stops growing, or appears to be distressed, then he will be delivered early, either through induction of labour or Caesarean section (see pages 66 and 67).

Twins

Although most twin pregnancies proceed smoothly, there's a higher risk of complications such as anemia, high blood pressure, pre-eclampsia, gestational diabetes, and premature delivery. The average length of a twin pregnancy is 36 to 37 weeks, but twin babies are smaller than a corresponding singleton of the same gestational age. Labour may

be complicated by the babies' positioning in the womb, and thus there is a higher chance of Caesarean section.

Treatment Pregnancy with twins means more frequent prenatal visits and ultrasounds to ensure that the babies are growing well. It is especially important that you eat well and gain enough weight. Twin pregnancy puts greater strain on your body, so watch your

posture and rest as much as possible, especially in the last few weeks. You may be more comfortable lying on one side rather than on your back. You may also want to look into resources to help you when you get home with your babies.

Vaginal bleeding

If you notice bleeding from your vagina at any time in

Twins
You may find this position more comfortable to rest in.

Common complaints

You may suffer from a variety of discomforts in pregnancy, which, although worrying at the time, are perfectly normal. Many are caused by hormonal changes or because your body is under extra pressure. A few symptoms, however, should be taken very seriously, so call the doctor if you have any of the complaints that have been highlighted in the box on page 38.

Complaint	Symptoms	What to do
Bleeding gums ❶ ❷ ❸ The gums become softer and more easily injured in pregnancy. They may become inflamed, allowing plaque to collect at the base of the teeth. This can lead to gum disease and tooth decay.	Bleeding from the gums, especially after brushing your teeth.	• Floss and brush your teeth thoroughly after eating. • See your dentist. You should avoid X-rays or any dental procedures under general anaesthetic wherever possible.
Breathlessness ❸ Late in pregnancy, the growing baby puts pressure on the diaphragm and prevents you from breathing freely. The problem is often relieved about a month before the birth, if the baby's head engages. Breathlessness can also be caused by anemia.	Feeling short of breath and panting excessively when you exert yourself.	• Rest as much as possible. • Try crouching if there's no chair around until your breathing slows down. • At night, use an extra pillow. • If the problem is severe, consult your doctor or midwife.
Constipation ❶ ❷ ❸ The pregnancy hormone progesterone relaxes the muscles of the intestine, which slows down bowel movements, making you more likely to become constipated. Approximately 30 to 40 percent of pregnant women suffer from constipation at some point during pregnancy.	Passing hard, dry stools at less frequent intervals than usual.	• Eat plenty of high-fibre foods and drink lots of water. Go to the bathroom whenever you need to. • Exercise regularly. • Take any iron supplements you have been prescribed on a full stomach, with plenty of fluid. • See your doctor if the problem persists. • Avoid laxatives.
Fatigue ❶ ❸ Caused by the extra demands that pregnancy makes on your body. Sometimes tiredness can be made worse as a result of worrying too much.	Feeling weary, and wanting to sleep in the day. Needing to sleep longer at night or even suffering from insomnia.	• Rest as much as possible and practise relaxation exercises. • Go to bed earlier. • Don't overexert yourself.
Feeling faint ❶ ❸ Your blood pressure is lower in pregnancy, so you are more likely to feel faint.	Feeling dizzy and unstable. Needing to sit or lie down.	• Try not to stand still for too long. • If you suddenly feel faint, sit down and put your head between your knees until you feel better. • Get up slowly from a hot bath or when sitting or lying down. Turn onto one side first, if lying on your back.

Complaint	Symptoms	What to do
Frequent urination ❶ ❸ Caused by the womb pressing on the bladder. The problem is often relieved in the middle months of pregnancy.	You need to urinate often.	● If you find yourself getting up in the night to go to the bathroom try drinking a little less in the evenings. ● See your doctor if you feel any pain or burning sensation when passing urine, as you could have an infection.
Heartburn ❸ The valve at the entrance to your stomach relaxes in pregnancy because of hormonal changes, so stomach acid passes back into the esophagus (the tube leading to your stomach).	A strong burning pain in the centre of the chest.	● Avoid large meals and highly spiced or fried foods. ● At night, try a warm milk drink, and raise the head of the bed or use extra pillows. ● See your doctor, who may prescribe a medicine to treat stomach acidity.
Hemorrhoids ❷ ❸ Pressure from the baby's head causes swollen veins round the anus. Straining to empty the bowels will make the problem worse. Mild hemorrhoids usually disappear without treatment, after the baby is born.	Itching, soreness, and possibly pain or bleeding when you try to pass stools.	● Avoid constipation. ● Try not to stand for long periods. ● An ice pack held against the hemorrhoids may ease any itching. ● If hemorrhoids persist, tell the doctor or midwife who may give you an ointment.
Leaking urine ❸ Caused by weak pelvic floor muscles (see page 45) and the growing baby pressing on your bladder.	Leakage of urine whenever you run, cough, sneeze, or laugh.	● Urinate often. ● Practise your pelvic floor exercises regularly. ● Avoid constipation and heavy lifting.
Muscle cramps ❸ May be caused by calcium deficiency.	Painful contractions of muscles, usually in the calves and the feet, and often at night. Commonly started by a leg stretch with the toes pointed down.	● Massage the affected calf or foot. Stretch the calf by pushing down your heel and flexing the foot up towards the ceiling. ● Walk around for a moment or two once the pain has eased to improve your circulation. ● See your doctor or midwife.
Nausea and vomiting ❶ Often one of the first signs of pregnancy, which can occur at any time of day. Tiredness can make the problem worse. Nausea usually disappears after week 12 but can sometimes return later.	Feeling sick, often at the smell of certain foods or cigarette smoke. Most women find there is a particular time of day when this happens.	● Eat plain crackers first thing in the morning. ● Avoid foods and smells that make you feel sick, and have small, frequent meals. ● Try ginger in any form or acupressure above your wrist. ● Consult your doctor or midwife for medications that are safe to use. ● Severe vomiting with dehydration requires intravenous fluids.
Rash ❸ Usually occurs in women who are overweight and who perspire freely. Can be caused by hormone changes.	Red rash, which usually develops in sweaty skin folds under the breasts or in the groin.	● Wash and dry these areas often. Use unperfumed soap. ● Soothe the skin with calamine lotion. ● Wear loose cotton clothes.

❶ ❷ ❸ The numbers in circles after each complaint relate to the trimester of pregnancy in which you are most likely to suffer from the problem.

Complaint	Symptoms	What to do
Sleeping difficulty ❶ ❷ ❸ You may have a problem because the baby is kicking, you have to go to the bathroom frequently, or the size of the baby makes it difficult to get comfortable in bed.	Having trouble going to sleep in the first place, and finding it hard to get to sleep after waking. Some women find they have very frightening dreams about the birth or the baby. Don't worry about dreams; they do not reflect what will happen.	• Reading, gentle relaxation exercises, or a warm bath before bedtime may help. • Experiment with extra pillows. If you sleep on your side, put a pillow under the top thigh. • Ask your partner for a head and neck massage, which may relieve tension. • Don't eat too close to bedtime. Try a glass of warm milk.
Stretchmarks ❷ ❸ These form if your skin stretches beyond its normal elasticity. Excess weight gain can also cause them. The marks seldom disappear altogether, but they may fade to thin silvery streaks after pregnancy.	Red marks that sometimes appear on the skin of the thighs, stomach, or breasts in pregnancy.	• Avoid putting on weight too rapidly. • Rubbing moisturizer into the skin may feel cool and soothing, although creams and ointments won't prevent or heal stretchmarks.
Sweating ❷ ❸ Caused by hormone changes and because blood flow to the skin increases in pregnancy.	Perspiring after very little exertion, or waking up in the night feeling hot and sweaty.	• Wear loose cotton clothes. • Avoid synthetic materials. • Drink plenty of water. • Open a window at night.
Swollen ankles and fingers ❸ Some swelling (edema) is normal in pregnancy, as the body holds extra water. This is usually no cause for concern.	Slight swelling in the ankles, especially in hot weather and at the end of the day. This shouldn't cause pain or discomfort. You may also notice stiff, swollen fingers in the morning and that your rings don't fit.	• Rest often with your feet up. • Try gentle foot exercises. Hold your hands above your head; flex and stretch each finger. • See your doctor or midwife. More marked swelling could be a warning sign of pre-eclampsia (see page 38).
Vaginal discharge ❶ ❷ ❸ You may notice some increase in the amount of mucus produced by the vagina because of the hormone changes during pregnancy.	Slight increase in clear or white discharge, without soreness or pain.	• Avoid vaginal deodorants and perfumed soap products. • Wear a light sanitary pad. • See your doctor or midwife if you have any itching, soreness, coloured or foul-smelling discharge.
Varicose veins ❶ ❷ ❸ You are more likely to have them later on in pregnancy, if you are overweight, or if they run in your family. Standing for too long, or sitting cross-legged, can worsen the problem.	Aching legs; the veins in the calves and the thighs become painful and swollen.	• Rest often with your feet up. Try raising the foot of your bed with pillows under the mattress. • Support stockings may help. Put them on before getting up in the morning. • Exercise your feet.
Yeast infection (candida) ❶ ❷ ❸ Hormone changes in pregnancy increase the chances of developing a yeast infection. After birth, yeast infections (thrush) can occur in the baby's mouth and be spread to your nipples, which can make breastfeeding difficult.	A thick white vaginal discharge and severe itching. There may also be soreness and pain when you urinate.	• Stop using soap if you are sore. Avoid nylon underwear, tight pants, and vaginal deodorants. • See your doctor or midwife to confirm that it is a yeast infection. • Most intravaginal yeast treatments are available without a prescription and are considered safe to use in pregnancy. Check with the pharmacist.

Keeping fit and relaxed

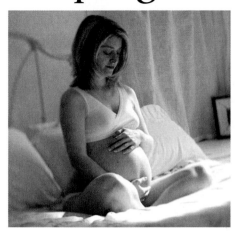

Pregnancy, labour, and birth will make great demands on your body, so the more you can prepare yourself physically, the better you will feel. You will also find it easier to regain your normal shape after the birth. Relaxation exercises are just as important – they will help you cope effectively during labour, and they are invaluable for relieving stress and increasing blood flow to the placenta. Begin exercising as soon as the pregnancy is confirmed or earlier if you wish.

Exercising sensibly

If you have always enjoyed sport, you can usually carry on during pregnancy, but remember that there are provisos. Pregnancy is not the time to launch into a fitness blitz – just continue with what your body is used to. If you want to keep on going to your dance or exercise class, make sure that the teacher knows you are pregnant. Don't exercise to the point where you get very tired or out of breath.

Avoid any contact sports or sports where there is a danger of hurting your abdomen, such as horseback riding, skiing, and water-skiing. Be extra careful towards the end of pregnancy, as you may overstretch your ligaments.

Swimming
This is excellent and perfectly safe throughout pregnancy; the water supports your body.

Looking after your body

During pregnancy, it's important to hold yourself well and avoid strain on your back. A good posture becomes increasingly important. You're far more likely to suffer from backache as the weight of the baby pulls you forwards, and so there is a tendency to lean slightly backwards to compensate. This strains the muscles of the lower back and pelvis, especially towards the end of pregnancy.

Be aware of your body, whatever you are doing. Avoid heavy lifting, and try to keep your back as long as possible. Wear low heels, as high heels tend to throw your weight even further forwards.

Protecting your back

To avoid back trouble, it's important to be aware of how you use your body when going about everyday activities, such as lifting a child or carrying heavy bags. The hormones of pregnancy stretch and soften the muscles of the lower back, so they are more easily strained if you bend over, get up too suddenly, or lift something the wrong way. You may need to support the small of your back when you are sitting or lying down.

Working at a low level
Do as much as you can at floor level, kneeling down to garden or clean instead of bending over. If you have younger children, have them climb up to your lap for a cuddle instead of lifting them from the floor.

Lifting and carrying
When lifting an object, bend your knees and keep your back as straight as possible, bringing the object close in to your body. Try not to lift something heavy from up high, as you may lose your balance. If you're carrying heavy bags, divide the weight equally on each side. Ask for help whenever possible. This is no time to be proud.

Getting up from lying down
Always turn on your side when you have been lying down. Then move into a kneeling position. Use the strength of your thighs to push yourself up; keep your back straight. During pregnancy you might suffer from bouts of dizziness due to the hormones, so always get up slowly from either sitting or lying down.

Standing well

Drop *your shoulders and keep them back*

Hold *your back straight*

Tuck in *your bottom*

Bend *your knees slightly*

Stand *with your feet a little way apart*

Getting it right
You can check that you are standing the right way in front of a full-length mirror. Lengthen and straighten your back, so that the weight of the baby is centred and supported by your thighs, buttocks, and stomach muscles. Try to drop your shoulders to prevent tension in your neck. Distribute your weight evenly on both legs. Lift your chest and ribs and tighten your stomach muscles. This will help prevent backache, and tone up your abdominal muscles, making it easier for you to regain your figure after the birth.

Bad posture
This is an example of posture commonly adopted during pregnancy. As the baby grows, its weight throws you off-balance, so you may over-arch your back and thrust your abdomen forwards. This can lead to discomfort and can strain or injure the lower back, so take care to maintain good posture while standing or sitting.

The pelvic floor

This is a hammock of muscles that supports the bowel, bladder, and womb. During pregnancy, the muscles go soft and stretchy, and this, together with the weight of the baby pushing down, weakens them, making you feel heavy and uncomfortable. You may also leak a little urine whenever you run, sneeze, cough, or laugh. So, to improve pelvic muscle tone, prevent incontinence, and aid the process of labour, it's essential to strengthen the pelvic floor.

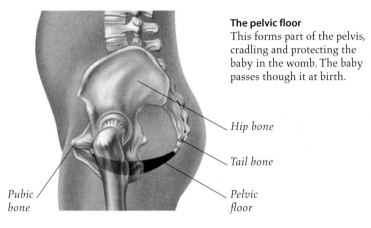

The pelvic floor
This forms part of the pelvis, cradling and protecting the baby in the womb. The baby passes though it at birth.

Hip bone

Tail bone

Pubic bone

Pelvic floor

Do this when:

- waiting for a bus or train
- ironing or cooking
- watching TV
- having intercourse
- you have *emptied* your bladder.

Strengthening the pelvic floor

Lie on your back, with your knees bent and your feet flat on the floor. Tighten the muscles, squeezing as if stopping a stream of urine. Imagine you are trying to pull something into your vagina, drawing it in slightly, then pausing, then pulling, until you can go no further. Hold for a moment, then let go gradually. Repeat 10 times. Practise this exercise often – at least three or four times a day. Once you've learned it, you can do it anytime, anywhere, lying down, sitting, or standing. You will also find it useful in the second stage of labour, when knowing how to relax the muscles can reduce the risk of a tear, by easing the passage of the baby through the pelvis.

Pelvic tilt

This exercise helps you move the pelvis with ease, which is good preparation for labour. It also strengthens the stomach muscles and makes the back more flexible. The pelvic tilt is especially helpful if you suffer from backache. You can do the tilt in any position; remember to keep your shoulders still.

Do this when:

- lying on your back
- standing or sitting
- kneeling
- dancing to music.

1 Kneel on the floor on your hands and knees. Make sure that your back is flat (you can use a mirror to check this). Your hands should be directly under your shoulders.

2 Pull in your stomach muscles, tighten your buttock muscles, and gently tilt the pelvis forwards, breathing out as you do so. Your back should hump up. Hold this position for a few seconds, then breathe in and let go. Repeat this step several times, so that your pelvis is rocking in and out of the position.

Tailor sitting

Tailor sitting strengthens the back and makes your thighs and pelvis more flexible. It will also improve the blood flow in the lower part of the body, and will encourage your legs to flop apart during labour. The main position below is far easier than it appears. This is because your body becomes more supple during pregnancy.

Thigh strengthener

Sit with your back straight, the soles of your feet together, and your heels touching also. To get used to the position, try to spend 10 minutes sitting like this 2–3 times a day while reading, meditating or simply relaxing. Grasp your ankles, and press your thighs down with your elbows. Hold them there for 20 seconds. Do this several times once you're comfortable. Breathe normally throughout.

Warning

When you are doing any exercise remember these guidelines.
• Don't push yourself beyond your own limits or exhaust yourself.
• If you feel any pain, stop.
• Try not to lie flat on your back in late pregnancy.

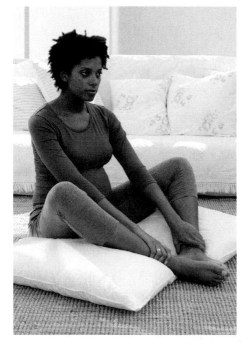

Sitting with cushions

If you find tailor sitting difficult, put a cushion under each thigh, or sit against a wall for support. Remember to keep your back straight.

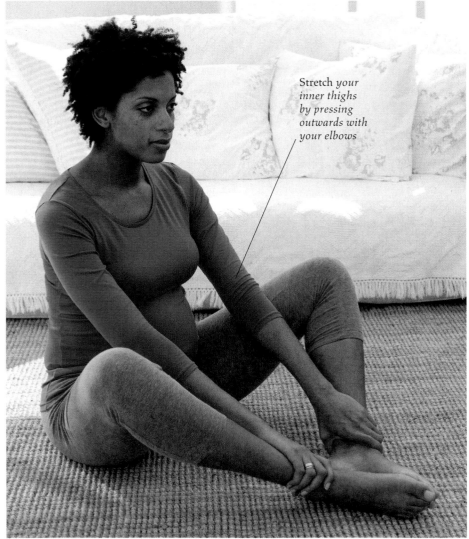

Stretch your inner thighs by pressing outwards with your elbows

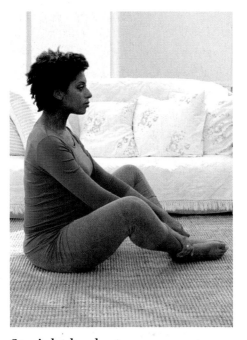

Straight back

Sit up straight and don't bend your back or slump. Look straight ahead, not down at your legs. You may use a wall to support your back if you have difficulty in keeping your back straight.

Squatting

Squatting makes your pelvic joints more flexible, and strengthens the back and thigh muscles. It can also protect your back if you squat down instead of bending over, and is comfortable if you experience backache. Squatting is also a good position to take up during labour.

You may find it difficult to do a full squat at first, so try holding on to a firm support, such as a chair or window ledge, and place a rolled-up rug or blanket under your heels. Get up slowly or you may feel slightly dizzy.

Do this when:

- picking up an object
- taking something from a low drawer
- on the telephone
- there's no chair around
- listening to music.

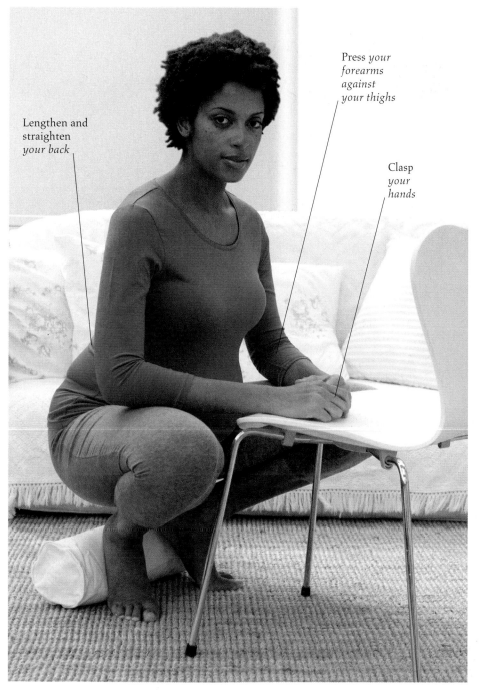

Lengthen and straighten *your back*

Press *your forearms against your thighs*

Clasp *your hands*

With a chair

Stand facing a chair with your feet slightly apart. Keeping your back straight, open out your legs, and squat down, using the chair to support you. Stay in this position as long as it is comfortable to do so. If you find it difficult to keep your feet flat on the ground, place a folded blanket under your heels.

Unsupported

Keeping your back straight, open out your legs and squat down, turning your feet out slightly. Try to keep the balls of your feet flat on the ground if you can, and stretch your inner thighs by pressing outward with your elbows. Stay in this position as long as you find it comfortable.

Relaxation and breathing

These relaxation and breathing exercises are among the most beneficial that you can learn to prepare yourself for childbirth. They are invaluable during labour. Proper breathing will help relax the muscles of your body, which will help you cope with painful contractions, and in doing so, you will conserve vital energy. Practise them regularly so that they become a natural response during labour. These exercises will also help you unwind any time you feel tense or anxious during your pregnancy.

How to relax

At first it's best to practise the following exercises in a warm and quiet room where you won't be disturbed. Later you should find it easy to relax anywhere.

Relax your body

Make yourself comfortable. Lie on your back, propped up by pillows, or on your side, with one leg bent and supported on cushions. Now, tense and relax each muscle of your body in turn, starting with the toes and working upwards. After doing this for several minutes, let your body go limp.

Lying on your side

You may be more comfortable, especially during later pregnancy, lying on your side with one leg bent and supported on cushions. Don't place too many pillows under your head because this is bad for your spine.

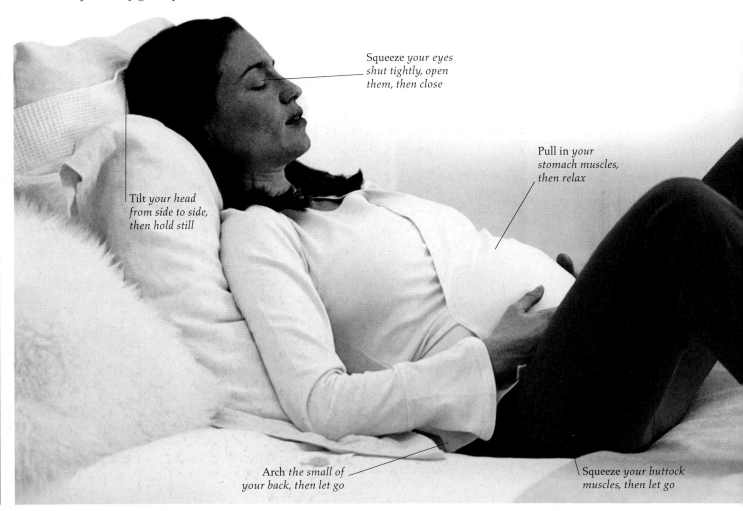

Tilt *your head from side to side, then hold still*

Squeeze *your eyes shut tightly, open them, then close*

Pull in *your stomach muscles, then relax*

Arch *the small of your back, then let go*

Squeeze *your buttock muscles, then let go*

Your partner's role
Lean back against your partner so he can support your weight and cuddle you.

Tighten *your thigh muscles, then let the tension go*

Tense *your calf muscles, then relax*

Bend *your feet at the ankles, then let go*

Curl *your toes, then relax*

Relax your mind
While relaxing your body, try to calm and empty your mind. Breathe slowly and evenly, sighing each breath out gently. Do not breathe too deeply. Alternatively, repeat a word or sound silently to yourself or concentrate on some pleasant or peaceful image. Try not to follow any thoughts that arise.

Breathing for labour

Practise the different levels of breathing on a regular basis in the weeks leading up to labour. Controlled breathing will help you remain relaxed and calm during labour, and can even control your body during contractions.

Breathing with a partner

Practising breathing exercises with your partner, a friend, or a family member will help you feel supported. Sit together in a comfortable position so that both of you have your hands over the baby. Take steady breaths focusing primarily on your birthing muscles and try not to tense any other part of your body unnecessarily.

Light breathing

This level of breathing will help you at the height of a contraction. Breathe in and out of your mouth, taking air into the upper part of your lungs only. A partner or friend should put his hands on your shoulder blades and feel them move. Practise making the breaths lighter and lighter, but take an occasional deeper breath when you need one.

Deep breathing

This helps to calm you at the start and end of contractions. Sit as comfortably as possible. Breathe in deeply through the nose, right to the bottom of your lungs. Your partner or friend should place his hands just above your waistline and feel your ribcage move. Concentrate on breathing slowly and gently out. Let the next in-breath follow naturally.

Panting

After the first stage of labour, you will want to push, even though the cervix may not be fully opened. You can resist this by taking two short breaths, and then blowing a longer breath out: say "huff, huff, blow" to yourself

Warning

Try not to lie flat on your back in the late stages of pregnancy as you can restrict the flow of oxygen to the baby in this position, and you may also feel faint.

Eating for a healthy baby

A baby has only one source of food – you. During pregnancy more than at any other time it is essential that you have as varied and balanced a diet as possible. You do not need to plan this specially, nor do you have to eat for two. Choose from the selection below to ensure that you get all the nutrients you need. Once you are, or know you want to become, pregnant think about how many healthy foods you eat regularly. Do you eat or drink anything that may harm the baby?

Essential nutrients

Calcium

This is important to ensure the healthy development of your baby's bones and teeth, which start to form from around week eight. You will need about 1000mg of calcium per day. Dairy products such as milk, cheese, and yogurt are the best sources of calcium, and you should aim for three servings per day. However, dairy products are high in fat so try to choose low-fat varieties. Other sources of calcium include leafy green vegetables, almonds, chickpeas, sardines, or fortified white bread. However, you would have to eat seven slices of bread to equal the calcium in two glasses of milk!

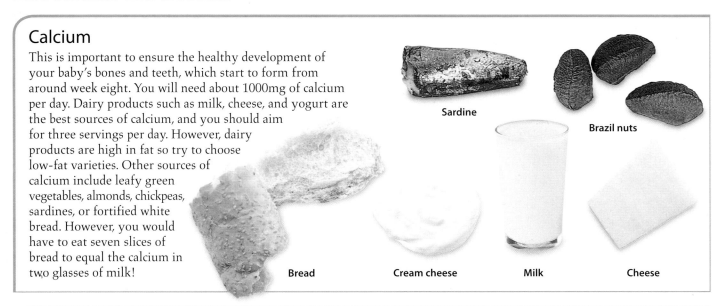

Sardine

Brazil nuts

Bread

Cream cheese

Milk

Cheese

Protein

Try to eat a variety of protein-rich foods because your needs increase during pregnancy. Fish, meat, nuts, legumes, tofu, and dairy foods all supply protein, but animal sources can also be high in fat so choose lean cuts of meat whenever possible. Avoid lightly cooked or raw eggs and make sure all eggs you buy are fresh.

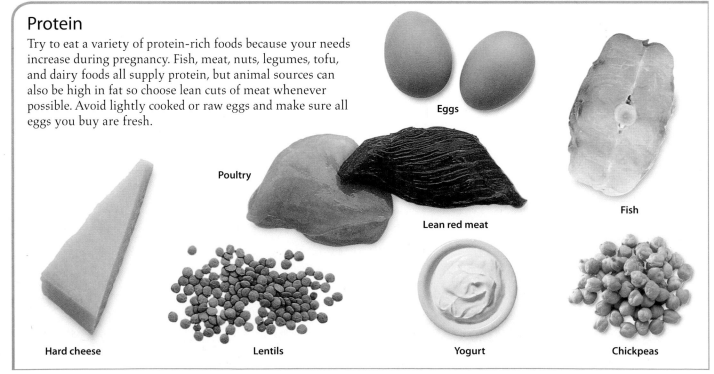

Eggs

Fish

Poultry

Lean red meat

Hard cheese

Lentils

Yogurt

Chickpeas

Vitamin C

This will help build a strong placenta, enable your body to resist infection, and aid the absorption of iron. It is found in fresh fruit and vegetables, and supplies of the vitamin are needed daily as it cannot be stored in the body. A lot of vitamin C is lost by prolonged storage and cooking so only eat fresh produce, and steam green vegetables or eat them raw.

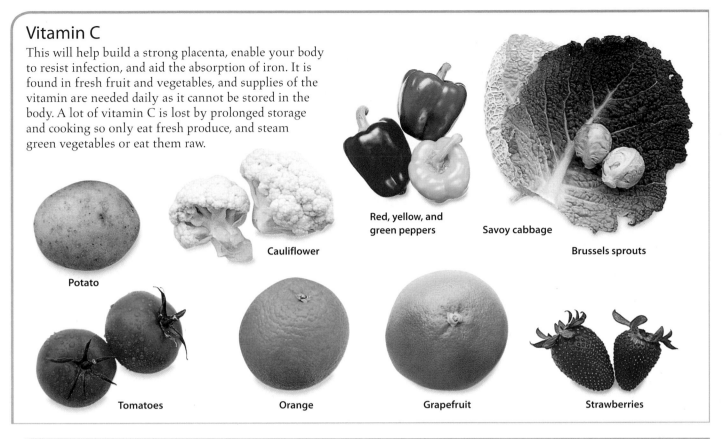

Potato

Cauliflower

Red, yellow, and green peppers

Savoy cabbage

Brussels sprouts

Tomatoes

Orange

Grapefruit

Strawberries

Fibre

Foods rich in fibre should form a large part of your daily diet since constipation (see page 40) is common in pregnancy and fibre will help prevent this. Fruit and vegetables are important sources as you can eat a lot of them every day. Choose wholegrain breads and breakfast cereals. Bran, in moderation, is useful.

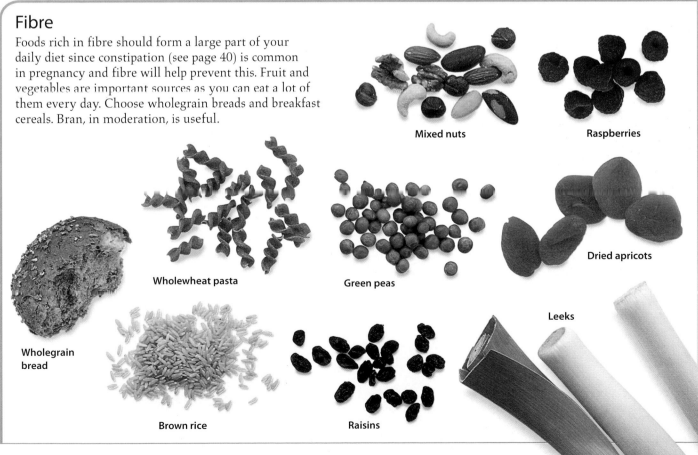

Mixed nuts

Raspberries

Wholewheat pasta

Green peas

Dried apricots

Wholegrain bread

Brown rice

Raisins

Leeks

Folic acid

Folic acid is a B vitamin that is needed for the development of the baby's central nervous system, especially in the first few weeks (see page 11). During the first three months of pregnancy you need as much as three times the amount of folic acid than normal. Folic acid is destroyed by over-cooking and by prolonged storage, but not by freezing. So, if you can't buy fresh vegetables daily, buy frozen ones instead. Look out for bread and cereals fortified with folic acid – they usually provide between 30 and 100mcg of folic acid in an average portion. Foods high in folic acid (50–100mcg/ serving) include: cooked beans (fava, kidney, pinto, soy, white, or navy), chickpeas, lentils, brussels sprouts, kale, spinach, broccoli, green beans, wholegrain bread, and hazelnuts. However, you cannot get enough folic acid from even the healthiest diet alone – it's essential to take a folic acid supplement as well, starting before you conceive and continuing throughout the pregnancy.

Wholegrain bread

Broccoli

Hazelnuts

Spinach

Iron

Pregnant women need increased amounts of iron to support the expanded blood volume that is needed for fetal development and to compensate for blood loss during delivery. Lean red meat and oily fish, such as sardines, are the most easily absorbed sources of iron. Baked beans, spinach, black-eyed beans, wholegrain bread, cereals, and legumes are all iron-rich too, though they are not quite as readily absorbed. Iron is absorbed more easily in the presence of vitamin C, while tea and coffee inhibit iron absorption. Avoid liver because it is too rich in vitamin A, which can be harmful in high doses.

Salmon

Spinach

Lean red meat

Dried apricots

Vegetarian diet

If you eat a variety of protein-rich foods and fresh fruit and vegetables every day, you should provide the baby with all the nutrition she needs to grow. The only nutrient you may lack is iron. This is because the body has more difficulty absorbing iron that comes from plant sources, so you may be given supplements of the mineral to compensate. If you are vegan and don't eat any dairy foods, you may be prescribed calcium, and vitamins D and B12.

Salt

Most people consume too much salt. Health Canada recommends that all Canadians reduce their salt intake. In pregnancy, excess salt can aggravate swelling.

Fluid

This is essential during pregnancy for keeping your kidneys healthy and avoiding constipation. Water is best.

Top foods

These foods are excellent sources of at least one nutrient. Eat some of them once a day:

● Cheese, milk, yogurt: *calcium, protein.*
● Dark green, leafy vegetables: *vitamin C, fibre, folic acid.*
● Lean red meat: *protein, iron.*
● Oranges: *vitamin C, fibre.*
● Poultry: *protein, iron.*
● Raisins and prunes: *iron, fibre.*
● Sardines: *calcium, protein, iron.*
● Fish such as flounder, salmon, and haddock: *protein, iron.*
● Wholegrain bread: *protein, fibre, folic acid.*
● Wholewheat pasta and brown rice: *fibre.*

Taking supplements

Folic acid supplementation of 0.4 to 1mg is recommended when you stop using contraception and throughout pregnancy. Most prenatal vitamins contain the recommended amount of folic acid and iron to complement a varied diet with plenty of fresh foods. Additional iron may be prescribed if you are anemic. Vitamin D is essential for calcium absorption and has other important roles in pregnancy. The ideal dose is unclear, but pregnant women should consider taking 1,000IU per day.

Protecting your baby

As the nutrients from your food can cross the placenta to the baby, so can many harmful substances that we regularly eat and drink.

Processed foods

Avoid processed convenience foods, such as processed meals and packaged mixes. Processed foods often have sugar and salt added, and they may contain a lot of fat, as well as preservatives, flavourings, and colourings. Read the labels carefully, and choose additive-free products.

Food safety
Pre-cooked foods

Avoid hot cafeteria foods, pre-cooked supermarket meals, and ready-to-eat poultry (unless served piping hot). These foods may contain bacteria that can be passed to your baby.

Cheese

Raw and unpasteurized milk and dairy products, and soft matured cheeses such as Brie, can be harmful because of the risk of listeria infection, so it's best to avoid them. Listeriosis may be a cause of miscarriage or stillbirth.

Fish

Sushi and other raw fish may be a source of parasites or listeriosis. Cook fish until it easily flakes with a fork.

Meat

Sliced meats, hot dogs, and refrigerated pâtés or spreads may contain bacteria such as listeria or toxoplasma. Avoid these products and make sure that all meats are well cooked. Avoid raw and lightly cooked eggs.

Fruits and vegetables

Wash all fruits and vegetables to remove any traces of pesticides or bacteria.

Coffee, tea, and hot chocolate

Caffeine, a substance found in all of these drinks, may affect your baby's growth if taken in high levels. Try to have no more than two cups of caffeine-containing drinks a day, and if possible, gradually cut them out altogether. Drink plenty of water instead.

Herbal teas

If you want to drink herbal teas in pregnancy, it is sensible to check first with your doctor or health advisor. Teas with citrus peel, lemon balm, rosehip, and ginger are considered safe in moderation. Health Canada lists several teas including chamomile that pregnant women should avoid.

Sugar

Sugary foods, such as cookies, jam, and soft drinks, are low in nutrients and can make you put on excess weight during pregnancy. It is best to get your energy from starchy carbohydrates, such as wholegrain bread and pasta, and cut down on sweet treats.

Alternatives to alcohol

Any alcohol that you drink during pregnancy is passed through the placenta into your baby's bloodstream, and can cause physical defects and developmental delay. So it's best to cut out alcohol altogether. Even beers and wines that claim to be alcohol free or low in alcohol are not necessarily free from undesirable additives and chemicals.

Essential fatty acids (EFA)

Essential fatty acids are vital for the development of your baby's brain, nervous system, and retina. The fetus can't manufacture these for itself, and relies on an efficient supply from the mother across the placenta, and after birth, from breast milk. Essential fatty acids aren't synthesized by the body, so it's important to include EFA-rich foods in your diet, especially during pregnancy. Oily fish, such as salmon, tuna, and mackerel, are by far the richest source. Health Canada recommends that pregnant women consume at least 150g (5oz) of cooked fish per week. However, large predator fish such as tuna (fresh or frozen), shark, marlin, swordfish, or orange roughy, may contain high levels of mercury, so limit your consumption of these fish to 150g (5oz) per month. Also limit canned albacore (white) tuna to two 170g (6oz) cans per week; however, there is no limit on "light" tuna such as tongol, skipjack, or yellowfin, which are low in mercury. Nuts, seeds, vegetable oils, and eggs are other sources of essential fatty acids.

Genetically modified (GM) foods

Genetically modified foods (also called genetically engineered or biotechnology-derived foods) are foods that have been modified by genetic manipulation. All GM foods are studied by Health Canada to ensure that they are safe prior to being introduced in Canada.

Cravings

It's common in pregnancy to find that you suddenly develop a taste for certain foods, such as pickled onions or ice cream. You can go ahead and indulge yourself within reason, provided it isn't too fattening, and doesn't cause indigestion.

Practical preparations

About a month before your due date, check that everything is ready for the baby, and buy food and other essentials to make life easier for you after the birth. Now is the time to pack for hospital, or to think about what you need if you are having a home birth. Some hospitals provide a list of what to take with you, and even some of the items on it, so check with your hospital before you start making your arrangements. Keep your bag packed and near the door.

Helpful things for labour

All the items below may be useful in labour and immediately after birth. Pack them separately as you will probably need them in a hurry.

Baggy T- shirt or an old nightgown
You will also need a front-opening nightgown for after the birth.

Thick socks
You may become cold in the later stages of labour.

Toiletries bag, toothbrush and toothpaste, lip balm

Small natural sponge
Moisten it, and suck on it if your mouth is dry.

Towel, facecloths, soap

Deodorant

Also

- your prenatal record
- a hot-water bottle
- books, magazines, MP3 player, or a personal stereo
- camera or video equipment
- cellphone and charger
- food and drink for your partner
- anything else that you have practised with at prenatal classes and would like to use during labour, such as a bean bag or birthing ball – check availability with your hospital first
- your own pillow.

For after the birth

You will need a few essentials after the birth, but your partner can bring these along later if you go into labour unexpectedly. The hospital may provide all you need for the baby during your stay.

Breast pads
Slip these inside your bra to absorb leaking milk. Shaped ones are best.

Also
- tissues
- face wash
- hairdryer
- two nursing bras
- sanitary pads, larger size
- baby clothes and supplies if the hospital does not provide them.

Brush, comb, shampoo, towel

Choose *large ones, with plenty of air holes*

6 pairs of cotton underwear in a dark colour, or, better still, disposable underwear.

Slippers

Front opening, *with buttons that undo well below the breasts, if breastfeeding*

Two to three machine-washable nightgowns and a bathrobe
These should be made of cotton or polycotton as the ward may be hot.

Home birth
There are several preconditions for a home birth (see page 32), so talk to your midwife if you are thinking about one. This includes a warm room, with easy access to hot water, a bathroom, and a telephone. You should also be within 30 minutes of the hospital, in case of complications.

What you will need:
- firm mattress
- two clean surfaces nearby, one for equipment, the other for the midwife's examination of the baby after birth
- clean towels, sheets, and blankets
- disposable bed pads
- small, bright lamp
- pillows
- plastic sheets to protect the bed and the surrounding floor
- one medium-sized plastic bowl
- large garbage bags
- two packages of sanitary pads, one superabsorbent
- baggy T-shirt or nightgown
- front-opening nightgown, bra, underwear
- diapers, undershirt, sleeper, hat, and blanket for the baby.

Making the bed
Put a clean fitted sheet on the bed. Cover this with a plastic sheet and another clean fitted sheet, which can be taken off after birth, leaving the bed freshly made underneath.

Coming home
You will need to leave out a set of clothes for your partner to bring when it's time for you to leave hospital. Don't choose anything too tight fitting; you will not be back to your pre-pregnancy size. The baby needs clothes for coming home in too, so set aside these things:

- two diapers (don't forget baby cleaning equipment)
- undershirt
- stretchsuit or nightgown
- sweater and hat
- blanket.

Labour and birth

At last, the labour is beginning. You will feel excited, yet apprehensive, about how your labour will progress. You will feel more confident if you have prepared yourself well so that you understand what is happening to your body at each stage of labour. Giving birth can be an immensely fulfilling experience, and keeping calm and relaxed is key. Practise your relaxation and breathing techniques beforehand to help you stay calm during the contractions and cope with the pain.

Knowing you are in labour

You may worry that you won't recognize labour when it comes. This is most unlikely. Although it is possible to confuse the first labour contractions with the contractions that may occur in the last weeks of pregnancy, you will probably be able to tell if labour is imminent, as it is heralded by a number of signs.

Signs of labour

A show
The plug of thick, blood-stained mucus that blocks the neck of the womb in pregnancy usually passes out of the vagina, either before or during the early stages of labour.
What to do The show may happen a few days before labour starts, so wait until you have regular pains in your stomach or back, or your waters break, before calling the doctor or midwife.

Your waters break
The bag of fluid that surrounds the baby can break at any time during labour. It may be a sudden flood, but it's far more common to notice a trickle of fluid as the baby's head has often engaged – this stems the tide.
What to do Call the hospital or your caregiver at once. You may need to go to hospital even without contractions, as there is a risk of infection. In the meantime, wear a sanitary pad to absorb the flow.

Contractions

These may start off as a dull backache, or you may have shooting pains down your thighs. As time goes on, you will probably have contractions in your stomach, rather like bad period pains.
What to do When the contractions seem to be regular, time them. If you think you are in labour, call the doctor or midwife. Unless contractions are coming very frequently (every five minutes), or are very painful, there is no need to go into hospital immediately. A first labour usually lasts about 12 to 14 hours, and it is often better to spend several hours of this time at home. Remain calm. Perhaps relax in a warm bath if your waters haven't broken, or eat a light snack. The hospital will probably suggest you wait until the contractions are strong and occurring every five minutes or so before you leave home.

False starts

Throughout pregnancy, the womb contracts. In the last weeks, these Braxton Hicks contractions become stronger, so you may think you are in labour. But true labour contractions occur very regularly and grow stronger and more frequent, so you should be able to tell when the real thing begins. Occasionally contractions start and then stop. Keep moving – in time they will get going again.

Timing contractions

10 minutes

Contraction

20 minutes

15 minutes

Interval between contractions

15 minutes

Time contractions over an hour, noting the length of each one. They should become stronger and more frequent, and last for at least 40 seconds as labour becomes established. The diagram shows the kind of intervals between contractions you may have in early labour.

The first stage

During this stage, the muscles of your womb contract to open up the cervix (neck of the womb) to allow the baby to pass through at birth. It takes an average of 10 to 12 hours for a first baby.

Don't be surprised if at some time in the first stage you suddenly feel panic-stricken. You may even find yourself rushing around trying to finish last-minute tasks. However well-prepared you are, the feeling that your body has been taken over by a process that you can't control can be frightening. Stay calm and try to go with your body. It is now that you will most appreciate having your partner or a good friend by your side, especially if they know about labour and have gone to prenatal classes.

During admission
A nurse will review your prenatal records and ask you about your contractions.

Admission to hospital

At the hospital, a nurse will carry out several routine admission procedures. Your partner can stay with you during this process. If you are having the baby at home, your midwife will probably prepare you for the birth in much the same way.

Admission questions
The nurse will check your records and will ask if you think your waters have broken and whether you have had a show. She will also ask you about your contractions: when they started, how frequent they are, what they feel like, and how long each one lasts.

Checking you
After you have changed into the hospital gown or your own clothes for the birth, the nurse will take your blood pressure, temperature, and pulse, and may give you an internal examination to check how far the neck of the womb has opened. If you are still in very early labour, she might suggest that you go home or walk around for a few hours.

Checking the baby
The nurse will check the baby's position by feeling your abdomen, and she will listen to his heartbeat with a fetal doppler or a stethoscope. She may attach a heart monitor to you for 20 minutes or so, to record the baby's heartbeat and to assess his well-being in labour.

Group B streptococcal infection
About 10 to 30 percent of women are carriers of Group B streptococcus, a bacterium that can cause serious infections in newborn infants. The risk of infection occurs in labour, particularly once the membranes have ruptured. You will be tested for Group B streptococcus (with a vaginal/rectal swab) at 35 to 37 weeks. If you are a carrier, or you go into premature labour, you will be given an antibiotic during labour to protect you and your baby from infection.

Internal examinations

Your care provider may give you regular internal examinations to check the position of the baby and how much the cervix is dilating (opening up). Ask how much you have dilated if you are not told – it is encouraging to find that the cervix is widening, but this may not happen at a completely steady rate.

The examination is usually done between contractions, so tell the nurse if you feel one coming so she can wait until it subsides. Try to relax as much as possible, and take slow deep breaths to minimize any discomfort.

The cervix in labour

This is normally kept closed by a ring of muscles. Other muscles run from the cervix up and over the womb. These contract during labour, drawing the cervix into the womb, and then stretching it so it is wide enough for the baby's head to pass through. The tough cervix is gradually softened by hormone changes.

1 Gentle contractions efface (thin) the cervix.

Lower segment of uterus

Cervix

2 Once the cervix has fully effaced, stronger contractions dilate it.

Cervix being drawn up by uterus

Cervix shortened

Positions for the first stage

Try a variety of positions during the first stage of labour as different positions will probably be comfortable at different times. Practise these positions beforehand so that you can follow your body's natural cues with ease.

Your birth partner

If you do not have a partner, or if he or she cannot be at the birth, choose your mother, sister, or a friend to be with you. Research shows that effective labour support can actually shorten labour and reduce the risk of complications.

Stay upright

As far as possible, try to maintain an upright position. This keeps pressure on the base of the uterus and helps to stimulate strong contractions.

Early labour
During early contractions, support yourself on a nearby surface, such as a wall, chair seat, or the hospital bed.

The birth partner's role

● During contractions give her plenty of praise, comfort, and support. Don't worry if she becomes annoyed with you; you are important.
● Remind her of the relaxation and breathing techniques she has learned.
● Mop her brow, give her sips of water, suggest a change of position, or do anything else that helps. Learn what sort of touch and massage she likes beforehand, but remember that she might not feel like having a massage during the birth. Always take your cues from her.
● Act as a mediator between her and the hospital staff, letting them know, for example, if she decides she needs pain relief.

Tubs and showers

Immersion in water, warmed to body temperature, can help you to relax and ease pain during labour. Some hospitals provide tubs, with or without water jets, for this purpose. If you want to use a tub in labour, check early in your pregnancy to see if the maternity unit you plan to attend has one available.

On all fours
Kneel down on your hands and knees on the floor (you may find a mattress more comfortable), and tilt your pelvis to and fro. Do not arch your back. Between contractions, relax forwards and rest your head in your arms.

Lower back massage/kneel forwards
This will relieve your backache. Your partner should massage you at the base of your spine, using the heel of his hand to make firm, circular movements. Kneel down with your legs apart and relax on a pile of cushions. Sit to one side between contractions.

Breathing for the first stage

Deep even breaths   Light breaths   Deep even breaths

IN

OUT

← Peak →

← Length of contraction →

At the beginning and end of a contraction, breathe deeply and evenly, in through the nose, and out of the mouth. When the contraction peaks, try a lighter, shallower kind of breathing – in and out breaths both through your mouth. Don't do this for too long as you will begin to feel dizzy.

Birthing balls

A birthing ball can help you find a comfortable, supported position during contractions. You may want to kneel and lean over it, or sit on it and lean forward over a stack of pillows on your bed so that you are virtually lying down and yet can still rock your hips backwards and forwards. This can be especially helpful during back labour. You can still use the birthing ball during fetal monitoring. Some hospitals also offer birthing balls when they administer light epidural anaesthesia.

Ways to help yourself
- Keep moving between contractions; this helps you cope with the pain. During contractions, take up a comfortable position.
- Try to stay as upright as possible, so the baby's head sits firmly on the cervix, making your contractions stronger and more effective.
- Concentrate on your breathing. This will calm you and take your mind off a contraction.
- Relax between contractions (see pages 48–9) to save energy for when you need it.
- Sing, or even moan and groan, to release pain.
- Look at a fixed spot or object to help take your mind off a contraction.
- Take one contraction at a time, and don't think about the contractions to follow. Perhaps see each contraction as a wave that you have to ride over to reach the baby.
- Urinate often, so your bladder doesn't get in the way of the baby.

Back labour
When the baby is facing towards your abdomen instead of away from it, her head tends to press against your spine, causing backache. To relieve pain:
- during contractions lean forwards with your weight supported, such as on all fours, to take the baby's weight off your back; rock your pelvis to and fro, and move around between contractions
- ask your partner to massage your back.

Transition

The most difficult time in labour is often at the end of the first stage, when contractions are strongest. They last about a minute and may be only a minute apart, so there is little time to rest after one ends before the next is upon you. This phase is known as transition. You will be tired, and may feel tearful, excitable, or just bad-tempered. You may also lose all sense of time and doze off between contractions. Feeling sick, vomiting, and shivering are common in this phase.

Eventually, you may experience a strong urge to push. However, if you start to push too early, before the cervix is fully dilated, it can become swollen. It's important that you tell the nurse or doctor when you first feel the urge to push. She will examine you to determine whether your cervix is fully dilated. If it is not, she may ask you to pant during contractions (see box, above right) to help you resist the urge to push until the cervix has dilated to about 10cm (4in). If you wish to change position at this stage, kneeling down and leaning forwards with your head resting on your arms and your bottom in the air can help you resist the urge to push.

If your waters have not yet broken, they will almost certainly do so during transition. You may feel a gush or only a trickle when this happens. Without the amniotic sac, the baby's head presses directly on the bottom of the uterus, and labour often speeds up.

Breathing for transition

Short breaths   **Short breaths**   **Short breaths**

IN

OUT

Blow   **Blow**   **Gently out**

If you want to push too early say "huff, huff, blow" to yourself, taking two short in- and out-breaths, blowing a longer out-breath. When the need to push fades, breathe out slowly and evenly.

The birth partner's role
- Try to relax her, encourage her, and wipe away any perspiration; if she doesn't want to be touched, stay back.
- Breathe with her through contractions.
- Put thick socks on her feet if they start to shake, and gently hold them still.

The cervix in labour

Cervix

At 7cm (2¾in), the doctor or midwife feels the cervix stretched out around the baby's head.

When the doctor or midwife can't feel the cervix (at about 10cm/4in), you are fully dilated.

The second stage

Once the cervix has dilated and you can push, the second stage of labour has begun. You can now add your own efforts to the powerful contractions of the womb to push the baby out. If the baby is lying in a slightly different position you may not feel this urge to push, but the doctor or midwife will guide you so that you push when it is most needed. She will also help you find the most comfortable position in which to push. Even though the contractions are stronger, they don't feel as bad as before. This stage usually lasts about an hour for a first baby.

Breathing for the second stage

Deep breaths   **Deep even breaths**   **Even breaths**

IN

Push   **Push**

OUT

When you want to push (this may happen several times during a contraction), take a deep breath and hold it for a short time as you bear down, if this helps the push; it's important to do what your body tells you. Between pushes, take a few deep calming breaths to relax.

Positions for birth

Try to remain as upright as possible when you are pushing during the second stage of labour, so you are working with gravity rather than against it. This will help the delivery process.

Squatting and kneeling

Squatting is an excellent position for delivery, because it opens the pelvis wide and uses gravity to help push out the baby. But unless you have practised it beforehand (see page 47), you may find it tiring after a while. If your partner sits on the edge of a chair with his legs apart, you can squat between his knees, resting your arms on his thighs for support.

Kneeling may be less tiring than squatting (see above), and is also a good position to push from. A helper on each side will make you feel more stable. You may also find kneeling down on all fours comfortable; keep your back straight.

Sitting upright

A common delivery position is to sit on the bed propped up by pillows, a beanbag, or a wedge. Keep your chin down, and grip your knees as you push. Relax between contractions.

Side lying

A side lying position is good if you have an epidural or are too tired to squat. Your partner can support your upper leg.

Ways to help yourself

- Push steadily during a contraction.
- Try to relax the muscles of your pelvic floor (see page 45).
- Keep your face relaxed.
- Don't worry about trying to control your bowels, or leakage from the bladder.
- Rest between contractions, so you save all your energy for pushing.

The birth partner's role

- Try to relax her between the contractions, and give encouragement.
- Tell her when you can see the baby's head emerging.

The birth

The climax of labour has now arrived, and you can actually touch your baby's head for the first time as she emerges. Your partner's company may calm you and give you confidence during the long hours of labour and delivery. If you have both been to childbirth classes you have trained together for this moment. Your partner can support you and remind you of breathing and relaxation techniques. The sheer force of the muscular contractions can make you feel like you have little control over your body – your partner can help by rubbing your back, sponging your brow, and counting you through the contractions so that you can push with them. His involvement will help him to feel that he is a more integral part of the birthing process. If your partner is not able to be there, you will appreciate the help of a close friend or relative, or even a doula. You will probably feel a great sense of physical relief once your baby is born. There may also be tears of joy, and a feeling of great tenderness towards your baby.

1 The baby's head moves nearer the vaginal opening, until eventually your partner will be able to see the bulge where it is pressing against the pelvic floor. Soon the head itself will be seen, moving forwards with each contraction, and perhaps slipping back slightly as the contraction fades. Don't be discouraged if this happens – it is perfectly normal.

When the head "crowns" (the top is visible), the doctor or midwife will ask you not to push because if the head is born too quickly your skin might tear. So, relax, and pant like a dog for a few seconds. If there is a risk of a serious tear, or the baby is distressed, you may have an episiotomy (see page 66).

As the baby's head widens the vaginal opening, there will be a stinging feeling, but this will only last for a short while, and will soon be followed by numbness because the tissues have been stretched so much.

2 The head is born face down. The doctor or midwife will probably check the umbilical cord, to make sure it isn't looped around the baby's neck (if it is, the cord can usually be slipped over the head before the body is delivered). If it is very tight, the cord might be clamped and cut at this time. Then, the baby turns her head to one side so that it is in line with her shoulders. The baby is usually able to clear her own nose and mouth.

3 The body comes sliding out within the next two contractions. The baby will usually be delivered onto your stomach, still joined to the cord. Your baby will probably look rather blue at first, covered in vernix, with streaks of blood on her skin. She may be crying. If she is breathing normally, you can hold her at once. Drying her off and keeping her "skin to skin" with you will help to keep her warm.

"I'm very worried about permanently damaging myself during the birth of my baby. Is there any danger of this occurring?"
You won't damage yourself as you push during the birth. The vaginal walls are elastic, and made of folds, so they can stretch to allow the baby through.

"Should I breastfeed my baby immediately after the birth?"
Try offering your baby the breast and leave the decision up to her. Although there won't be any milk yet, a newborn baby's urge to suck is often strong, and she will find the sucking comforting.

Q&A

The third stage

During, or just after, the birth you will probably be given an injection in your thigh or intravenously, of a drug called oxytocin, which makes the womb contract strongly, and delivers the placenta quickly. Giving oxytocin reduces postpartum bleeding significantly. If you are concerned about this, talk to the doctor or midwife beforehand.

To deliver the placenta the doctor or midwife puts her hand on your stomach and gently pulls the umbilical cord with her other hand to help the placenta detach. Later, she will check the placenta to ensure it is complete.

After the birth

Once the baby is born, the umbilical cord will be clamped and cut. However, exactly when that occurs varies among care providers. Studies suggest that delaying cord clamping for about two minutes or until the cord stops pulsing may increase the amount of blood that goes to the baby, preventing anemia and low iron levels. This may be especially important for smaller or preterm babies. If you have strong feelings about when you would like the cord clamped, speak to your doctor or midwife.

The baby will be given a shot of vitamin K to prevent a rare bleeding disorder and antibiotic eye ointment.

The Apgar score

One minute after birth, the doctor or midwife will assess the baby's breathing, heart rate, skin colour, movements, and response to stimulation, and give her an Apgar score of between 0 and 10. Most babies score between 7 and 10. The test is done again at five minutes, which is a more accurate reflection of her adjustment to life outside the womb.

Becoming a family
After the birth, you and your partner can relax and spend a few quiet moments with your baby.

Pain relief

Although labour is not usually pain free, the pain does have a purpose: every contraction brings you one step nearer the birth of your baby. However determined you may be not to have pain relief, do try to keep an open mind. Whether you need it or not depends very much on your labour and your ability to deal with pain. You may be able to cope better during labour using the self-help methods on pages 59 and 61. Remember that pain is always worse if you try to fight it. But if the discomfort is more than you can bear, ask for pain relief. There are several options that are available to you.

Epidural

An epidural is an anaesthetic that relieves pain by temporarily numbing the nerves in the lower body. It can be especially good in a back labour. Most hospitals offer epidurals.

Epidural techniques and the medications used have changed over the past decade to allow women more mobility and more sensation. This is important for the second stage of labour, which can be affected by epidural use.

What happens

An epidural takes about 20 minutes to set up. You will be asked to tuck your knees up under your chin, so that your back is rounded. The anaesthetic is injected through a tube into your lower back. This is left in place, so that you can be given top-ups (either through a pump, which you control, or by the nurse) as necessary; the anaesthetic wears off in about two hours. Your movements may be restricted, however most women are able to walk, at least with support.

Effects

You If the epidural works properly, you should feel no pain, and remain fully aware of what is happening. You may feel faint, experience itching, or have a headache that may last for a few hours afterwards. Serious complications are rare.
The baby None.

Nitrous oxide
(laughing gas)

A mixture of oxygen and nitrous oxide can take the edge off the pain for many women. It is easy to administer, quick-acting, and safe for your baby.

What happens

You inhale the gas through a hand-held mask, so you control it. It takes about half a minute to reach a peak so you need to breathe deeply when a contraction starts.

Effects

You The medication may not provide enough pain relief. You may feel light-headed or sick while inhaling the gas.
The baby None.

Opioids

Drugs such as morphine and fentanyl can be given by injection early in the first stage of labour and by patient-controlled intravenous drip in later stages. The pain-relief effect is small but it will help to relax you during labour.

What happens

The medication will be given by injection in your buttock or thigh. It takes about 20 minutes to work and its effect lasts about two to three hours.

Effects

You Some women may feel out of control, confused, or "high," while others feel relaxed and drowsy. Vomiting may occur.
The baby If given too close to the birth, it can slow the baby's breathing and make her sleepy.

Vertebra   *Epidural space*

Hollow needle

Spinal cord

Giving the anaesthetic
A hollow needle is inserted between the vertebrae of your spine. A fine tube is passed through the needle, and local anaesthetic fed directly into this. The picture (far left) shows a woman in labour being administered an epidural.

TENS

This treatment lessens pain and stimulates the body's natural system of pain relief by delivering impulses of electrical current into your body. It helps to practise with the TENS machine in the last month before the birth. TENS units are available at health-care supply stores.

What happens

Four pads containing electrodes are stuck on your back, over the nerves that supply the womb. These pads are joined by wires to a hand-held control with which you regulate the strength, frequency, and duration of the electric current to suit yourself.

Effects

You TENS can lessen the pain considerably for some women, especially if used from early labour. If labour is very painful, TENS probably won't be sufficient.
The baby None.

Press the switch on the control box to change the intensity of the current

The pad delivers the electric current into your body

Using the machine
With TENS you are in total control, and mobile.

Monitoring

Throughout labour your baby's heartbeat will be monitored to make sure she is coping well during the entire process. This can be done by intermittent auscultation (listening) or continuous electronic fetal monitoring. Intermittent auscultation is the preferred method in low risk labours.

Intermittent auscultation

The nurse or midwife uses a special stethoscope or fetal doppler to listen to the baby's heartbeat at regular intervals throughout labour.

Electronic fetal monitoring (EFM)

This is a way of recording the baby's heartbeat and your contractions using sophisticated electronic equipment. Some hospitals routinely monitor women throughout labour, others only at intervals unless:

- your labour is induced (see page 66)
- you are having an epidural
- you have a problem or condition that puts you or your baby at risk
- the baby is distressed at any time.

EFM is not painful. The procedure is safe for both you and your baby. If you are unsure as to why it is being used, ask your doctor or midwife.

Your baby's heart rate is monitored with a small plastic circular device. One or two elastic belts are placed around your abdomen to secure the monitors. Fetal monitoring can restrict your freedom to move around; however, you should be able to stand, sit, or squat with the monitors in place. Some hospitals even have monitors that allow you to walk around and be monitored by radio signals.

How Electronic Fetal Monitoring works

Your baby's heartbeat is recorded, measuring both the baseline rate and variation in heart rate. The heart rate rises and falls naturally with contractions; unusual variations can indicate fetal distress.

A separate reading records the frequency and duration of each contraction. This can detect infrequent or irregular contractions and can be useful with an epidural when you can't feel contractions.

Continuous monitoring
Two monitors strapped to your stomach continuously monitor the baby's heart rate and your contractions.

Special procedures

Episiotomy

This small cut widens the vaginal opening and prevents a tear. Some hospitals perform episiotomies more often than others, so speak to your doctor or midwife about the trends in your hospital.

When used
An episiotomy may be needed if:
- the baby is breech, premature, distressed, or has a large head
- you have a forceps delivery
- the skin around your vaginal opening hasn't stretched enough.

What happens
Your pelvic floor area will probably be frozen with an injection of local anaesthetic, and a small cut will be made from the bottom of the vagina, either in the middle or slightly out to one side, at the peak of a contraction. If there is no time for an injection, the stretching of the tissues also numbs them, so you shouldn't feel any pain.

Stitching up after an episiotomy or a tear may take some time, as the different layers of skin and muscle have to be carefully sewn together. It can be painful, too, so ask for more anaesthetic if you need some. The stitches will dissolve and do not have to be removed.

Effects
Some discomfort and soreness is normal after an episiotomy, but the pain can be quite severe, especially if an infection develops. The wound should heal within 10 to 14 days, but if you are sore after this time, go to see your doctor. There is usually less pain with a natural tear.

Assisted delivery

Sometimes the baby has to be helped out with forceps or by vacuum. Your doctor will explain the reasons for the procedure and why she has chosen a particular instrument.

When used
You may have an assisted delivery if:
- you cannot push the baby out, perhaps because he has a large head or is positioned in an awkward way
- you or the baby show signs of distress during labour
- you have a condition (e.g. some heart conditions) which makes prolonged pushing dangerous.

What happens
If you do not have an epidural, you will need anaesthetic for a forceps delivery. This is not necessary for a vacuum-assisted delivery. The doctor uses the forceps or a vacuum to deliver the head while you help by pushing. The rest of your baby's body is delivered normally.

Forceps
These form a cage around the baby's head, protecting it from pressure and damage.

Vacuum
A small plastic cup, connected to a vacuum pump, is passed into the vagina and attached to the baby's head. The baby is gently pulled through the birth canal as you push.

Effects
- If forceps are used to deliver your baby, they may leave pressure marks or bruises on either side of the baby's head, which will disappear within a few days of the birth. Very rarely, there may be serious injuries to the baby's face or head. You may have an episiotomy or vaginal tears.
- The vacuum cup will cause slight swelling, and later a bruise, on the baby's head. This gradually subsides. Very rarely, there may be retinal bleeding or bleeding within the baby's head.

Induction

Induction means that labour is started artificially. Ask your doctor or midwife what their policy is on induction.

When used
Labour may be induced if:
- it is more than 7 to 10 days past the baby's due date or he shows signs of being distressed, or the placenta starts to fail
- you have high blood pressure, or another problem or condition that puts you or the baby at risk
- your waters have been broken for several hours and you are not in labour.

What happens
Induction is always planned in advance, and you will be asked to go into the hospital. Four methods of induction may be used alone or in combination:
1 Inserting a gel or other preparation of prostaglandin, a hormone that softens the cervix, into the vagina. This is done to soften the cervix before labour starts, although sometimes it does put you into labour.
2 Using a catheter to stretch the cervix. The catheter is inflated with water and usually left inside for 12 to 24 hours or until it falls out.
3 Breaking your waters (amniotomy). The doctor uses a special instrument to make a small hole in the bag of waters surrounding the baby Most women don't feel any pain. Contractions nearly always start soon afterwards.
4 Giving you a hormone (oxytocin) that makes the womb contract. This medication is administered through an intravenous drip which is controlled.

Effects
Discuss the method of induction recommended with your doctor or midwife. An induced labour may bring on contractions that are stronger and more painful, with shorter intervals between them than in labour that has started naturally. Your mobility is restricted if you have an intravenous drip.

Breech birth

A breech baby is born bottom first. About four in 100 births are breech. As the largest part of the baby (the head) is born last, there is always the risk that it will be trapped in the birth canal, which has not been sufficiently stretched by the buttocks. Because of this and other potential complications of breech presentation, it is the policy of many hospitals to deliver all breech babies by a Caesarean section.

However, it is possible to deliver a breech baby vaginally if your baby is in the right position, is a reasonable size, and you have a care provider who is experienced and comfortable with vaginal breech deliveries. In some situations, an external cephalic version (ECV) can be used to turn your baby from breech to head first before labour.

Twins

It is essential to have twins in hospital. There is a higher chance of Caesarean section, and the babies may be small and need special care afterwards that would not be available at a home birth.

In a vaginal twin labour there is only one first stage, but you will have two second stages as you push one baby out, and then the other usually 10 to 30 minutes after the first.

Caesarean section

With a Caesarean birth, the baby is delivered abdominally. You may know you are going to have a Caesarean in advance, or it may be an emergency operation because of problems in labour. If a Caesarean is planned you can have it under an epidural or spinal anaesthesia (see page 64), so you are awake throughout and can hold your baby straightaway. This may also be possible if you are told in labour you need the operation, but rarely a general anaesthetic is necessary.

It's only natural to feel disappointed, and perhaps cheated of a normal delivery, if you need a Caesarean. But these feelings can be minimized if you prepare yourself thoroughly, and seek support from your birth partner. Ask your hospital if your birth partner can be with you throughout.

The incision
The "bikini" cut is usually made horizontally, just above the pubic hairline, and it is almost invisible when it heals.

Stitching the wound
You or your partner can hold the baby, while the doctor stitches you up.

What happens

An intravenous drip will be put in your arm, and a catheter inserted into your bladder. You will most likely have an epidural or a spinal anaesthetic. There is a screen set up between you and the surgeon. The cut is usually made horizontally, and the underlying muscles are separated gently to reach the uterus. The baby is lifted out through the uterine incision. You can hold him as the placenta is delivered. The whole procedure takes about 45 minutes.

After the operation

You will be encouraged to walk soon after the birth. The incision will be painful for a few days, so ask for pain medications. Continue to take them as long as you need pain relief. Moving around won't open the wound up. When walking, stand tall, and cup your hands over the wound. Approximately two days after the operation, the dressing will be removed, and you can have a shower. You may also begin gentle exercises (see page 72). The stitches or staples will be removed three to five days after birth, unless dissolvable. You will feel much better after a week. Avoid straining yourself for at least six weeks. The scar usually fades in three to six months.

Breastfeeding after a Caesarean section
Support your baby on one or two pillows beside you, so he is not resting on the wound.

Your new baby

Your baby will probably look very different from what you expected. He may seem smaller than you imagined, the shape of his head may seem strange, and you are bound to notice spots, blotches, and changes of colour – this is all perfectly normal. Ask your doctor or midwife if anything worries you. You may love your baby immediately. But if you don't feel this strongly at first, allow yourself time. Once you start caring for your baby, the bond will deepen, and love will grow naturally.

First impressions

Don't be dismayed if your baby doesn't look perfect – few babies do at birth. You may notice the following imperfections, but most of these will disappear within two weeks. Below and facing is a rundown of how different parts of your baby's body may appear after birth.

Head
A cone-shaped head is usually caused by the pressure of birth. The head should look normal within two weeks.
On the top of the head is a soft spot (fontanelle), where the bones of the skull have not yet joined together. They should fuse by the time the child is 18 months old.

Eyes
True eye colour may not develop until the baby is about six months old.
Puffy eyelids are usually caused by the pressure of birth, but ask the doctor to check your baby's eyes, as it could be an infection.
Cross-eye is common in the first months.

Tongue
This may seem anchored to the floor of the mouth and might look slightly forked when the baby sticks the tongue out. The tip will grow forwards in the first year.

Hands and feet
These may be bluish because the baby's circulation is not working properly. If you move your baby into another position, they should turn pink.
The fingernails are often long at birth; carefully trim using special baby scissors.

The fontanelle *cannot be damaged through everyday handling*

Your baby *may have a good head of hair, or he may be bald*

His hands *will be clenched*

Red marks *are caused by pressure from the birth, or because the baby's skin is still immature*

The umbilical cord *stump drops off in about 10 days*

The baby's legs *often look bowed because he has been curled up in the womb*

Your baby can see *you at birth if you hold him about 20cm (8in) away from your face*

Breasts

Your baby's breasts may be swollen and even leak a little milk. This is normal in both sexes. The swelling should go down within two days; do not squeeze the milk out.

Genitals

These appear large on both male and female babies.
A baby girl may have discharge from her vagina. This is caused by the mother's hormones and will soon disappear.
The testicles of a baby boy are often pulled up into his groin. If worried, see your doctor.

Skin

Spots and rashes are very common, and should vanish of their own accord.
Peeling skin, especially on the hands and feet, should disappear in a couple of days.
Downy body hair (lanugo) may be visible, especially if the baby was born early. This rubs off within two weeks.
Greasy white vernix covers and protects the baby's skin in the womb. It can be wiped off.
Birthmarks usually vanish. These include:
● red marks (stork bites) often found on the eyelids, forehead, and at the back of the neck; they take about a year to go
● strawberry birthmarks, which gradually increase in size; they usually disappear by the time the child is five
● blue patches (Mongolian spots), often found on the lower backs of babies with dark skin
● port wine stain, a bright red or purple mark, which is permanent.

Stool

At birth, the baby's bowel contains a dark, sticky substance called meconium.

Checks on the baby

Your baby will be examined several times in the first week. The doctor or midwife will weigh him regularly, and check him for any problems or signs of infection. This is a good time to discuss any worries that you may have.

General examination
The doctor will check the baby from head to toe to make sure there is nothing abnormal.

1 The doctor measures the head. He checks the fontanelle, and feels the roof of the mouth to make sure it is complete.

2 He listens to the heart and lungs to see if they are normal. Heart murmurs are common among newborn babies, and do not usually indicate any kind of defect.

3 By putting his hand on the baby's stomach, the doctor checks that the abdominal organs are the right size. He also feels the pulses in the baby's groin.

4 The genitals are checked for abnormality. If you have a boy, the doctor checks if both testicles have descended.

5 He moves the baby's limbs to see that the lower legs and feet are in alignment and legs are the right length.

6 The doctor checks the hips for any dislocation, by bending the baby's legs up and gently circling them.

7 He makes sure that all the vertebrae are in place along the spine.

8 The doctor checks the baby's eyes and hearing.

Newborn screening
After 24 hours, all Canadian babies have a blood test (from a heel prick) which tests for three rare but serious disorders: phenylketonuria (a cause of mental handicap), thyroid deficiency (which causes poor growth and developmental problems) and galactosemia (a cause of blindness, developmental delay, and death). These conditions can be treated if diagnosed early. Several provinces test for up to 25 other hereditary conditions. Ask your care provider which tests are done in your area. All newborns are also tested for hearing loss before leaving the hospital.

Babies needing special care

Premature (born before 37 weeks) or small for dates (see page 38) babies need extra care after birth. They are more likely to have problems with breathing, feeding, and maintaining their temperature, and so need special treatment and monitoring. If your baby needs intensive medical care, she will have to spend her first days in an incubator, but once this is no longer necessary, you will be able to give her "kangaroo care," the prolonged skin-to-skin contact that has been found as effective as an incubator in keeping a premature baby warm and safe. Research shows that babies given kangaroo care sleep better and gain weight more quickly, and it even improves the chance of successful breastfeeding.

Getting to know your baby

Even if your baby is in an incubator, she needs as much love and attention as any other baby, so it's important to spend as much time with her as possible, and take part in her daily care. All babies respond to loving handling, and even if she can't be taken out of the incubator and cuddled, you can still talk to her and stroke her through the portholes in the side.

Asking questions

Ask the doctor or nursing staff about anything that worries you. Often parents don't ask questions because their baby looks so frail that they are afraid of the reply. But with modern intensive care, even babies born before 28 weeks can survive.

Feeding

If your baby can suck, you may be able to feed her normally. Otherwise, she will be fed through a tube, which is passed through her nose or mouth and down into her stomach.

Jaundice

Many newborn babies develop very mild jaundice about three days after birth, which turns their skin and the whites of their eyes slightly yellow. This happens because a baby's liver is still immature, and a pigment called bilirubin accumulates in the blood faster than the liver can dispose of it.

Jaundice usually clears up in a few days of its own accord, although the baby may be more sleepy than usual, so wake her up often and encourage her to feed. It also helps if her crib is near a window, so she is exposed to sunlight. Sometimes jaundice has to be treated with a special light (phototherapy). This can usually be done in your hospital room, and only in a few severe cases is the baby taken into special care. If the baby is still jaundiced after two weeks, the doctor may refer her back to the hospital for a check up.

Kangaroo care
You – or even your partner – can give this skin-to-skin contact, either propped up in bed or sitting in a chair, holding your baby against your chest.

Control, *to regulate the temperature inside the incubator*

Portholes, *so you can touch your baby and talk to her*

Feeding tube, *which passes into the baby's stomach; you can express your own milk to be fed to the baby*

The baby in the incubator
Even with all the extra medical care available in the special care unit, your baby needs just as much love and attention as any normal baby.

Stillbirth

Very rarely, a baby is born dead. The exact cause for stillbirths remains uncertain as it can be a number of different factors. What makes this so hard to bear is that you never knew your child. It's probably a good idea to see her after birth; by holding her, and giving her a name, you can grieve for her as a person, and it's important to do this. You will probably feel angry, and want to know what went wrong, and find something or someone to blame. Shame and guilt are also quite common. But you should know that it is not your fault. Ask your doctor to put you in touch with a therapist or self-help group.

Getting back to normal

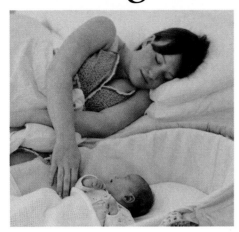

For the first week after delivery try to rest whenever you can. Don't be tempted to try to catch up on everything you have not had the time to do. Call your doctor if you have any problems before your postpartum check-up. You may be rather disheartened when you see your body after birth. Your stomach won't be flat, your breasts will be large, and the tops of your legs will feel heavy. But if you practise your postnatal exercises as soon as possible after birth, you will begin to look and feel better.

How you will feel

As the initial rush of excitement of your baby's birth settles down, you will probably experience some discomfort, and even pain, in the first days. Ask the doctor or midwife if anything worries you.

After pains
You may feel cramping pains in your stomach, especially when breastfeeding, as the womb contracts back to its pre-pregnant size. This is a good sign that your body is returning to normal. The pains may last several days.
What to do If contractions are severe, a mild painkiller such as acetaminophen or ibuprofen may ease them.

Bladder
It's normal to urinate more often in the first days, as the body loses the extra fluid gained in pregnancy.
What to do Urinating may be difficult at first because of soreness, but try to do so as soon as possible after birth.
● Get up and about to encourage the urinary flow.
● Soak in a warm bath. Don't worry if you pass urine into the water as urine is sterile; wash yourself well afterwards.
● If you have stitches, try pouring warm water over them as you pass urine to stop your skin stinging.

Bleeding
You may have vaginal bleeding for anything from two to six weeks. This usually stops more quickly if you are breastfeeding. The bright-red discharge is heavy at first, but over the next few days it decreases and gradually becomes brownish. Often the discharge continues until the first menstrual period.
What to do Wear sanitary pads to catch the flow; don't use internal tampons, because they may be uncomfortable.

Bowels
You may not need to empty your bowels for a day or more after the birth.
What to do Get mobile as soon as possible: this will start your bowels working.
● Drink plenty of water and eat high-fibre foods to stimulate your bowels.
● When you want to empty your bowels, do so at once, but don't strain too hard.
● It is most unlikely that any stitches will tear when you move your bowels, but holding a clean sanitary pad against the area while you do so may help you feel more confident.

Stitches
These may be very sore for a few days. Most dissolve in about a week.
What to do The following suggestions will help the recovery process.
● Practise pelvic floor exercises as soon as possible after birth to speed up healing.
● Keep the stitches clean by relaxing in a warm bath. Dry the entire area thoroughly afterwards.

Coping with the blues
Many women feel low a few days after delivery, usually when the milk comes in. One cause is the sudden change in hormone levels, another is the feeling of anticlimax that sometimes occurs after birth. These postpartum blues usually vanish. If you feel depressed for more than four weeks, or your depression is severe, see your doctor immediately.

Thinking positively
The sheer pleasure and delight of finally having your newborn baby will probably more than compensate for the after effects of the labour and birth process.

● Soothe soreness by applying an ice-pack to the area.
● Lie down to take pressure off the stitches, or sit on a rubber ring.

Shaping up after birth

With some gentle exercising every day your figure can return to normal in as little as three months after the birth, although your stomach muscles may not be as firm as before. Build up your exercise program slowly at first as your ligaments are still soft and stretchy, and always stop immediately if you feel pain or tiredness. It's best to exercise a little, but on a regular basis. You may want to join a local postnatal exercise class.

Warning

If you have had a Caesarean, you won't be ready to start the exercises for your stomach muscles described in *week one* or the *week two* daily routine until much later after birth. Check with your doctor first before practising these exercises, and stop immediately if you feel any pain.

Week one

You can begin to strengthen the stretched, and possibly weakened, muscles of your pelvic floor and stomach from as early as the first day after birth. The pelvic floor and foot pedalling exercises are also good if you have had a Caesarean but delay doing them until you have no more wound discomfort.

Pelvic floor exercise
from day one

Practise gentle squeezing and lifting exercises (see page 45) as often as possible every day to stop yourself leaking urine involuntarily. It's important to do this before you go on to the exercises in week two. If you have had stitches, strengthening the pelvic floor will heal them.

Foot pedalling
from day one

This will guard against swelling in the legs and improve circulation. Lie down and bend your feet up and down at the ankle. Practise hourly.

Stomach toner
from day one

A gentle way to strengthen stomach muscles is to pull them in as you breathe out, hold them in for a few seconds, then relax. Try to do this as often as possible.

from day five after birth

If you feel fine, practise the following exercise twice a day, too:

1 Lie on your back with your head and shoulders supported on two pillows and your legs bent and slightly apart. Cross your arms over your stomach.

2 Lift your head and shoulders, and as you do this, breathe out and press gently on each side of your stomach with the palms of your hands, as if pulling the two sides together. Hold this position for a few seconds, then breathe in, and relax. Repeat three times.

Week two

Introduce the following exercises into your daily routine, and continue for at least three months. Repeat each exercise as many times as is comfortable. Remember to keep practising the exercise for your pelvic floor.

Cat arching exercise

1 With knees and hands slightly apart, kneel on all fours. Your back, head, and neck should be absolutely straight.

2 Clench your buttocks and arch your back upwards slowly. Your arms should be straight, but remember not to lock your elbows. This exercise helps you to relieve stress from your lower back.

Curl ups

1 Lie flat on your back on the floor, with your knees bent and your feet slightly apart. Rest your hands on your thighs.

2 Breathe out, and lift your head and shoulders, stretching forwards to touch your knees with your hands. Don't worry if you can't reach far enough at first, you will with practise. Breathe in and relax.

3 When this is easy, try lifting yourself up more slowly and holding the position for longer, placing your hands on your chest as you lift your head and shoulders, or you could clasp your hands behind your head as you lift yourself up.

Side bends

1 With your arms by your sides, stand straight with your feet apart and the palms of your hands resting on the outsides of your thighs.

2 Bend sideways slowly at the waist, stretching your leg outwards at the same time. Come back to the initial position and repeat on the other side. Remember to exhale on the effort and inhale when you relax.

Checking your pelvic floor

By three months after birth these muscles should be strong again. Test them by skipping. If any urine leaks, practise the pelvic floor exercises for another month and try again. If leaking is still a problem, see your doctor.

How your body recovers

Your body won't be fully recovered for at least six months after the birth of your baby. However, by the time you have your six-week check-up, your body should be getting back to normal. Your womb may have shrunk back to its pre-pregnant size and you may have started your periods again. If you have been practising your postnatal exercises regularly, your muscles should be in far better shape.

The six-week check-up

About six weeks after the birth, you will have a check-up with your doctor or midwife. It is a good time to discuss any worries with the doctor or nurse who performs the check-up.

What happens
- Your blood pressure and weight will be checked.
- Your breasts and stomach will be examined. The doctor will check if any stitches have healed.
- You may have an internal examination to check the size and position of the womb, and may be given a Pap smear test.
- The doctor will discuss contraception; you can be fitted with a diaphragm, or discuss an IUD or the pill.

Your periods

The first period after the birth is often longer and heavier than usual. When it arrives depends on how you are feeding your baby. If you are breastfeeding, your periods may not start until after your baby is weaned. If you are bottle-feeding, the first period usually comes four to six weeks after the birth.

Q&A

"When can we resume our sex life?"
The best time to start making love again is when you both are ready. You may feel too sore and tender to resume sex until after the postnatal check-up, or you may want to try sooner – it's entirely up to you.
   When you resume your sex life, take it slowly. Relax as much as you can, and use extra lubrication as your vagina may be slightly drier than normal.

"I'm breastfeeding my baby; do we still have to use contraception?"
Even if you are breastfeeding or haven't started your periods again, you need to use contraception. The doctor or midwife will discuss this with you soon after the birth. If you want to go on the pill, make sure the doctor knows you are breastfeeding; if you previously used a diaphragm, you must have a new one fitted, as your tissues may have changed.

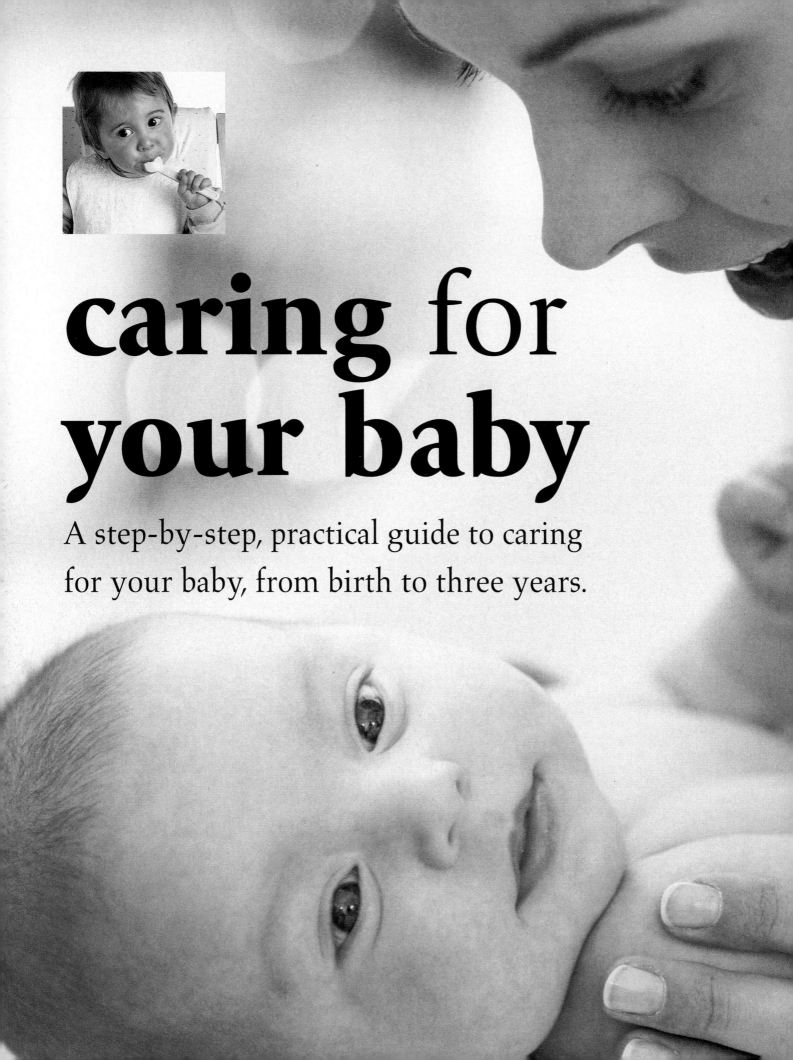

caring for your baby

A step-by-step, practical guide to caring for your baby, from birth to three years.

The first weeks of life

Nothing can prepare you for the reality of having a child. The first weeks of your baby's life will seem like a whirlwind of new experiences as you adapt to being a parent. Looking after a new baby involves providing lots of warmth and attention, and although some of this will be instinctive, some has to be learnt by both of you. The early phase of adjustment won't last long. You'll quickly learn new skills and before long eating one-handed while your baby feeds will be second nature. Here is how one couple and their baby, Amy, coped in the first few weeks.

"The first weeks weren't easy. You think you're a capable, confident person, then you have a helpless baby to look after, and you feel like jelly!"

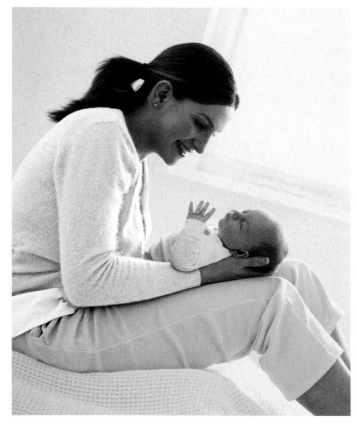

First days at home

Life with your new baby will take you by surprise. Her apparent vulnerability produces powerful feelings within you, while a turmoil of emotions makes you burst into tears for no known reason. You may become distressed by, for example, the television news. Don't fight your feelings; concentrate on the new life that you are nurturing.

Amy at one week

Amy's navel *is already well healed – her cord stump dropped off on the fifth day*

Her arms and legs *wave aimlessly: she has little control over her limbs*

She lies curled up just as she was in the womb. Her fists are usually tightly clenched, and when she lies on her back, she can't stop her head from lolling to one side. If her hand comes into contact with her mouth she sucks it. As happens with almost all newborn babies, her weight has dropped, from 3.54kg (7lbs 13oz) at birth to 3.4kg (7lbs 8oz) now. She should be back to her birthweight by about 10 to 14 days.

Becoming a family

Now there are three of you and everything changes. Your partner is no longer just your lover, he's your companion and ally in this new adventure of parenthood – and the baby is as much his as she is yours. Your tried and tested family relationships will subtly change, too – you're not just a son or a daughter anymore, you're a parent, with a new life depending on you.

Often it's the new father who is most shell-shocked in the days immediately after the birth. But for a while you'll both be tired, sleep deprived, anxious, and possibly even shorter tempered than usual. Make allowances for each other and try to support and make time for each other, too. It's easy to make your partner feel sidelined and useless at this time if you behave as though the baby is your exclusive domain. Talk to each other about your feelings and share babycare as much as you can – it will be very much to your advantage if your baby has a hands-on father. At first he may be more nervous than you of handling her floppy little body, but he will soon grow more confident.

Above all, relax and enjoy your baby. New parenthood may seem like an island of anxiety surrounded by good advice, but remember that there are very few absolute rights and wrongs about baby care. Babies can survive inexperienced parents; what they need most if they are to thrive are happy and loving ones. So have the confidence to rely on your own intuition, and do things in the way that seems right to you – the chances are that it will be right for your baby, too.

"The first days were such a tangle of conflicting feelings – elation and overwhelming pride at being a father, anxiety about Ruth, exhaustion from the round-the-clock demands of our new baby, even a tiny regret that our happy, carefree life together seemed to be at an end."

Amy's day

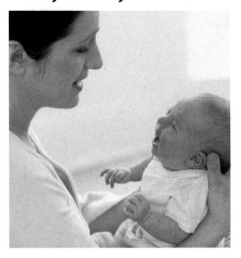

"Amy seemed insatiably hungry and sometimes in the evening she would cry inconsolably for hours at a stretch. I was worried that it was because I didn't have enough milk, but my family doctor assured me that this was probably evening colic and would only last for about three months. Despite the disturbed evenings, this was a huge relief because I loved breastfeeding her and would have been so sad if I'd had to stop. I felt that it was making us really close. Meanwhile, it did at least mean that Tim got to see more of Amy because she was awake so much in the evening when he was home."

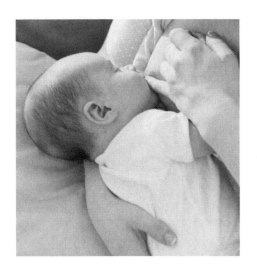

Building a loving relationship

Right from the beginning, your relationship with your new baby is an intense, two-way one that will grow into a real and lasting love. Bring her up close to your face to talk and coo to her – she will look intently back at you, gazing raptly at your face. Eye contact always plays a big part in falling in love, and it is the same with you and your baby. Try sticking the tip of your tongue out when you are looking at each other; she will quickly learn to respond by doing the same – this is real two-way communication. She will reward your efforts to calm her by quietening at the sound of your voice. And when she's miserable, she will want you to hold and comfort her.

Amy crying
Crying is your baby's way of expressing her need for love and comfort. Always respond – don't leave her to cry.

A typical day at around three weeks old

9:00am	**Ruth is woken** by Amy's crying. She had her last feed at 6am (breaks between feeds at 3 weeks should be 3 hours normally, with one 4 hour stretch at night), then they both fell asleep again. It is time for Amy to have another feed now.	1:00pm	**Ruth has** some lunch and then dozes.
10:00am	**Ruth takes Amy** into the bathroom to change her diaper and clothes, and sponge bathe her. Then she puts Amy in the bassinet, and chats to her while she dresses herself.	3:00pm	**A friend** comes to visit and the doorbell wakes Ruth and Amy. The friends have a cup of tea, share baby stories, and admire Amy. The friend is an experienced mother who nursed both of her children. She is able to give Ruth some breastfeeding and "new mom" tips.
11:00am	**Amy falls asleep.** Ruth puts the laundry in the washing machine, and tidies up. Then she puts her feet up, but doesn't sleep.	4:00pm	**The friend** leaves, but Amy is cross from being woken abruptly from her afternoon sleep, so Ruth feeds her to soothe her. It doesn't take long before Amy settles down once again.
11:30am	**Amy cries** for a feed, and then dozes off after she is fed. Ruth takes the opportunity to have a nap, too.	5:30pm	**Ruth puts Amy** in her carriage, and walks to the bus stop to meet Tim. The movement of the carriage soothes Amy, and she drops off to sleep within a few minutes.

Amy asleep

Newborn babies sleep an average of 16 hours a day, but Amy sometimes slept as little as 10 or 11 hours in total, with a long, stormy period from late afternoon to late at night when she only dozed for very short periods. Within five weeks Amy had adopted a more sociable sleep pattern, with a longer sleep during the night, and an earlier bedtime.

"Rubbing her tummy was a good way to soothe her, provided we rubbed fast and firmly – despite my instincts to be very gentle. You soon learn how tough babies are."

6:15pm	**Home again**, and Amy starts to cry. Ruth feeds her, changes her, then rocks her in her arms. Feeding is the only thing that really soothes Amy at this time of the day, but Ruth is sore so it's painful. After feeding, Ruth leaves her nipples exposed to the air for as long as possible. Tim snatches some sleep.	**10:00pm**	**Amy is still crying;** she will be soothed for a while, then cry again. Tim and Ruth let her suck, walk her around, and push her to and fro in her carriage.
		1:00am	**Amy falls asleep** at last. Tim and Ruth are exhausted, and go to bed immediately.
8:30pm	**Tim wakes up,** and he and Ruth take turns carrying Amy around and preparing some food. Amy dozes off for a few minutes at a time, then wakes and cries – so supper is interrupted by short feeds at the breast. Tim helps out as much as possible with the preparation of the food.	**3:00am**	**Amy wakes** and cries, Ruth gets up and feeds her. Tim wakes up too, and helps to rock Amy back to sleep again after her feed.
		7:00am	**The alarm goes off** and Tim gets up to go to work while Ruth tries to snatch some more sleep before Amy wakes for her morning feed.

Involving other family members

Your parents, sisters, brothers, and other members of your family will all be extremely keen to meet the new baby, but don't feel guilty about limiting visitors if you want to.

Getting plenty of rest

Every new mother has to learn how to cope with too little sleep. Plenty of rest whenever you can snatch it is the only answer – and this is especially important if you're breastfeeding your baby. Rest whenever your baby is asleep, even if you don't go to sleep yourself. Your body isn't strong enough yet for strenuous work, and the housework can go undone for now.

Amy wakeful
Held against your shoulder, your baby has a good view of the world around her, and will enjoy her wakeful times.

Six weeks old

"By six weeks Amy was a real person – nothing like the greedy, screaming bundle she had been only weeks before. She responded to each of us in her own way: her first crooked smiles were just for me, usually when I changed her, but at times only Ruth would do. We were lucky – Amy was very perky, and she helped us to love her. You certainly learn fast when you have a new baby reliant on you for her every need."

Amy at six weeks

Amy has a *range of facial expressions*

She has a round stomach *in relation to the rest of her torso*

Amy has much more control over her limbs now, and enjoys the sensation of kicking them around in the air. She's no longer curled up and her fists are unclenched. When she lies on her stomach, she may lift her head momentarily. She doesn't cry as much as she used to – she has a definite wakeful time during the day, when she will sit happily in her bouncing chair, and loves to be entertained by Ruth and the world around her.

Premature babies

Your baby's first six weeks at home may be especially difficult if she was born prematurely. She may cry incessantly and refuse to be comforted, or be very sleepy and reluctant to feed. In addition to your natural anxiety about your new baby, you may feel rejected by her – she doesn't make you feel that she loves you, so it's that much harder to love her in return. Your pre-term baby will need extra care from you – she loses heat quickly, so you need to keep your home warm, especially when bathing or changing her, and she will need frequent feeding to help her grow. Even though she may have a small appetite and be a troublesome feeder, you should offer her a feed at least every three hours, letting her take as much as she wants at each feed. Concentrate on giving the care she needs and in time your baby will grow more responsive to you, and you will learn to understand her better. Be patient. Her growth and development will eventually catch up to the babies who are born at full term.

Amy's check-up

Amy's first month includes several visits with the doctor or midwife to make sure that she is growing well. The one-month or six-week check-up is the first of the major developmental checks.

1 **General assessment** The doctor discusses Amy's general well-being and demeanour with Ruth. She wakes Amy, and talks to her to assess how she responds to the stimulus of a new face. The doctor is looking for that magical early smile, a sure sign that Amy is developing a normal, sociable personality. She looks at Amy's retina through an ophthalmoscope to check that the retina is healthy, and moves a rattle across her field of vision. Amy follows it with both eyes, demonstrating healthy eyesight with no sign of cross-eyes.

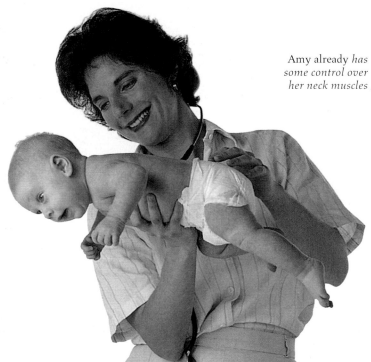

Amy already has some control over her neck muscles

2 Limbs and muscle tone The doctor undresses Amy, so she can observe her muscle tone and how she moves her limbs.

3 Head control The doctor holds Amy in the air to see that she holds her head in line with her body. Then the doctor lays Amy on her back and observes as she pulls her into a sitting position.

4 Grasp reflex A baby at birth can grasp hold of a finger put into her palm and hold on strongly. By six weeks, it's normal for her birth reflexes to begin to disappear, as Amy's have.

5 Head circumference Amy's head is measured, to check for normal growth. Her head is now 38cm (15in). The doctor also checks Amy's facial features for shape and symmetry.

6 Heartbeat The doctor listens to Amy's heart with a stethoscope to make sure that it has a steady rhythm – about 120 beats a minute is normal for the first year.

7 Internal organs A good feel around Amy's stomach reassures the doctor that her liver, stomach, and spleen are all growing normally, and none is too big or in the wrong shape.

Amy's weight is recorded on her personal chart

8 Hip check Hip dislocation is a possibility still, so the doctor tests the joints' action with her middle fingers, as she manipulates Amy's legs. She checks for hip symmetry, too.

9 Weighing Amy has been weighed naked at regular intervals up to now, and will be weighed at every visit to the doctor's office, or whenever Ruth requests. Normal weight gain means a healthy baby. Amy's weight will be plotted on a centile chart to ascertain her growth in comparison to length and weight averages. The chart will be an important record for months to come.

Handling your baby

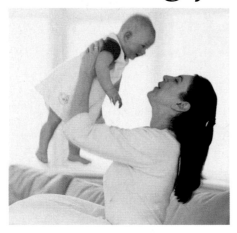

Your baby needs closeness and the comfort of your reassuring voice, so talk to her as you handle her. Until she is about eight weeks old she cannot hold up her head, and needs you to support her body. Careful handling won't hurt her, but you may startle her if you pick her up suddenly. By five months she'll enjoy more boisterous games, and may love to be swung above your head or perched on your shoulders. If she's timid, handle her gently until she's more confident.

Picking up a newborn baby

If you are a first-time parent you might find picking up and holding a newborn baby a little daunting at first because your baby seems too delicate to handle. But as long as you provide proper support, you'll find that she's perfectly safe and loves being held.

Always put your baby on her back to sleep. She will be at lower risk of crib death and choking than if she sleeps on her tummy or her side (see page 123). However, when she is awake, she should spend some time each day lying on her tummy.

1 To pick up your baby, slide one hand under her lower back and bottom and the other under her head and neck.

2 Lift her gently and slowly so that her body is supported and her head can't loll back.

3 Carefully transfer her head to the crook of your elbow or your shoulder so that it remains supported.

Cradling your baby in your arms

Your baby will feel secure cradled in the crook of your elbow, with her head and limbs well supported.

Holding your baby face down

Your baby may like being held face down in your arms, her chin and cheek resting on your forearm.

Holding your baby against your shoulder

Your baby feels secure when held upright like this. Take her weight with one hand under her bottom. Make sure you support her head with the other hand.

Putting your baby down

1 Put one hand underneath her head and neck, then hold her under the bottom with the other. Lower her slowly, gently supporting her until the mat or mattress is taking her weight. Make sure her head is fully supported.

2 Slide your nearest hand out from under her bottom. Use this hand to lift her head a little so you can slide out your other hand, and lower her head down gently. Don't let her head fall back on to the surface, or jerk your arm out quickly.

Laying your baby on her back

Recent research has shown that it is much safer for a baby to sleep on her back than on her side or tummy. Babies who sleep on their backs have reduced risk of crib death, although we don't know exactly why (see page 123). And although it used to be thought that if a baby in this position vomited there was a danger that she might choke, childcare experts now believe that babies sleeping on their back have no difficulty turning their heads if they are sick. Once your baby is old enough to begin turning over by herself, she may well turn over during the night. Continue to put her to bed on her back as usual, but don't worry if she turns over later. There is no need to turn her back during the night.

Safety first

You will often want to lay your baby down for a few moments, either for her own amusement, or because you need to do something. Whether in your own home or visiting family or friends, follow the simple precautions given below to ensure that your baby keeps safe and sound at all times:

● Never leave your baby unsupervised – even for a single second – on a bed, sofa, chair, or changing table.
● Never place your baby's infant seat, basket, or bassinet on a raised surface – only the floor will be completely safe.
● Never put your baby next to a radiator, fire, or open window. She may burn herself or overchill.
● Never leave your baby alone with a dog, cat, or any other animal.
● Never place your baby within reach of unstable furniture or other heavy objects. She may pull them over and seriously hurt herself.
● Leaving your baby's favourite toys with her will keep her entertained – but take care never to leave anything sharp in her reach. Avoid toys that are small enough to fit into her mouth, or heavy enough to hurt her.
● Until your baby is a little older and her immune system has had time to develop, it is a safe practice not to expose her to a large group of people or other small children to minimize the risk of infection.

Infant carriers

An infant carrier is an excellent way of carrying your baby around in the first three months. The contact with your moving body is comforting to her and your arms are left free. Soft slings are also popular for carrying young babies. However, it is essential that the infant's face is never covered due to the risk of possible suffocation by the sling's fabric.

Putting on an infant carrier

1 Slip the carrier straps over your shoulders so that the two metal rings hang down at the front.

2 Attach the padded triangular section by snapping the circular fasteners on the straps into place.

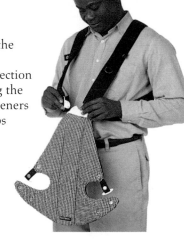

3 Close one side of the carrier by feeding the toggle through the ring and snapping it securely closed.

4 Hold your baby so that she faces you. If she is very young, support her head with your hand. Feed her leg through the hole on the fastened side of the carrier. Keep your arm around her on the open side to ensure that she doesn't fall.

5 Support your baby in the seat of the carrier with one hand while you fasten the toggle and snap under her arm with the other.

6 Close the top fasteners so that an arm hole is created on each side. The back flap supports a younger baby's head and neck.

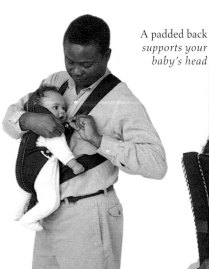

A padded back *supports your baby's head*

Wearing the carrier

After three months, your baby may prefer to face forwards. Follow the same sequence, but start with your baby facing forwards. With the front flap folded down, she can get a better view of the world around her.

Wide shoulder straps *are the most comfortable*

A machine-washable fabric *is a good idea*

Handling and physical play

Let him kick
It's best not to let your baby become too dependent on being held. Let him spend some time kicking on the floor – you can get down to his level, too.

Play bouncing games on your lap
Your four-month-old baby will love the feeling of being jogged up and down by your knees, in time to a favourite rhyme. Hold your baby carefully, in case he jerks.

Sit him on your shoulder
Sit your six-month-old baby on your shoulder, so that he's taller than you are: he'll be exhilarated by this new perspective. Remember to hold him carefully.

Let him look around
Your baby will love to see the world. Hold him securely in your arms and perch his cheek gently on your shoulder. Twirl around slowly and let him enjoy the view.

Eye-to-eye contact
Your baby will love you to swing him up high. Your face is always the best entertainment of all. You must be very careful not to jerk your baby's neck or head. Never throw him up in the air.

Play rocking games
Rock your baby to and fro, going higher if he likes the game. This type of rocking motion is a good way to soothe him, too. Make sure you hold your baby properly, so he doesn't slip from your hands.

Winding down
However boisterously you play with your baby, have a few minutes of gentle cuddles afterwards. Always take your cue from your baby; forget rough-housing for today if he's not responding with his usual giggles.

Feeding your baby

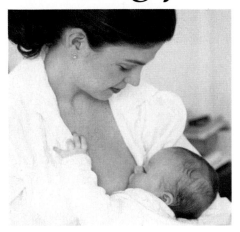

Breastfeeding is recommended for all infants with very few exceptions, because breastfed babies are generally healthier, with fewer ear, chest, gastrointestinal, and urine infections. They also suffer fewer allergies, and suffer less from asthma, eczema, diabetes, and obesity. Breastfeeding also has benefits for you. Nursing your baby immediately after delivery reduces the risk of excessive uterine bleeding, and continuing to breastfeed helps you return to your pre-pregnancy weight more quickly.

What mothers say about breastfeeding

Some women know early on in pregnancy that they want to breastfeed. Others are unsure. It is natural to have questions about which method might be the best option for you. Even if you have made your decision, it is best to learn about breastfeeding before your delivery. You can talk to other mothers who breastfed, your doctor, your midwife, lactation consultants, and your local breastfeeding support group. Breastfeeding clinics are also useful if you have any particular concerns. The La Leche League may also be helpful – go to www.lllc.ca.

"I knew that by breastfeeding I was giving my baby the best milk he could have. I could tell he was digesting it easily, and I knew it had exactly the right blend of nutrients."

Breast milk contains substances that help protect your baby from disease until his own immune system has matured. These also protect against allergies, which is important if there is an allergy in your family.

"I loved the convenience of breastfeeding my baby: the milk was always there, always sterile, always at the temperature he liked."

If you are out visiting friends, travelling, or just enjoying a day in the park, breast milk is the ultimate convenience food.

"The breast was always the best method of soothing my baby whenever he cried."

Breastfed babies are less fussy than bottle-fed babies. They have less constipation, less gas, and suffer fewer illnesses. Breastfeeding also allows you and your baby to come closer physically and emotionally, and this strengthens the bond between you.

"I was extremely worried that my breasts would become saggy with breastfeeding, but my obstetrician told me that if the breasts are going to go saggy, the changes already happen during pregnancy."

During the first few months, breasts will be fuller as feeding time nears. After that, you'll notice only occasional feelings of fullness, such as after your baby has had a longer sleep.

"I was tired and sore after my Caesarean section and the baby was nursing often. My mother and husband helped a lot, and it worked out very well."

All mothers need help in the weeks after delivery. They need the time to focus on the baby, and to get the hang of breastfeeding.

"I was convinced that I wouldn't be able to breastfeed – my bust was so small. But I had plenty of milk, and my baby certainly didn't mind my small breasts."

All mothers have enough milk for feeding their babies. If your baby is not gaining weight adequately, review your technique, feed more frequently, and discuss the issue with your healthcare providers.

"At first, I found it really hard nursing at night, but then the lactation consultant showed me how to nurse lying down. He sleeps in his bassinet beside our bed so he can nurse whenever he needs to."

Nursing lying down is restful – however, it is dangerous for babies under six months of age to sleep with their parents, either in an adult bed or on a sofa, especially if either parent is a smoker, using sedating medication, alcohol, or recreational drugs. Co-sleeper products are not recommended because of risks of suffocation and entrapment. Instead, use a crib or a cradle beside your bed. If you do let your baby sleep in your bed, take precautions to make it safer (see p.126).

"My husband was a great help after the baby came, but said he felt left out when I was breastfeeding. I told him how good he made me feel by all the things he was doing, and how much I loved him. It was a special moment for both of us."

Fathers and mothers are both important in their children's lives. The father's support is essential for the child's development and well-being.

Demand feeding

Feeding on demand simply means giving your baby a feed whenever he is hungry, without following a timetable. His digestive system is too immature to cope with large meals at infrequent intervals; little and often must be the rule at first. There is nothing to be gained by keeping your baby waiting for a feed once he has cried to be fed – he will only get so distressed that he will refuse to suck. In the early weeks, his hunger is the usual reason for waking and crying. As his digestive system matures and his stomach grows, he'll take more at each feed, and the intervals between feeds will become longer.

How often will he demand food?

Your baby will demand food whenever he needs it, and to begin with this will be often. Newborn babies will have no discernible pattern of feeding. By day three or four, feeds will be every two or three hours, and there may be eight or so feeds a day, with a lot of short feeds during the evening. At night you may be feeding your baby two or three times because few babies under the age of six weeks are able to sleep for more than five hours without waking with hunger. Breastfed babies need more frequent feeds than bottle-fed babies, because breast milk is more easily and quickly digested than formula.

By three months, your baby may be settling into a regular feeding routine. Do bear in mind that babies don't grow at a regular rate; they have growth spurts, and their hunger fluctuates accordingly.

Special cases

Premature babies Your pre-term baby may have a small appetite, but he will need frequent feeds. Pre-term babies tend to sleep a lot, and may not wake and demand food even though they need it, so when applicable, wake your baby every three hours, and offer a feed.

If you have managed to express milk for your baby while he's been in hospital, you will be able to breastfeed once you get him home. It isn't always easy for a baby to adapt to taking milk from a human nipple. To help him, express a little milk before a feed (see page 94) so that the nipple stands out, and rub breast milk over it to give him the taste.

Twins It's possible to breastfeed twins successfully. It's fine to feed them one at a time. When you have gained more confidence, you might find it possible to feed them both at the same time, their legs tucked under each arm, and their heads lying in your hands.

Burping your baby

Whether your baby is breast- or bottle-fed, give him chance to burp up swallowed air when he pauses for a rest; the gas may be making him feel full. If he cries or doesn't burp after about half a minute, give up: he probably doesn't need to bring up any gas.

Your newborn
To help your baby bring up gas, put him against your shoulder and rub his back. Make sure his head is supported. He may bring some milk up too, so keep a clean cloth handy.

Sit him up
By about three months, when your baby can sit up for short periods, jiggling him gently on your lap while you rub his back will help him burp up swallowed air. Make sure you still support his head.

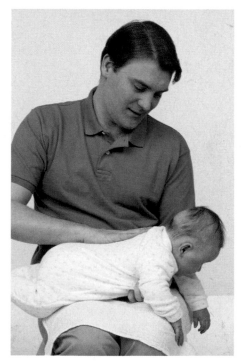

Hold him face down
At any age, holding your baby face down across your lap or in your arms may help him bring up gas. Rub or pat his back gently, but rhythmically, to help him to burp.

Breastfeeding your baby

Breastfeeding can be a very rewarding aspect of caring for your baby, and you'll be giving her the best nourishment – so don't be deterred if you encounter a few problems in the early days. You and your baby have to learn this new skill together, so if at first she doesn't seem to know how to suck, or doesn't suck for very long, be patient with her. She doesn't need a lot of food just after the birth. If breastfeeding seems difficult at first, your midwife or doctor will be able to help you, and there will be plenty of friends and relatives to offer advice. Several breastfeeding associations also provide support. Once you're over the first few weeks, you can look forward to months of successful and satisfying feeding.

Getting comfortable

Settle yourself comfortably. The more relaxed you appear to your baby, the easier she will settle to feed. If you're in private, take your top off: with no clothes in the way, you will give her plenty of opportunity for skin contact, and might find it easier to get her "latched on" – that is, properly positioned on your breast and sucking efficiently.

Make sure your *baby has a hand free to touch and stroke your breast*

A pillow *takes the weight of your baby's body*

Your young baby's early feeds

Sit comfortably in an upright position with your back supported. A low chair without arms is ideal, or sit up in bed with plenty of pillows propping your back. Your baby should be held close, chest to chest. Lift her up to your breast, rather than bending over her.

Your older baby's feeds

Once you are both adept at feeding, you will find you can nurse in almost any relaxed position. Sitting cross-legged on the bed or floor is excellent, especially if you can prop your back against pillows or furniture.

Your first breastfeeds

Finding the nipple

1 Your baby has an instinctive reflex that makes her search for your nipple to find food – this is called the "rooting" reflex. You can alert this reflex by stroking the cheek nearest you.

2 If your baby doesn't turn her head instinctively, try gently squeezing just behind your areola until a few drops form on your nipple. Touch her lips with this to encourage her to open her mouth.

3 Bring her head up close to your breast, so her chin is against it, and her tongue is underneath your nipple. Lift your baby to your breast, and let her latch on properly (see below).

Latching on

1 Once latched on, your baby doesn't just suck, she "milks" the breast with her jaws by pressing on the reservoirs of the milk at the base of the areola. If your baby just sucks on the nipple, you will get sore and she won't get any milk. If you feel a momentary piercing pain, breathe deeply to help you relax.

2 From your viewpoint, your well latched-on baby will have her jaws very wide and her mouth full of your breast. You can tell she is feeding properly when you see her temples and ears moving, showing her jaw muscles are working hard.

The let-down reflex

Your baby's sucking action stimulates your breasts to release the milk they have stored. You may feel the warm rush of milk – the let-down reflex – as a tingling sensation soon after your baby has latched on. The stimulation sends a message to the pituitary gland to release oxytocin, which contracts the muscles around the mammary glands. Not everyone feels it though, so don't be surprised if you don't. If the reflex makes milk leak out of the other breast too, hold a breast pad over your nipple to catch drips, or use a breast shell (see page 96).

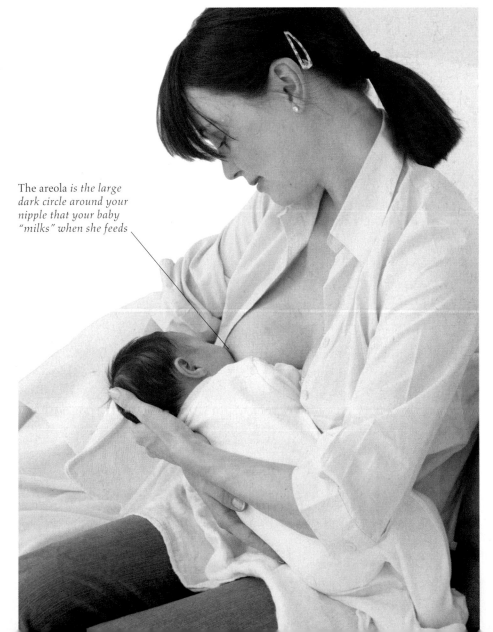

The areola *is the large dark circle around your nipple that your baby "milks" when she feeds*

Offering the other breast

Use your clean *little finger to break your baby's suction*

1 Let your baby feed for as long as she wants to at the first breast, so she drains it – your breast will look smaller, and feel lighter when all the milk has gone. Your baby will often pause during her feed and just suck for a while. After a pause of several minutes when she is no longer taking in any milk, remove her from the breast, and burp her. Don't pull your nipple away – this will hurt. Slip a finger between her jaws to break the suction.

2 When your baby is off the nipple, slip a tissue or breast pad into your bra to catch any drips. Sit your baby up to burp her. Make a note to start her next feed on the other breast, so that they get equal stimulation.

How your breasts produce milk

In the first few days after the birth, your breasts produce colostrum, a protein-rich food that supplies your baby with valuable antibodies against infection. Once you begin to produce milk on around the fourth day, your baby will naturally stimulate your body into producing a plentiful supply for her dietary needs.

The key to a good milk supply is feeding your baby when she wants to be fed – and in the early days that may mean at one- or two-hourly intervals. Breast milk production works on a demand and supply system: the more often your baby nurses, and the more she takes, the more your breasts will produce. Supplementary bottles of formula milk will undermine this system: if your baby's hunger is satisfied by a bottle, she won't be eager to suck and your breasts won't get the stimulation they need.

Breast milk isn't all the same. At the beginning of the feed, your baby takes foremilk, which is watery and thirst-quenching. Then she gets to the hindmilk, rich in calories and more satisfying. This is why it's important to let her suck for as long as she wants to at each feed: otherwise she will soon be hungry again.

What you need to do
All you need to do to produce enough milk is to eat a good, balanced diet with plenty of protein, to drink whenever you are thirsty – have a glass of juice or milk on hand while you nurse – and to rest as much as you can. Your baby's natural appetite will do the rest.

Breastfeeding and vitamin D
Most medical organizations recommend exclusive breastfeeding for the first six months because it is the perfect food for babies. However, breast milk contains only small amounts of vitamin D, which is needed for bone development. Canadian health agencies currently recommend that breastfed babies receive 400 IU of vitamin D per day for the first year. These are available as infant drops and should be started within the first month.

3 After a burp or two, and perhaps a short sleep, you can offer your baby the other breast. She may be hungry enough to drain this one, too, or she may just suck for comfort. She needs this as much as she needs the milk – so let her carry on.

4 When your baby's had enough to drink, she will fall fast asleep in your arms and let your nipple slip from her mouth. Don't worry if you think she has not taken a full feed; you can trust your baby to know how much she wants and needs at any time. If she feels hungry again, she will wake and let you know.

When your milk comes in

Normal breast **Engorged breast**

The areola is swollen and firm, so it may be hard for your baby to grasp; and the nipple is flattened

Draw your fingertips down towards the areola

1 On about the fourth day of breastfeeding your breasts start to produce mature milk, as well as the colostrum that you've fed your baby up to now. You may wake up to find your breasts big, hard, and heavy and they can be quite uncomfortable. This is engorgement, and it may last for up to 48 hours. Your baby will find it hard to latch on because the nipple isn't sticking out, but is flattened by the swollen areola. The following tips should help her to feed, clear the engorgement, and ease your discomfort.

2 Before you try to breastfeed your baby, soften your breasts by laying warm washcloths over them for several minutes. Or you may prefer to stand in the shower and splash warm water over your breasts.

3 Massage your breasts gently with your hands, and try to express some milk to relieve the swelling and help your baby get the nipple in her mouth (see page 94). Don't worry if you can't get the hang of expressing at this stage – you will soon.

4 When you put your baby to the breast, put your free hand on your ribcage under your breast and push gently upwards: this should help the nipple to protrude so your baby can get the areola in her mouth. Her sucking will quickly relieve the engorgement and discomfort.

"My baby son cries a great deal; could it be that he isn't getting enough milk from me to satisfy his hunger?"
When you are breastfeeding you can't actually see how much milk your baby is taking, so it's natural sometimes to worry that he is not getting enough. However, as long as you offer a feed whenever your baby cries, and he is gaining weight normally with occasional spurts, you have no need to worry that he will be undernourished. Remember that your baby will probably lose a little weight during the first days of life, and may not regain his birthweight immediately. It could also be that your baby is suffering from colic (see page 118).

"Will breastfeeding alter my figure for life?"
Your breasts may be slightly smaller after you have weaned your baby from the breast, because some of the fatty tissue in the breasts has been replaced by milk glands. Otherwise, you will probably regain your pre-pregnancy figure more quickly if you breastfeed. This is because the hormones released during breastfeeding encourage the uterus to shrink back to normal quickly, and the fat reserves that your body laid down during your pregnancy are used in the production of breast milk. Your waistline will also contract sooner than if you bottle-feed, and your pelvis returns to normal more quickly.

Q&A

"When I am breastfeeding, do I have to be as careful as I was when I was pregnant about the drugs, medications I take, as well as my caffeine and liquor intake?"
What you eat and drink can be passed on to your baby through your milk, so it's still vital that you tell your pharmacist or doctor that you are breastfeeding before they prescribe any medicines for you. It's sensible to avoid stimulants such as alcohol and caffeine, too. If your baby won't sleep well, it may be worthwhile cutting coffee and tea out of your diet for a few weeks to see if the situation improves – the caffeine may be keeping him awake.

Expressing milk by hand

At some point, you might need to be separated from your baby, and will need to have breast milk available for him. By experimenting, you will find the best way for you to express milk – some mothers find manual expression works best, others like pumping, and some find both work well. It takes time and experience to learn how to stimulate the let-down reflex, so expressing only small amounts of milk does not mean that you don't have enough. Before you express by hand, sterilize the equipment, and wash your hands. Encourage the flow of milk by having a warm bath, or hold warm washcloths over your breasts. Make yourself comfortable at a high surface, with the bowl in front of you.

Hand expressing

1 Support your breast in one hand and start to massage, working downwards from above the breast. Use your whole hand to massage the breast.

2 Work your way all around the breast, including the underside. Complete at least 10 circuits – this helps the flow of milk through the ducts.

3 Stroke downwards towards the areola with your fingernails several times. Use a rolling motion and avoid pressing on the breast tissue.

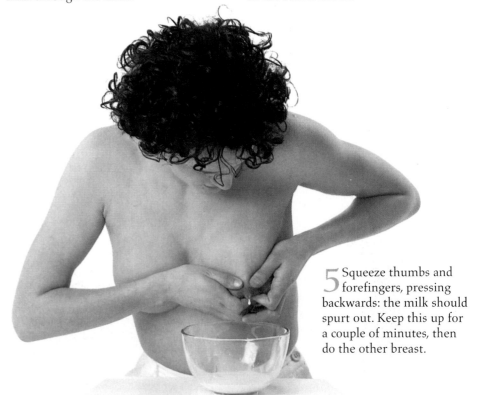

4 Apply gentle downward pressure on the area behind the areola with your thumbs and fingers, and rotate them gently to help access reservoirs.

5 Squeeze thumbs and forefingers, pressing backwards: the milk should spurt out. Keep this up for a couple of minutes, then do the other breast.

Expressing milk using a pump

Using a pump to express milk is often quicker and less tiring than expressing it by hand. Ease of use, durability, and suction adjustment are things to consider when choosing a breast pump. Ask your midwife, nurse, or doctor for advice. Your own personal circumstances are likely to dictate the pump you choose to some extent. For example, if you are frequently separated from your baby, or if you have twins, you might consider a double-sided electric pump, which will allow you to express milk in a shorter time. Or, if you plan to express milk only occasionally, a hand- or battery-operated pump may be the best option. In addition, the more expensive and powerful electric pumps can usually be rented. When pumping, it is important to make yourself as comfortable as possible in a chair with good back support. Relax as much as you can to ensure the best flow of milk.

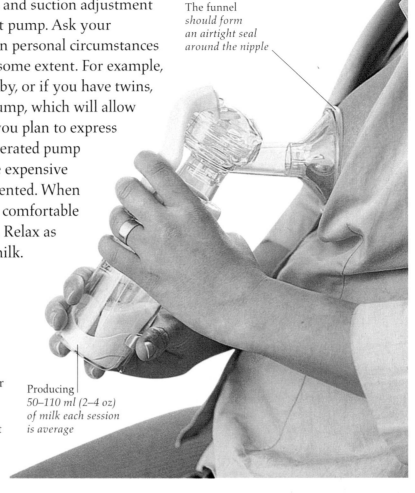

The funnel *should form an airtight seal around the nipple*

Producing *50–110 ml (2–4 oz) of milk each session is average*

Preparing your pump

Pumps can vary, so read the instructions carefully. Stimulate your breasts beforehand, as described for expressing milk manually on the facing page. This is important for stimulating the let-down reflex, and pumping efficiently. Place the funnel of the pump over the areola to form an airtight seal. Your nipple should be positioned so that it is in the middle of the funnel. Once attached, start the pump. It is recommended that you don't go for longer than 20 minutes per breast. Ideally you should swap between your breasts as soon as milk flow from one begins to decrease.

Pumps

Manual pump

This type of pump has improved in recent years, and is now more effective and easier to use. A manual pump allows you to control the rate of pumping, but some women still find the device tiring.

The funnel *must be the right size for your nipples*

Handle

Storage lid

Storage cups *can be used to store your expressed milk in the fridge for up to three days, or in a freezer for up to three months. To avoid wastage, freeze small amounts.*

Battery pump

Battery-operated pumps take the work out of pumping, but the rate is not as easy to control as it is with manual pumps. Some battery pumps come with an adaptor so that they can also be operated by plugging into a wall outlet if desired.

Battery

Integral *container can be used to store milk*

Breastfeeding problems

Get professional help quickly if you have any problems with breastfeeding: struggling on alone is discouraging, and something minor such as a blocked duct can lead to mastitis if it doesn't clear. Don't stop feeding if you encounter the problems below: you will only become engorged with milk, and make any problem worse. Take good care of your breasts.

Wear a comfortable nursing bra, both day and night for the early weeks: don't wear one that is too tight, as it may constrict the milk ducts. Be gentle when you massage your breasts. Let the air get to your nipples as often as possible, and wash them with water, not soap as it dries the skin. Dry thoroughly. You may even use a hair dryer on a low setting to do this.

Leaking breasts

Your breasts may leak copiously between feeds in the early weeks.
Treatment Breast pads inside your bra will absorb some drips, but change the pads frequently as wetness near your skin may make you sore. If you leak a lot, try using a plastic breast shell, and, in extreme cases, wear breast pads over it.
Prevention None, but leaking breasts are proof of a good milk supply, and help prevent engorgement. Don't be too concerned because the leaking will diminish as your milk supply matches the demands of your baby.

Blocked ducts

A small, hard, tender, red lump in the breast usually means that one of the milk ducts has become blocked.
Treatment Bathe the breast in hot water and massage it gently, then put your baby to the breast. You might want to apply a heat pack on the affected side while you breastfeed. You may get a moment's intense pain when your baby latches on, but the duct should clear. If it doesn't clear, see your doctor that day.
Prevention Make sure your breastfeeding technique is sound and your baby is latching on properly.

Mastitis

A blocked milk duct may become infected, producing flu-like symptoms. Seek medical help urgently: if untreated, mastitis may lead to a breast abscess, which may need surgery.
Treatment Your doctor will prescribe antibiotics, and you must finish the course. Continue to feed your baby from both breasts as normal.
Prevention Regular feeding from both breasts will help prevent mastitis. Never let a tender lump in your breast go longer than a day without treatment.

Sore or cracked nipples

Prevention is always better than cure – sore nipples are nearly always caused because your baby is not correctly positioned or latching on properly. Make sure she takes a large mouthful of breast and not just the nipple into her mouth. If your baby doesn't latch on properly don't pull your nipple out – that will hurt even more – but break the suction by putting your finger into the corner of her mouth, take her from the breast and start again. Sometimes the problem can be a badly fitting bra that puts pressure on your nipples, and breast pads and bra linings can make it worse by trapping moisture.
Treatment for sore nipples Try the following suggestions:
• Ask your healthcare provider to help you make sure your baby latches on properly.
• Try expressing a little colostrum or breast milk and then rubbing it gently onto your nipples – many people find that this works wonders.
• Dry your nipples after a feed using a hairdryer on a cool setting.
• Let the air get to your nipples for several hours a day. A cracked nipple may cause a sharp, shooting pain in your breast as your baby sucks. Rest the breast for a day by expressing milk with the same frequency as your baby feeds. A crack will usually heal within a few days.
Prevention Make sure that your baby takes the areola into her mouth. Keep your nipples dry between feeds.

Cracked nipples
A purified lanolin cream formulated for breastfeeding might help the healing process.

Disposable breast pad
A breast pad will absorb drips and small leaks and can help you stay dry and comfortable if you experience leaking. You can use disposable or washable nursing pads.

Your emotions and the let-down reflex

Your let-down reflex is strongly associated with your emotional state of being. When you are embarrassed, irritated, exhausted, or anxious, your breast milk doesn't always appear as readily as when you are relaxed. A few minutes of quiet cuddling with your baby in private should help relax both of you and make you and your baby ready to nurse.

Feeding the older child

Until the age of about six months, babies need only milk. After that, they are ready and able to start complementary foods. Milk will still be the most important food for the first year of life and remains an important food afterwards. Talk to your healthcare provider about how to introduce solids. Remember that you can easily and inexpensively make your own healthy foods for your baby. Start by offering your baby solids in small amounts, ideally at the same time as you have your own family meals if practical, so that her routine will coincide with that of the rest of the family. In the meantime, she will continue to nurse whenever she needs to, and for as long as she needs to.

How often will she nurse?

As your baby grows, her feedings will become more varied in duration and frequency. She'll nurse for hunger, thirst, when cold, tired, and when she just wants a cuddle. Remember that her varied nursing pattern does not mean that your milk is drying up. This is a perfectly normal pattern for a growing baby. There will be still more changes when you introduce her to solids.

How do I wean?

Gradually replace one breastfeeding at a time with milk by bottle or cup (depending on the age of your child). See page 106 for suggested guidelines when switching to bottle-feeding. If your baby is less than 12 months of age, replace breast milk with formula; otherwise, check with your doctor.

You may want to stop the night-time breastfeeding last, especially if this is a time for you and your baby to bond.

Going back to work

It is perfectly possible to return to work and continue breastfeeding, but it means planning ahead. While you are away, your baby will have to take milk from a bottle or, if she is over six months, from a trainer cup with a soft spout. So aim to get her used to it before you return to work.

If you want your baby to have breast milk only, you will need to express milk at work during the day to keep your milk supply stimulated. Or you may want her to have formula milk during the day but continue to breastfeed when you are at home. Your milk supply will respond to your baby's changing needs.

• Stock up on expressed milk in your freezer for a few weeks before you go back to work. Let it thaw naturally and warm it by putting the container in a bowl of warm water (not a microwave).
• At work you will need sterile equipment and a private place to express milk during the day, plus access to a fridge to store it. Transport the milk in a cooler bag with an ice pack.
• If necessary, boost your milk supply by giving extra feeds during the evening and night.
• Ask your baby's caregiver to delay the late afternoon feed so your baby will be ready for a breastfeed when you get home.
• Leave formula ready to be made up in case your baby demands an extra feed while you are away.

How long should I nurse for?

No international group or organization has put a limit on the duration of breastfeeding and all encourage extended breastfeeding. The World Health Organization recommends two or more years, or as long as mutually desirable. When your baby is ready to stop, she will just nurse less and less.

Continuing breastfeeding
You can continue to nurse your baby for as long as you feel comfortable doing so. The more breast milk a baby gets, the healthier she will be.

Bottle-feeding your baby

Bottle-feeding has two advantages – your partner can also do it, and you can see how much milk your baby is taking. It is important to follow the manufacturer's instructions closely when making up a formula feed: formula that is too weak or too concentrated is harmful to your baby. Infant formulas are fortified with iron and vitamin D, so a formula fed baby does not need supplements. If you have concerns, speak to your doctor or midwife.

Equipment for bottle-feeding

For a baby who is fully bottle-fed, you will need at least eight full size (250ml/8oz) bottles. Buy extra nipples, and keep them ready in a sterile jar in case one gives an inadequate flow of milk (see page 100).

Some bottles come with discs that seal them, while the more modern, wide-necked bottles can be sealed with the protective cap. Disposable bottles are also available for travelling.

Bottles and other equipment

125ml (4oz) bottle

Disc
Placed over nipple to keep the bottle sealed

Nipple
Placed upside down in the bottle: don't let any milk touch the nipple

Cap
Seals bottle and protects the sterile nipple

Ring
Screws on to secure the nipple

Nipple
Find the type that suits your baby best

Bottle
Shapes vary, choose one you find comfortable to hold

250ml (8oz) bottle

How to store a bottle when not in use

How the parts of the bottle fit together when in use

Bottle with disposable liner

Bisphenol A (BPA)

Bisphenol A is a chemical used in the production of polycarbonate, a clear, hard plastic used to make many products including baby bottles. In some circumstances – if the bottles are heated or scratched through repeated washing – the chemical can leak into the milk. Although the dose the baby receives is very small, there is some uncertainty surrounding the potential of bisphenol A to cause neurological and behavioural effects in early stages of development. For this reason, Canada has prohibited the advertisement, sale, or importation of polycarbonate baby bottles that contain bisphenol A, effective March 2010. The safest bottles are made of glass or softer plastics. Throw out any old bottles made of clear, shatter-proof plastic, which may have the number "7" within or the letters "PC" near the recycling triangle.

Nipples

The holes must point toward the roof of your baby's mouth

Wide neck

Narrow neck

Valve in rim lets air under the teat and into the bottle

Nipples for young babies have a short nipple

Natural-shaped nipple
The nipple must go into your baby's mouth with the hole facing upward, so that the milk sprays over the roof of his mouth. This nipple is good for babies who are otherwise breastfed, as it mimics the shape of the mother's nipple more closely, and may be more acceptable. The shape may also promote correct development of the baby's mouth.

Standard nipple
The standard shape of this nipple gives a sucking action that is not really like sucking from your breast, and babies who are otherwise breastfed may find them difficult to use. Nipples are available with different rates of flow: slower flow rates are better for newborns and breastfed babies, while faster rates are more suitable for older bottle-fed babies.

Anti-colic nipple
An anti-colic nipple lets air into the bottle as your baby sucks the milk out. This stops the nipple from collapsing, so enabling him to get a steady stream of milk, and perhaps lessening the likelihood of him developing colic from swallowing air. Like standard nipples, anti-colic nipples are available with different flow rates to suit your baby's needs.

Wide-based nipple
This type is not interchangeable among different makes of bottle. As your baby sucks, his lips press against the squashy base and the nipple moves in and out of his mouth. This mimics the feel of the mother's breast. Fit nipple and ring together before assembling the bottle ready for filling.

Q&A

"There are so many different types of formula – how do I know which one to buy?"
A cow's milk-based, iron-fortified formula remains the most acceptable alternative to breast milk. Some babies have problems digesting standard formula. If you think that your baby is having a problem with a milk-based formula, ask your doctor or nurse practitioner for advice. If your healthcare provider identifies a problem, you may be advised to buy an alternative formula that is not milk-based, but do not do this without seeking professional advice first.

"Formula is expensive. When can I switch to regular milk?"
Cow's milk is very different in composition from breast milk, and a poor source of iron. It should only be introduced as a drink when your baby is eating a wide range of other foods, usually at about 12 months of age.

"The rest of my family uses low-fat milk products – when can my baby use these?"
Low-fat milk products (skim, 1 percent fat, and 2 percent fat) should not be used until your child is at least two years old. Low-fat milk products have excessive amounts of minerals and protein, are low in fat content, and lack essential fatty acids. Although popular with adults, they are not appropriate for very young children.

"Should I warm the formula?"
It is not necessary to warm the bottle of formula. If your baby prefers warm formula (and that might be only because that is what he has become used to), heat the bottle in a pan of hot water or hold it under the hot water tap for a few minutes. Never heat baby formula in the microwave and always check the temperature before feeding your baby.

Formula: what's in it?
Formula is sweeter than ordinary cow's milk, and as close in composition to breast milk as manufacturers can make it. Cow's milk is not well suited to your baby's needs – it doesn't contain all the nutrients essential for growth, and it can be difficult for him to digest. Most infant formulas are adapted from a cow's milk base, but are well supplemented with many other ingredients. Vegetable oils are added to replace cow's butter fat, and lactose is used to sweeten the mixture. Make sure the formula you choose is iron fortified. Use soy-based formulas only if your healthcare provider has recommended them. If your baby vomits after a bottle; has diarrhea, cramps, or excessive gas; wheezes; develops a rash; or is irritable, call your doctor immediately, and discuss the problem. Babies can dehydrate very quickly.

Washing your baby's feeding equipment

Your baby's nipples, bottles, and other feeding equipment must be kept scrupulously clean. They can be cleaned either by hand, in hot, soapy water, or you can put them into your dishwasher to save time and energy. For babies under four months old, it will also be necessary to sterilize all equipment before use. Pacifiers and teething rings will also have to be thoroughly cleaned before use.

Using a dishwasher

An efficient way to wash your baby's feeding equipment is to put it in your dishwasher, making sure it goes through the hot drying cycle. The high heat is usually sufficient to kill any bacteria. Nipples may have to be boiled separately, because dishwashers can turn them into unusable sticky blobs.

Dishwasher-proof nipples should be put upwards within the cutlery compartments

Dishwasher basket *holds bottles, rings, and caps, and has grippers on top to keep nipples in place*

Hand-washing

1 Put the rinsed-out bottles, nipples, caps, rings, discs, jug, funnel, spoon, and knife into hot soapy water, and wash them thoroughly.

2 Scrub inside the bottles with the bottle brush to remove all traces of milk. Make sure that you scrub carefully around the necks and the screw heads.

3 Make sure that you rinse the bottles, nipples, and any other equipment thoroughly under running water. Use a pin to clear the holes in the nipples.

Taking care of nipples

Your baby can only feed happily if the nipple allows him to suck out formula at the right rate. When you tip the bottle up, you should see one drop a second: too small a hole will mean that your baby gets frustrated in his efforts to suck out enough formula; too large and the formula will gush out. Nipples do deteriorate, and the holes clog up. Have some spare sterile nipples stored in a jar, so you can easily swap an imperfect nipple for a fresh one. Throw away nipples if the holes are too large; holes that are too small can be enlarged with a needle. Check the flow again afterwards.

A nipple brush *should be used to clean the bottles thoroughly*

Good hygiene and sterilizing

Warm formula can provide a breeding ground for bacteria that cause vomiting and diarrhea, which can be serious for a young baby. For this reason, the Canadian Paediatric Society recommends that water and equipment used to feed babies be sterilized until babies are three to four months old. However, many experts feel that in developed countries with safe drinking water, it is not necessary to boil the water used to reconstitute formula, and that it is acceptable to clean bottles and nipples in a dishwasher, particularly if the nipples are scrubbed first. If you choose to sterilize, here are some different methods to consider.

Equipment for sterilizing

Microwave unit
This unit works as a steam sterilizer in the microwave.

Steam sterilizer
You can sterilize a large number of bottles at once.

Sterilizing tank
You must incorporate a float to keep the items fully submerged.

Sterilizing tablets
You can use tablets to sterilize your equipment.

Sterilizing your baby's feeding equipment

You can sterilize all your baby's feeding equipment either by using a sterilizer or a steam sterilizer.

The occasional use of the boiling method will also sterilize, although repeated use will spoil the quality of the nipples. If using the boiling method, wash the equipment and boil for five minutes. Use tongs to remove the hot bottles, and leave them until they are quite cold before filling.

If using tablets, fill the sterilizing tank with cold water, and add the tablets. When they have dissolved, put the equipment in, filling the bottles so they can't bob up. Leave for at least the minimum time, then take out items as needed and rinse in boiled water. Drain on paper towels.

All items must be fully submerged during the boiling period

The boiling method

Sterilizing with tablets

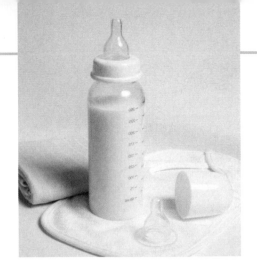

Making up your baby's bottle

Your baby needs a fresh bottle for every feed. You can have a supply of bottles ready in the refrigerator or carry a sterile empty bottle and fill it with measured cooled boiled water and powdered formula whenever your baby is hungry. Until your baby is at least one year old, give him an iron-fortified infant formula. Most are made with modified cow's milk. Once you and your doctor decide on the type of formula that is right for your baby, you can choose the brand as they are all similar.

Infant formula is available as ready-to-feed, and as a concentrated liquid or powder. Choose the format that best meets your budget.

Ready-to-feed formula

Some brands of infant formula are available ready-mixed in 250ml (8fl oz) sealed cans. You do not need to add water to the milk. If the brand of formula you are feeding your baby comes in this form, then you have a very convenient – but expensive – option.

Concentrated formula

The instructions on the cans tell you the correct amount of liquid or number of level, loosely filled scoops to add to each measure of water. It is important to maintain these proportions precisely. If you add too much formula, the feed will be dangerously concentrated: your baby may gain too much weight, and his kidneys may be damaged. If you consistently add too little formula, he may gain weight too slowly. Once the formula is made up, let your baby take as much as he wants at each feed.

Always use fresh, cold tap water to make your baby's feeds, and boil it only once. Before using well water, have it tested to ensure that it's safe. If you live in an older house that has lead pipes, run the water for two minutes before collecting water to mix with formula, even if you plan on boiling it. Some types of water should never be used to mix formula: water that has been repeatedly boiled or left standing in a kettle, water from a tap with an attached domestic softener or domestic filter, or mineral water. These types of water may contain salt and minerals or bacteria that may be harmful for your baby.

Storing formula

Store unopened cans of liquid or powder formula in a cool place, and do not use after the "best before" date. Once opened, cans of powder should be used within a month. Open cans of ready-to-feed and concentrated liquid formula may be stored for up to 48 hours in the refrigerator.

How much will my baby want?

On average, your baby needs 150ml of formula per kilogram (2½fl oz per 1lb) of body weight every 24 hours. As your baby gets bigger, the size of the feeds will increase while the number of feeds per day will decrease. This means that he will go from 8–10 feeds of 60–90ml (2–3fl oz) as a newborn but quickly progress to 4–5 feeds of 210ml (7fl oz) when he is six months. His appetite will help you to determine how big to make his bottles.

Should I give anything else?

While your baby is taking iron-fortified formula, extra supplements are not necessary.

Is my baby allergic to cow's milk?

Formula is modified cow's milk and can, in very rare cases, cause an allergic reaction. If this happens, go back to breastfeeding if possible or see your doctor to discuss alternatives. She may suggest a specially prepared formula, which contains proteins that have been broken down so that they do not cause an allergic response.

The right milk to give your baby							
Type of milk		Birth	6m	9m	12m	18m	
Infant formula	Cow's milk modified to resemble human breast milk. Supplements are not necessary.						
Follow-up formula	**Optional.** Modified cow's milk, intended for babies of six to 12 months. Less expensive than, but not inferior to, starter formula. Supplements are not necessary.						
Full fat cow's milk	Introduce as main milk drink from 12 months.						

Making up powder formula in the bottle

1 Fill a bottle with freshly boiled water. Open the tin of formula, and use the scoop inside to scoop up some powder. Level each scoop with the back of a clean knife: do not heap the scoop, nor pack the powder down inside it.

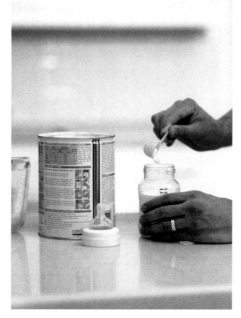

2 Drop each scoop of powder into the bottle. Add only the number of scoops recommended for that amount of water. The powder will dissolve quickly in hot water. Always add one scoop at a time; never add extra.

You will need

- Can of powder formula
- Bottles and nipples
- Paper towel

DHA and ARA supplemented formulas

DHA and ARA are fatty acids that are found naturally in breast milk and are added as supplements to some formula mixtures. There is some evidence that they may boost eyesight and language development in the first year, but by the age of three no difference has been found between these babies and those who were not given a supplemented formula. The supplemented formulas are more expensive, and are not generally recommended at this time.

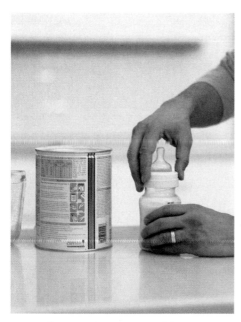

3 Make sure that you've added the right amount of formula. Put the disc, ring, and nipple on the bottle. Screw on tightly. Put the lid on the top before shaking.

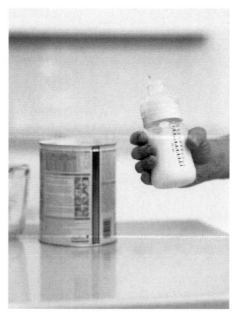

4 Shake the bottle to make sure the formula mixes thoroughly in the water. Cool the bottle in a bowl of cold water or under a cold running water tap.

5 Check the temperature of the milk before offering it to your baby by shaking a few drops on to your wrist. The milk should feel neither hot nor cold against your skin.

Using ready-to-feed formula

1 Rinse the can lid by pouring boiling water over it. Shake the formula can well to ensure the contents are evenly mixed.

2 Open the can using a clean punch-type opener. Then make a second opening very carefully so the formula doesn't spill.

3 Pour the formula into a bottle. Attach the nipple and ring. Shake the bottle, test the temperature, and feed (see page 102 for storage of this type of formula).

You will need

- Can of ready-to-feed formula
- Bottles and nipples
- Scrubbing brush
- Punch-type can opener

Protecting your baby from an upset stomach

If you take the precautions listed below, you should be able to protect your baby from the bacteria that cause stomach upsets (gastroenteritis).
- Sterilize all feeding equipment before you use it, even if it is brand new.
- If you do not have a fridge, make up each feed only when you need it.
- If your baby doesn't finish his bottle at a feed, throw the formula away as his saliva will have contaminated it.
- Throw away any formula warmed for your baby, even if he doesn't touch it; the process of warming the formula encourages bacteria to grow.

- Store bottles of made-up feeds in the main part of the fridge (not in the door). Don't keep the feed for longer than 24 hours.
- Leave the bottles in the sterilizing solution until you need them (it's effective for 24 hours) so that they can't be contaminated by bacteria in the air. Take the nipples out after the minimum time, drain on a paper towel, then store in a sterile jar.
- Don't drain sterilized equipment on your draining board or dry it on a dish towel. Drain only on a paper towel.
- Wash your hands well with soap and water before touching the sterile feeding equipment.

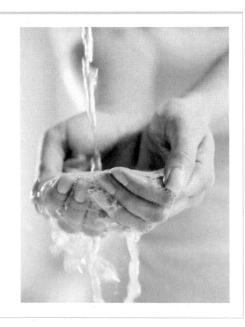

When away from home

If you're going out for more than a couple of hours, take cooled boiled water in a sterilized bottle and the measured formula powder in a dry container, and mix when your baby needs a feed. You can then take a thermos filled with hot water, and warm your baby's bottle in this. Never carry warm formula in a thermos: bacteria will grow in the formula, and may cause a stomach upset. Cans of ready-to-feed formula are even more convenient when you're away from home: the milk has been ultra-heat treated (UHT), so it needs only to be stored in a cool place to stay safe. Take sterile bottles and nipples in a sterile container and pour out each feed as your baby needs it.

Adjust the amount *to suit your baby's appetite*

Powdered formula *and sterile water can be mixed on the spot*

Powder dispenser and bottle of water

Formula *can be heated on the go*

Thermos with bottle

Formula *can be warmed easily when you're away from home*

Travel bottle warmer

Ready-to-feed *formula has been ultra-heat treated*

Can of formula

Giving your baby a bottle

Feeding your baby is the most important thing you can do for her – but don't make the mistake of thinking that the milk in the bottle is all she needs, or that "anyone" can feed her. Your love, your cuddling, and your attention are just as important to your baby as the formula itself. Always hold her close and cuddle her against you, smile and talk to her – just as you would if you were breastfeeding. Never, under any circumstances, leave your baby alone with her bottle: she may choke.

Right from the beginning, give your baby as much control over feeding as you can. Let her set the pace, pausing to look around, touch the bottle, or stroke your breast if she wants to – it may take as long as half an hour to empty the bottle, if she's feeling playful. Above all, let her decide when she's had enough milk.

Make yourself comfortable, put a bib on her, and have a cloth at hand for when you burp her, in case she brings up any milk.

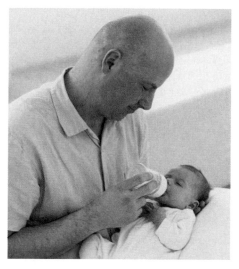

Bottle-feeding your baby
Your partner can now share in the joy and closeness of feeding your baby.

From breast- to bottle-feeding

If you have to change over to bottle-feeding from breastfeeding for any reason, remember that the transition needs a gradual approach and professional advice. Replacing one breastfeed with the bottle every third day is the best method – or you can go more slowly. You may start by replacing a lunchtime breastfeed with a bottle. If your baby won't take it, try again at the same feed the next day – you could offer a different type of nipple (see page 99), or moisten the nipple with a few drops of breast milk to encourage her. After three days with one bottle-feed, replace a second daytime feed with a bottle, and wait another three days before tackling a third feed. Your baby may accept a bottle more readily from someone other than you.

Getting the bottle ready

1 Always prepare a fresh feed. If the milk requires cooling, do so by keeping the bottle under a running cold water tap or standing it in a bowl of cold water.

2 Check the flow of milk: it should be about one drop a second. A small hole makes sucking hard; a large one lets the milk gush out. If the nipple isn't right, get another sterile nipple, and test the flow.

Q&A

"My baby never seems to finish her bottle: is she getting enough?"
If your baby is feeding poorly, it could be a sign of illness, or of a serious underlying condition that needs medical attention. Check to see how much milk your baby should have for her weight (see page 102), and see if that matches what she actually takes. If you are at all concerned, talk to your doctor about the problem, and make sure your baby is weighed regularly at the doctor's office, where her weight will be plotted on a growth chart (see pages 254–257). Poor feeding, if combined with inadequate weight gain, is always a cause for concern.

3 Test the temperature by tipping a few drops on to the inside of your wrist – it should feel tepid. Cold milk is safe, but your baby may prefer it warm.

4 Unscrew the ring to let the air into the bottle. Then screw it back before giving to your baby as he sucks milk out. This will stop the nipple from collapsing and halting the flow.

Giving your baby her bottle

1 Stroke the cheek nearest you, she should turn and open her mouth. If she doesn't, or is older, let some drops of milk form on the nipple, then touch her lips with it to give her the taste.

2 Hold the bottle firmly so that she can pull against it as she sucks, and tilt it so that the nipple is full of milk, not air. If the nipple collapses, move the bottle around in her mouth to let air back into the bottle.

3 When your baby has finished all the milk, pull the bottle firmly away. If she wants to continue sucking, offer her your clean little finger: she will soon let you know if she wants more milk.

If she won't let go

If your baby doesn't want to let go of the bottle even after a long suck, slide your little finger between her gums alongside the nipple.

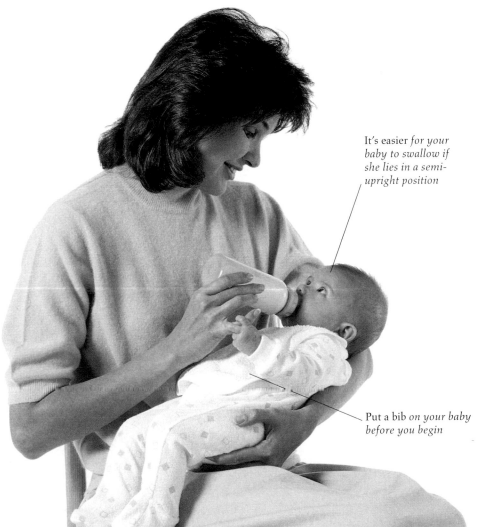

It's easier *for your baby to swallow if she lies in a semi-upright position*

Put a bib *on your baby before you begin*

Sleeping during a feed

If she dozes off during her feed, she may have gas, which is making her feel full. Sit her up, and burp her for a couple of minutes, then offer her some more milk.

Introducing solid food

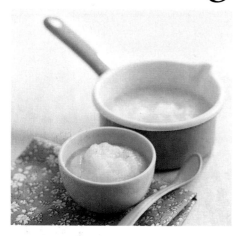

From the age of six months, your baby will be ready to try some solid food. Getting him used to unfamiliar tastes and textures may help him to avoid becoming a picky eater when he gets older. Let him eat as much as he reasonably wants – you want mealtimes to be enjoyable. Allow his own appetite to dictate how much he eats, and avoid confrontations. Including your baby in family mealtimes from an early age will help him learn essential social skills.

Equipment for first solids

The essential items you'll need for feeding your baby his first tastes include a clean plastic spoon, a bowl, and a bib to keep his clothes clean. Soon he will need sippy cups for drinks, and once he's sitting up steadily you will need a high chair. You don't need to sterilize equipment for solid food, just wash it well in very hot water, rinse, drain, and dry with paper towels.

Plastic bowl

Spoon for first tastes

Hand blender

Spout *prevents the drink from spilling if the cup tips over*

Plastic cups

Spill-proof bowl

Some plastic feeding bowls are fitted with a suction cup to anchor them firmly on the table or the tray of a high chair.
These are useful when your baby begins to feed himself and it's inevitable that he will try to throw the bowl on the floor.

Bibs

Plastic-backed cloth bib
This is the best type in the early months. Plastic backing and ties at the sides ensure that your child's clothes are protected.

A bib *that covers your baby's front and arms is ideal as he gets older*

Bib with sleeves

Plastic bib

Chairs

High chair

Your baby needs a high chair from the age of about six months, or from when he can sit up steadily. Always strap him into the chair with a safety harness, and never leave him unsupervised. Put the chair on a plastic sheet to protect the floor, and involve your child in family meals by sitting him next to the table.

Some chairs *have reclining seats for infants*

A rim around the edge *of the tray will stop at least some food from falling on the floor*

Make sure *the tray can be wiped clean*

A restraining strap *or bar is important to stop your baby from slipping down between the tray and seat*

The frame must *lock rigid, so your child's fingers can't get pinched*

A chair that folds *up is useful in a small kitchen*

An easy-care seat cover *is advisable, because food will go everywhere*

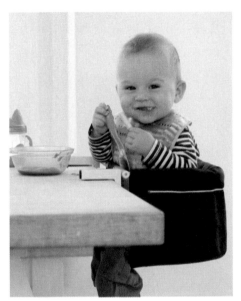

Clip-on chair

A seat that clamps onto a table is convenient when you're away from home – but follow the manufacturer's guidelines carefully, because there are several types of tables on which this chair must not be used. Use a safety harness, and protect the floor underneath.

Booster seat

From the age of about 18 months, your child can reach the level of the table with a booster seat strapped securely to an ordinary chair. Adjust the height by turning the seat over. It's harder for a child to fall off a booster seat than just a cushion placed on the chair.

Why wait to feed your baby solids?

In the past, babies used to be fed puréed foods from a very early age. But we now know that the digestive system of a very young baby isn't ready for solid foods. His gut and kidneys can handle formula or breast milk, but not much else. Indigestion, constipation, diarrhea, and obesity are less likely if you wait until your baby is six months old before starting to give solids. Very young babies cannot easily move food from the front to the back of their mouth, and have such poor head control that it is difficult to hold them securely to feed them semi-solid foods. By six months, most can sit supported in a chair and swallow food from a spoon. They may have only one or two teeth, but their gums are hard, and they can chew. A seven-month-old baby will turn his head away or grab the spoon to indicate that he wants to self-feed.

Food tastes and preferences

Food smells, tastes, and feels different from breast milk or formula, and it comes in mouthfuls, rather than a continuous stream. Don't worry if your baby refuses or spits out food at first. Let him play with his food, and as soon as he has teeth, give finger foods he can hold himself. All this will encourage your baby to experiment with this strange new way of feeding.

What to feed your baby

The best foods to give your baby are fresh foods that you prepare and cook yourself.

First solid foods Start with iron fortified single grain cereals such as rice, oats, or barley. When she tolerates these, start adding new foods as suggested below.

Texture Tailor the texture of the food to what she can happily cope with. Make her food wet and easy to swallow. Moisten puréed, mashed, or minced foods with boiled water, breast milk, formula, the cooking liquid (if unsalted), fruit juice, or yogurt.

Temperature Always let the food cool to lukewarm.

Introducing a new food Offer each new food on its own, and wait for at least 24 hours before giving it again. If diarrhea, sickness, or a rash follows, don't offer it again for several months.

Seasoning Don't use salt. It can damage young kidneys, and your baby won't mind bland flavours.

What to avoid Avoid hard, small foods such as nuts, popcorn, raw carrots, or whole grapes as they may choke her. Do not give honey in the first year. Fish that are high in mercury (such as canned albacore tuna) should be given only once a month.

First foods (6 months)

Texture Give your six-month-old baby semi-liquid purées, bland and smooth, and without any lumps.

Preparation

- peel carefully
- cook: steam or boil
- remove seeds and stems
- purée or sieve.

Other good foods

Other cereals, other well-cooked vegetables and fruits such as peas, beans, cauliflower, and pears.

Baby rice   Puréed carrot   Puréed apple   Puréed potato

7–8 months

Texture Foods can be minced or mashed to the texture of cottage cheese, adding liquid or yogurt. Give plenty of finger foods that are easy for your baby to pick up so she feeds herself. For example, sticks of soft vegetables, bite-sized pieces of peeled fruit.

Preparation, fruit/vegetables

- peel carefully
- remove ends and stems
- purée or sieve.

Preparation, meat/fish

- remove fat and skin
- cook: grill or poach
- remove all bones
- mince to fine consistency.

Other good foods

Mixed infant cereals, other cooked vegetables and fruits, tofu, beans, chickpeas, lentils, egg yolks (hard boiled).

Foods to avoid Cookies, cake, ice cream, fried foods, peanut butter, low-fat dairy foods, egg whites (wait until one year to introduce egg whites).

Minced chicken   Minced white fish   Mashed egg yolk   Plain yogurt   Finger foods

How to store your baby's food

Have nutritious, home-cooked food for your baby always on hand by making up batches of purées and freezing them. Purée fruits and vegetables separately, and cool them quickly by standing the bowl in cold water. Pour the purée into ice-cube trays, cover them well with plastic wrap, and then freeze. When frozen, empty the cubes out, and store in sealed freezer bags, one type of food per bag. Label with the name and date, and don't keep for longer than one month.

Half an hour before a mealtime, put some cubes in a bowl to thaw – one or two will be enough at first. Stand the bowl in hot water to heat the purée, then transfer it to your baby's bowl, ready to feed her. Stir to make sure it is warmed evenly.

You can keep prepared food for your baby in the fridge for up to 24 hours; always cover it first. After your baby has finished her meal, throw away any food that her spoon has been dipped into, including commercial baby foods if you have fed her straight from the jar. Never keep, as saliva may have contaminated the food.

8–9 months

Texture Introduce your child to chunkier textures now, so you can chop food rather than mashing it. Give plenty of finger foods to encourage feeding skills. Stay nearby when she is eating these in case she chokes.

Preparation, fruit/vegetables
- peel carefully
- remove seeds and stems
- give in slices or sticks or grate, if raw
- chop or mash, if cooked: leave plenty of lumps.

Preparation, meat/fish
- remove fat and skin
- cook: grill, stew, or poach
- mince lumpily.

Other good foods
Toast, meat, cubes of soft cheese, cottage cheese, home-cooked dishes such as soup or lasagna (cooked without salt).

10–12 months

Texture Your child is eating almost everything the family eats, chopped into bite-sized pieces. Continue to avoid salt in your cooking; you can salt your own food at the table.

Preparation, fruit/vegetables
- peel carefully
- remove seeds and stems
- if cooked, steam whenever possible.

Preparation, meat/fish
- remove fat and skin
- cook: grill, stew, or poach
- chop into small pieces.

Other good foods
Tinned light (yellow fin or skipjack) tuna, stronger-flavoured green vegetables, (cabbage, green pepper), whole peeled tomato.

Foods to avoid Spicy, fatty, or salty foods (ham, weiners, bologna), sugary foods, fruit punch, honey, unpasteurized cheeses, raw berries.

Lean ground beef or lamb   Pasta   Mashed lentils   Brown rice

Finger foods

Steamed broccoli   Green beans   Fruits

Chopped chicken

Develop a water habit

Many children drink too many high sugar beverages such as fruit juices. Some derive as much as a third of their daily calorie requirements from these drinks, which reduce their appetite and give no real nutrients. If they are sweetened, these drinks contribute to tooth decay, too. Offer water when your child is thirsty between meals, so she doesn't develop a "fruit juice habit." Colas and similar carbonated drinks aren't suitable for young children, and neither are "diet" soft drinks, which contain high levels of artificial sweeteners.

Iron and vitamins

The best way to make sure your baby gets the nourishment she needs is to offer her a wide range of foods. The store of iron she was born with will begin to run out when she is about six months old. Good sources of iron include: red meat, liver, iron-fortified infant cereals, lentils, egg yolk, and green vegetables, such as peas and spinach. Your baby will be able to absorb more iron if she eats foods containing vitamin C (found in fruit and vegetables) at the same time. Don't give her tea – it will reduce the amount of iron she absorbs from her food.

Warning

Never give a pre-school child peanuts. Apart from a risk of choking, it's easy for a small child to inhale a fragment accidentally, and if this happens, the oil the peanuts contain can cause severe irritation in the lungs.

Introducing first tastes

At around six months, your baby is probably ready to try small amounts of solid food. Even if she seems content on milk alone, she needs to learn this new skill, so don't wait too long to start solids. Remember that for the first weeks you're simply introducing her to the idea of eating solid food from a spoon; breast milk or formula is still providing her with all the nourishment that she needs. Start at breakfast or lunchtime, so you will have time to watch for any reactions to the food before she goes to bed for the night. Your baby will most likely be more co-operative if you let her partially satisfy her hunger first, so "sandwich" a teaspoon of baby rice or fruit purée between two halves of her normal breast- or bottle-feed. The whole process might take as long as an hour.

Give a feed first

Sit down comfortably with your baby's bowl of food within reach. Put a bib on her, then give her half her usual breast- or bottle-feed: let her empty one breast, or give her half her bottle, and then burp her. She will go on needing her milk feeds for several months to come. Your baby's digestive system is still developing, so it may be advisable to mix approximately one tablespoon of baby rice, for example, with enough breast milk or warm formula to give it a watery consistency. Babies over six months old are generally able to cope with thicker texture.

Commercial baby foods

Baby foods in jars or cans can be useful, especially when you're away from home or in a hurry. But your baby will be better off if you can keep them to a minimum in her diet. If you want to store some commercial food, avoid those with a list of ingredients that includes sugar, dextrose, sucrose, or salt, or that show water as the first item – this means that it's the largest ingredient, so the food may not be as nutritious as your home-made equivalent. Always check the expiry and packaging dates.

You will need

- Bib
- Small plastic bowl or egg cup
- Small plastic spoon
- About a dessert spoonful of iron-fortified baby rice cereal
- Damp tissue or washcloth

Giving your baby her first tastes

1 Scoop a little food on to her plastic spoon – enough to coat the tip. At first, she will probably eat only a teaspoonful or so. You can offer her more, but when she loses interest it is best to carry on with the rest of her milk feed.

2 Try sitting her on a high chair at first, but if she resists, sit her on your lap. Put the spoon between your baby's lips, so she can suck the food off. Don't try to push the spoon in, she will gag if she feels food at the back of her tongue. She may be surprised at the taste and sensation at first, so be patient and talk to her encouragingly.

3 She may quickly discover that she enjoys this new experience. If she pushes the food out, scrape it up, and put the spoon between her lips again. When she's had about a teaspoonful of baby rice cereal, wipe her mouth and chin, and resume her milk feed.

Your baby's nutritional needs

The World Health Organization recommends exclusive breastfeeding (no solids) until 6 months. How you manage the transition from exclusive breast milk or formula feeds to mixed feeding with solid foods will depend on your baby's temperament and your own lifestyle. The most important thing is not to rush her. The chart below is just one way you might approach feeding: it assumes you start at about six months. She will still need her milk feeds, so start slowly and drop one feeding at a time.

A stage-by-stage guide to infant feeding

Stage/age	What to do	Drinks	Early am	Breakfast	Lunch	Dinner	Bedtime
Weeks 1 and 2 **Age 6 months** (ages are guidelines only)	Give small tastes of baby cereal at lunchtime, halfway through the breast- or bottle-feeding. Give the same food for three days for your baby to get used to it.	If you are bottle-feeding, offer your baby occasional drinks of water if she is thirsty.	■	■	■ ■ ■	■	■
Weeks 3 and 4 **Age 6½ months**	Introduce solid food at breakfast, halfway through the feeding: baby cereal or other single-grain cereal is ideal. Increase the amount of solid food at lunchtime to 3–4 teaspoonfuls.	Offer water in a bottle. Don't worry if she doesn't want any.	■	■ ■ ■	■ ■ ■	■	■
Weeks 5 and 6 **Age 7 months**	Introduce solid food at dinner, halfway through the feeding. A week later, offer two courses at lunch: follow a vegetable purée with a fruit one, giving 2–3 teaspoonfuls of each.	Introduce a sippy cup, but don't expect her to be able to drink from it yet – it's just a toy.		■ ■ ■	■ ■ ■ ■	■ ■ ■	■
Weeks 7 and 8 **Age 7½ months**	Offer solid food as the first part of lunch, then give breast or bottle to top up. She can have two courses at dinner now: some chicken, a vegetable, and a piece of banana, for example. At breakfast and dinner continue giving the feeding first. She may eat 5–6 teaspoonfuls of solid food at each meal now.	You can start to give your baby drinks in her cup, but hold it for her as she drinks from it.		■ ■ ■	■ ■ ■	■ ■ ■ ■	■
Weeks 9 and 10 **Age 8 months**	After lunch solids, offer a breastfeed or a drink of formula from a cup. After a few days with no lunchtime breast or bottle, offer solid food as the first part of dinner.	Offer formula or breast milk in a cup at each meal and water at other times.		■ ■ ■	■ ■	■ ■ ■	■
Weeks 11 and 12 **Age 8½ months**	Offer your baby breast milk or a drink of formula in a cup instead of a full feeding after her dinner. You may find she often refuses her breast- or bottle-feeding after her breakfast solids now.	As for weeks 9 and 10.		■ ■	■ ■	■ ■	■
Week 13 onwards **Age 9 months**	Offer a drink in a cup instead of the feeding before breakfast: now your baby is having solids at three meals a day. Breast milk or formula should be the main drink until one year. She can have cow's milk only from 12 months.	As before. Your baby may possibly be able to manage her own trainer cup now.		■	■ ■	■ ■	■

Key
■ feeding   ■ solid food

How your baby learns to feed herself

Your baby will be eager to try and feed herself long before she's able to do so efficiently. However messy an experience this is, be prepared for food to end up all over her face and clothes, in her hair (and yours!), and on the floor. Regardless of how drawn out it makes mealtimes, try to encourage her as much as you can – it is her first real step towards independence. Try to maintain a calm and relaxed attitude at mealtimes, and don't rush your baby: if she finds them interesting and enjoyable occasions, you are less likely to encounter problems over food and eating in the future.

At seven months

Your baby may be making determined efforts to feed herself by this age, but she won't be co-ordinated enough to get all the food she needs into her mouth. Feed her yourself, but don't stop her from playing with her food. Smearing it all over her face may be messy, but it's the first step in learning to feed herself; have a clean washcloth handy to wipe her with when she's finished. Give her plenty of different finger foods, too. They're easy to handle, so she will gain in confidence and dexterity.

1 She will be hungry at the start of the meal. Keep the bowl out of her reach, and spoon-feed her.

2 Once you've satisfied her initial hunger, let her join in, but continue feeding her yourself.

Your baby won't be very skilful yet, but will love the challenge

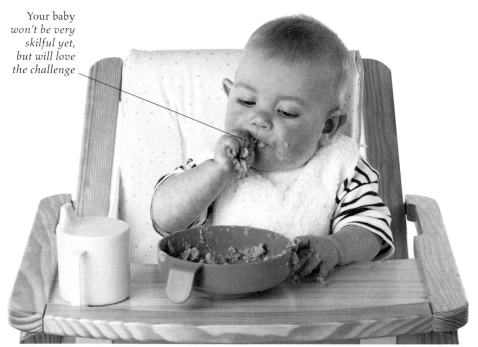

3 Your baby may get so absorbed in the pleasure of dabbling her fingers in her bowl and pushing the food into her mouth that she will lose interest in you feeding her with a spoon. If she's still hungry, she may cry and wriggle out of frustration because she can't get the food in quickly enough, so offer some more spoonfuls. Otherwise let her practise her feeding skills: feeling "I can do it myself" is important to her. The practice will also help her to develop a pincer grip. She knows when she's had enough.

Tips to help

● If she grabs your spoon, use two spoons at the same meal. Fill one and put it in her bowl, so she can pick it up. Keep your spoon ready. When her spoon turns over on the way to her mouth, pop your full spoon in, and fill hers, so she can try again.
● Have clean spoons ready for when she drops hers on the floor.

4 Solid food may make her thirsty, so offer formula, and tip the cup for her – she won't be able to hold it herself yet. Introduce cow's milk from one year.

"How much food should I offer my baby?"

Let your baby decide how much food he wants at each meal. At six months, start with no more than four teaspoonfuls of food in his bowl, and offer more if he eats it all. Follow his cues for quantity of food. Some days he will eat voraciously, others hardly anything. If he is gaining weight normally, there's no need to worry. Even if you think your baby isn't getting enough food, he is.

"My child will only eat cheese and sandwiches. What can I do?"

Food fads are extremely common in young children, and thankfully usually don't last for more than a couple of weeks. Don't stop offering your child other things at mealtimes, but don't worry or get frustrated with him if he won't eat them; he won't suffer unless the fad goes on for several weeks. If you are concerned that he is missing vital nutrients, ask your doctor for advice.

"Should I make him eat things he doesn't seem to like?" **Q&A**

Respect your child's opinions. If he doesn't like something, don't mix it with something he likes: he will end up disliking both. Try varying the form in which you give a particular food. For example, if he doesn't like vegetables, he might eat them raw or liquidized in soup; or scrambled eggs might be a good alternative to hard-boiled eggs, if he always refuses to eat those.

At 15 months

Your child will be making a good attempt to feed himself with a spoon or fork with rounded prongs, so cut his food into bite-sized pieces. Give him his own special bowl, spoon, and fork. He may need your help on some days.

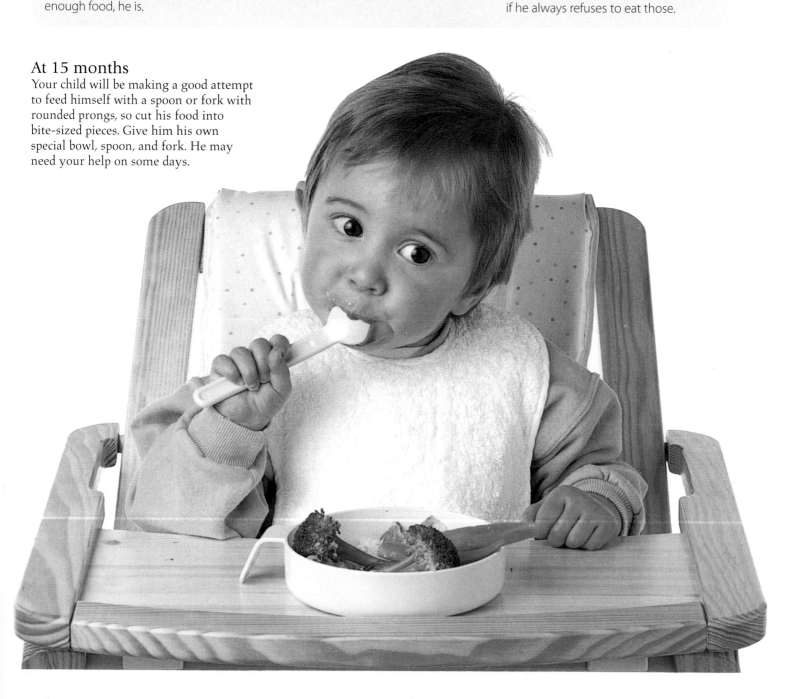

Eating and your older child

Around the age of two years, your child will probably be ready to graduate out of his high chair, and join the rest of the family at the meal table. Mealtimes are extremely important social occasions, and learning how to participate as a member of the family is a vital part of your child's continuing social development. What he eats is obviously important as well, but as long as you provide your child with enough nutritious food, you can leave it up to him to decide whether he eats it or not. Your child won't starve himself, and he knows best how much food he wants at any particular time.

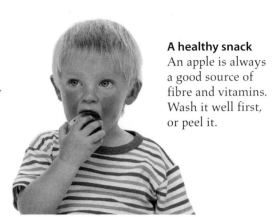

A healthy snack
An apple is always a good source of fibre and vitamins. Wash it well first, or peel it.

Avoiding mealtime problems

The secret of avoiding mealtime problems is to keep your own attitude relaxed and friendly. From the very beginning, make your child feel that eating is a pleasurable way to satisfy his hunger. It is always a mistake to turn eating into a battle of wills – you will end up upset, and he will refuse more strongly next time. Instead, keep the eating issue in perspective for both of you, for it should be an enjoyable experience:

● Give your toddler a varied diet, and give him some choice over what he eats. He will soon make his likes and dislikes clear to you.
● Don't punish him for not eating a particular food, and don't reward him for eating something either. "Eat up your carrots and you can play on your tricycle" will make any child think there must be something terrible about carrots if he has to be rewarded for eating them.
● Don't spend a great deal of time preparing food especially for him: you will only feel doubly resentful if he doesn't eat it.
● If he dawdles over his food, don't rush him to finish it. He's bound to be slower than you. If you would expect him to stay at the table while you finish your meal, then you must do the same, and wait for him to finish when he's being slow.
● Don't persuade him to eat more than he wants. Let him decide when he has had enough. He won't starve, and if he's growing normally, you know he's eating sufficient amounts to fulfil his dietary needs.

The right diet

Variety is the keynote of a good diet: if you offer different foods throughout the week, you can be sure that your child is getting the nutrients he needs. His diet will only be unhealthy if for long periods he eats too much of some kinds of food, such as cookies and cakes, or highly processed foods, such as sausages or hamburgers – to the exclusion of others.

Does my child need vitamin supplements?

Vitamins are important for your body to work well. But if your child is eating a healthy diet based on Canada's Food Guide, he won't need any extra vitamins.

Snacks and sweets

Your child will often need a snack to give him energy between meals. Rather than cookies, offer him healthy, nutritious snacks, such as a piece of wholegrain bread, an apple, a carrot, or a banana. If he's not very hungry at the next meal, he won't have missed out nutritionally.

Sweets can be a battleground, but it's up to you to make the rules and stick to them. Certainly it's not fair or realistic to ban sweets altogether; he may learn to covet them even more. But sweets provide few nutrients and lots of empty calories, and they are also very destructive for your child's teeth. Control your child's love of anything sweet by keeping sugary and sweetened foods to a minimum:

● Provide fruit or unsweetened yogurt for dessert at most meals. Cheese is excellent, too, because it neutralizes the acid that forms in the mouth and attacks tooth enamel.
● When you do let your child have sweets, offer them at the end of a meal, not between meals, so that he won't be filling up on empty calories.
● Limit diluted fruit juices to half a cup per day, and give them only at meals; offer milk or water at other times.
● Don't use sweets as your main way of rewarding or punishing your child: they will become intensely valuable to him, so harder to control.

Ways to improve your family's diet

A healthy diet is one that includes a wide variety of foods. Although a low-fat diet is healthiest for adults, a child should be given full-fat foods until the age of five.
● Use fresh rather than processed foods – fresh foods will contain more nutrients, and less salt and sugar.
● Keep the amount of red meat in your diet to a minimum.

● Eat chicken or fish at least three times a week.
● Steam vegetables rather than boil them to preserve nutrients, or serve them raw.
● Buy wholegrain bread and avoid sugary cereals.
● Fruit has a lot of nutritional value. Feed your child a wide variety of fruit as it contains essential vitamins helpful in the growth of your child.

Crying and your baby

Until he is about three months old, and more aware of the world around him, your baby may seem to cry for much of the time he is awake. Your instinct will be to pick him up and cuddle him, and this is exactly what he needs – you need not worry that by doing so you are spoiling him or encouraging him to cry more. Your baby needs to know that he can rely on you. If he cries so much that you feel your patience running out, seek help from your healthcare provider.

Ways to soothe your baby

The important thing when your baby cries is to respond quickly and calmly, without making a lot of anxious fuss: leaving him to cry will agitate him more. If your baby is crying for no obvious reason, try one of the methods below to soothe him. However, your baby should not become dependent on any of them. Never shake your baby, no matter how tired or angry you feel.

Seven ways to soothe your crying baby

 Offer a feed In the first few months, hunger is the most likely reason for your baby crying, and offering a feed is the most effective way to soothe him – even if that means frequent feeds throughout the day, and also at night. If your baby is bottle-fed, and sucks hungrily at his feeds with short gaps between bottles, try offering him cool boiled water in a sterile bottle – he may be thirsty.

 Cuddle him Very often this will be just the sort of loving contact your baby needs to calm down and stop crying. If he quietens when you hold him upright against your shoulder or face down in your arms (see page 83), it may have been gas that was making him cry. If he has been passed around for friends and relatives to hold, he may have become overstimulated, and just wants a few quiet moments being cuddled by you or your partner.

 Rock him rhythmically Movement often comforts an irritable baby, and may send him off to sleep. Rock him in your arms, and if he doesn't quieten, try rocking faster. Or just jiggle him up and down by shifting from foot to foot, perhaps with your baby in an infant carrier on your chest (see below). Or rock with him in a rocking chair, if you have one. You can also put him in his carriage and push him back and forth, or take him for a walk.

 Carry him Often you will be able to soothe your baby simply by putting him in the infant carrier and carrying him around with you. This leaves your hands free, and your baby will be soothed both by the close physical contact and the motion as you move around. If your baby is crying because of something you've had to do to him – changing his diaper, bathing, or dressing him, for example – this may be the best way to calm him, and will probably even send him off to sleep.

 Pat him Rhythmically patting and rubbing his back or tummy will often calm him down, and may help him to bring up gas. It may comfort him when you first put him down to change his diaper, too.

 Give him something to suck Almost all babies are soothed by sucking. Your clean little finger will probably work like magic. He may well suck his own fist from an early age. You could even use a natural-shaped pacifier, but remember to keep it clean.

 Distract your baby Something to look at may make your baby forget why he was crying. Bright, colourful patterns may fascinate him: he will often gaze intently at postcards, wallpaper, or your clothes. Faces and mirrors are also excellent distractions.

Seven reasons your baby might be crying

Often you won't really know why your young baby is crying or why he stopped. If you've tried the simple remedies, such as feeding and a cuddle, and you've tried the soothing tactics that have worked in the past (see previous page), all without success, then there may be another reason. Listed below are some other possible causes of his crying.

Illness may be making your baby cry, particularly if his crying sounds different from normal. Always call your doctor if your baby shows any symptoms that are unusual for him. A blocked nose from a cold may stop him feeding or sucking his thumb, so he can't comfort himself in the way he's used to, even though he may not be very ill. Your doctor can suggest strategies to help him breathe easily (see pages 180–1).

Diaper rash or a sore bottom may make your baby cry. Take his diaper off, clean him thoroughly, and leave him without a diaper for the rest of the day: just lay him on a towel or cloth diaper. Take steps to stop the rash worsening (see page 150).

Colic, often called three-month or evening colic, is characterized by a pattern of regular, intense, inconsolable screaming at a certain time each day, usually the late afternoon or evening.

The pattern appears at about three weeks, and continues until 12 or 14 weeks. The crying spell may last as long as three hours. Always ask for medical advice the first time your baby screams inconsolably. Colic isn't harmful, but you might misdiagnose it and miss other serious symptoms.

His surroundings may make your baby cry. He might be too cold: your baby's room temperature should be about 18–20°C (65–68°F), a temperature comfortable for lightly clothed adults. Avoid overheating – don't pile on too many bedclothes. If the back of your baby's neck feels hot and damp, he's probably too hot; remove some bedclothes, and undo some clothes to help him cool off. If he is sweating, a towel under the crib sheet may make him more comfortable. Bright lights can make him cry too, so make sure neither an overhead lamp above his changing mat, nor the sun, are shining in his eyes.

Activities he hates can't always be avoided, however loudly he voices his dislike. Dressing and undressing, bathing, having eye or nose drops are all activities a new baby commonly dislikes, but all you can do is get them over with as quickly as possible, then give your baby a cuddle to calm him down.

Your own mood may be a reason for your baby's distress. Perhaps it's evening and you're feeling tired; perhaps your baby's crankiness is making you irritable. Knowing that your baby is often just reacting to your own emotions may help you to be calmer with him.

Too much fussing can sometimes make an upset baby cry all the more. Passing him between you, changing a diaper unnecessarily, offering a feed again and again, discussing his crying in anxious voices, may all make him more agitated. If there's no obvious reason for his crying, don't keep trying to find one: he probably just wants a calming cuddle.

Soothing your baby
Bounce your baby gently in your arms and talk or sing to him – most babies are soothed by both sound and movement (see previous page).

Coping with colic

All you can do if your baby has evening colic is learn to live with it, in the certain knowledge that he isn't ill and that the colic will eventually pass. See your doctor regularly to ensure that your baby is gaining weight and doing well.
- Gripe water is harmless and comforts some babies. Don't resort to any other medication. Remember colic can't be cured.
- If you are breastfeeding, try excluding dairy products from your diet and avoiding caffeine.
- If you are bottle-feeding, anti-colic bottles may be effective in reducing bouts of colic.
- Rarely, colic may be due to a milk allergy, so ask your doctor's advice about changing to a hypoallergenic formula.
- Try to have an evening out. Leave your partner or a relative in charge, and enjoy some time to yourself.

Your crying older baby

From about three months of age, you may notice a real change in your baby. Now he's much more aware of what goes on around him, he's responsive and interested in everything; he's much more of a person altogether. He'll still cry a lot, and will continue to do so for many months to come, but by now you'll have a better idea of why he is crying.

Six reasons why your older baby might be crying

Hunger is still an obvious reason for your baby to cry. As his first year progresses, and he becomes mobile and moves on to solid food, he will often get tired and cranky between meals – his life is a busy one, as he is led by his own curiosity. A snack and a drink may restore his energy, and cheer him up.

Anxiety will be a new reason for crying from the age of seven or eight months, because by then your baby will have discovered his unshakable attachment to you. You are his "safe base"; he'll be happy to explore the world, provided he can keep you in sight. He may cry if you leave him, or if he loses sight of you. Be patient with him, and gently encourage him to get used to new people and situations.

Pain, from bumps as he becomes mobile, will be a frequent cause of tears. Often it will be the shock that makes him cry, rather than any injury, so a sympathetic cuddle and a distracting toy will usually help him forget it quickly.

Wanting to get his own way will often be a cause of friction and tears, particularly from the age of two. It's worth asking yourself if you're frustrating him unnecessarily, or perhaps trying to assert your own will; but sometimes he will need to be checked for his safety. If he gets so angry that he throws a tantrum, don't shout at or try reasoning with him, or punish him afterwards. It's best to ignore the tantrum completely. Wait until the fit of temper has passed, then continue with whatever you were going to do (see also page 176).

Frustration will become an increasingly common reason for your baby crying, as he tries to do things currently beyond his capabilities. You can't avoid this, although you can make life easier for him by, for example, putting his things where he can reach them. Distraction is the best cure: introduce a new game or toy, and his tears may soon be forgotten. Or help him, if he's struggling, but don't take over completely.

Overtiredness will show itself in whining, irritability, and finally tears. By the end of his first year, your child's life is so full of new experiences that he can run out of energy before he's run out of enthusiasm. He needs you to help him relax enough to get the sleep he needs. A quiet time sitting on your lap listening to a story may work, and a calming, enjoyable bedtime routine (see pages 124–5) that you stick to every evening will help, too.

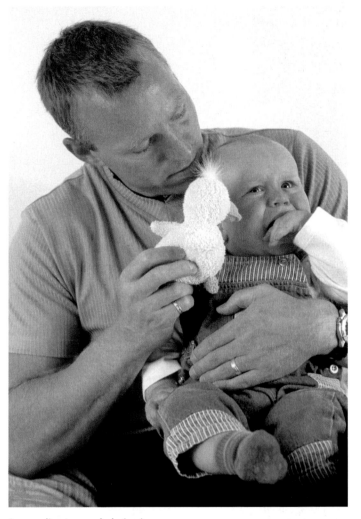

Responding to your baby's cries
All babies thrive on the company of their parents. When he's upset, put your baby on your lap and distract him with his favourite toy.

"Every new tooth my toddler cuts is preceded by days of crying. What can I do to help him?" Q&A

The first teeth shouldn't cause your baby any trouble, but the back teeth, which are usually cut during the second year, can be painful. Your child will probably dribble a lot, and have a red cheek for a couple of days. There are ways you can help him cope with the discomfort:
- Rub his gums with your little finger.
- Give him something to chew on: a cold wet washcloth or a refrigerated teething ring can be soothing.
- If you use a water-filled teething ring, put it in the fridge, not the freezer: frozen rings can cause frostbite.
- Occasional use of acetaminophen or ibuprofen is fine, but avoid giving repeated doses of medicines or teething gels.

Sleep and your baby

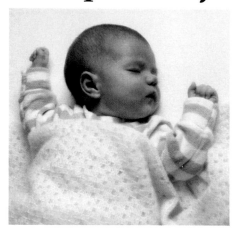

Lack of sleep for you will be a fact of life for many weeks before your baby settles into a routine that coincides more closely with yours. Until your baby is about three months old, she may not sleep longer than three or four hours at a stretch. However, as she grows and matures, she will be awake more often and be more aware of day and night. Her napping schedule and bedtime start to become more consistent. A relaxing bedtime routine that is exactly the same every night will give her the sense of security she needs.

Equipment for sleep

All cribs sold, advertised, or imported into Canada must comply with safety standards among the strictest in the world. Cribs made before September 1986 do not meet current safety regulations and should not be used. The mattress should be firm and not more than 15cm (6in) thick and should be tight against all four sides of the crib. The space between the mattress and crib should not be more than 3cm ($1^3/_{16}$in). Health Canada is currently considering a prohibition on drop-side cribs due to safety concerns.

What to sleep in

Moses basket A newborn baby may feel more secure in a Moses basket than in a larger crib. A Moses basket is also easily portable, and can be taken with you from room to room. However, it can only be used for the first few months, until your baby outgrows it.

Handles *enable you to transport your baby easily while asleep*

The spaces *between the bars should be no wider than 6cm (2½in)*

A fitted sheet *made of 100% cotton is easy to put on, and is comfortable for your baby*

Preventing "baby flat head"

The successful campaign to decrease Sudden Infant Death Syndrome (SIDS) by putting babies to sleep on their backs has caused an increased incidence of positional plagiocephaly, or flat head. This is not serious, but can lead to a noticeable difference between one side of your baby's head and the other. To prevent this, give her supervised tummy time when she is awake. You can also regularly change her orientation in her crib so that she is not always turning in the same direction to see interesting things in her room.

Your baby's bedding

Sheets and blankets

Cotton sheets and cotton cellular blankets are the best options for your baby's bedding. Babies should not have pillows, bumper pads, or comforters. These kinds of bedding, along with stuffed toys or soft objects, have shown to increase the risk of Sudden Infant Death Syndrome (SIDS).

Baby sleeping bag

Sleeping bags are worn over a sleepsuit, and must only be used without any other covering (see page 125).

Quilt

Quilts and comforters, while attractive, should only be used for babies over the age of one year. This is because older babies can easily kick them off, if they become too hot in the night.

Toys for the crib

Mobile

Hang just out of reach above your baby's crib; a colourful mobile will amuse her.

Teddy bear

Keep soft toys out of the crib for the first 12 months.

Your baby's room

● Keep the room warm, but not hot: 18–20°C (65–68°F) is ideal. At this temperature, a sheet plus one or two layers of cellular blankets is enough.
● Install a dimmer switch or nightlight, so you can check on your baby while she's asleep without disturbing her.
● A baby monitor is useful to have in your baby's room, unless you live in a small apartment. The type that can be plugged in wherever you are is the most flexible (see below).

Follow exactly the instructions on what size mattress to buy. It must fit snugly all round, so your baby can't get her face or head trapped

The mattress base should be at least 60cm (2ft) from the top edge of the crib, so your baby cannot climb out. You should be able to lower the base

Your baby will be sleeping in a crib from around three months to around three years, so it's worth investing in a sturdy, well-made one. Safety is paramount; choose a crib that conforms to Health Canada safety standards

Baby monitors

A baby monitor allows you to sit anywhere in the house and know your baby isn't crying. Many monitors come with additional features such as an integrated nightlight and even motion sensors. There is no proof that using a baby monitor that measures movement or breathing reduces the risk of SIDS. In fact, they can increase anxiety in families and result in less sleep for both babies and parents due to false alarms.

Always make sure that the equipment conforms to Canadian safety standards.

Daytime and nighttime sleep

Your newborn baby will sleep as much as she needs to; the only trouble is she may not take her sleep when you would like her to. In the early days, she will sleep in short bursts randomly throughout the day and night. The chart below shows how her sleep pattern might develop. As the months pass, her longest period of sleep aligns itself with the hours of night, and her wakeful times become longer. However, babies vary. Don't worry if yours takes longer than you expected to sleep through the night.

Emphasizing day and night

Right from the newborn stage, make a clear distinction between how you treat daytime and nighttime sleep to help your baby learn which time is for play and which for sleep. During the day, put her to sleep in a cradle, carriage, or Moses basket; if you're using a crib already, save it for nighttime only. A carriage can go outside with you, in a shady spot, always covered with an insect net, and with the brakes on. When indoors, make sure pets can't get into the room where your baby is, but there is no need to keep the house especially quiet for her. When your baby cries, pick her up, and make the most of her waking time: help her to associate the daylight hours with play and wakefulness.

At night, cover your baby lightly or use a sleeping bag, and put her to sleep in her crib, if you're already using one. Keep the room dark. When she wakes and cries for a feed, pick her up and feed her quietly, talking as little as possible, and changing her diaper only if she's very wet or dirty. She will gradually learn that nighttime feeds are business only, not social times, and her sleep pattern will become more like yours as the weeks go by.

Your toddler's naps

From the age of about six months, bedtime becomes a more and more important ritual in your baby's day, and she needs to be tired and ready for bed if she is to sleep through the night. She needs some daytime sleep to give her energy for her active life, and will go on needing it throughout toddlerhood, but don't let her nap for too long. Give her two hours for each nap (she may wake earlier), then wake her. She may be grumpy and confused if she was deeply asleep, so give her plenty of time before introducing the next activity.

Q&A

"My 13-month-old baby wakes up at 6am, and won't go to sleep again. Is there anything we can do?"

Early-morning waking probably just means your baby has had enough sleep. Leave a few toys in her crib each night to occupy her when she wakes. When she calls out for you, changing her diaper and offering some new toys in her crib may gain you an extra hour's sleep.

If early waking is a regular pattern, adjust the baby's sleep times through the day so she has a later bedtime. You could try putting thick curtains up in her bedroom, so the sun won't wake her up too early in the morning. Don't worry, when she's older she will probably wake up later.

How much will my baby sleep?

Age of baby	Nighttime							Daytime													Nighttime			Key
	1	2	3	4	5	6	7	8	9	10	11	12	1	2	3	4	5	6	7	8	9	10	11	12	
4 weeks																									
3 months																									Nighttime sleep
6 months																									
12 months																									
18 months																									
2 years																									Daytime sleep
3 years																									

Getting the temperature right

The risk of crib death is increased when a baby is overwrapped or overheated, especially if she is feverish or unwell. And yet it is important not to let your baby become chilled. The ideal room temperature should be between 18 and 20°C (65–68°F) – a comfortable temperature for a lightly clothed adult. If the room is at this temperature, a baby who is wearing a sleepsuit and an undershirt should not need more than one or two lightweight blankets to cover her. To prevent restricted chest expansion, wrap your baby from the waist down. Wrapping a baby snugly in a blanket stops her limbs jerking, and often helps her settle more easily. Whatever method you use, make sure your baby doesn't get too hot or cold. Don't add extra bedding if your baby is unwell, and don't expose her to direct heat from a hot water bottle, electric blanket, or heater.

Sleeptime safety

- The safest place for your baby to sleep is in a crib close to your bed.
- Never let your baby sleep with a duvet or a pillow until she is at least two years old.
- Put your baby to sleep on her back. Doctors now know this is the safest position. Babies who sleep on their front run an increased risk of crib death (SIDS).
- Use a firm mattress with a fitted sheet.
- Don't let your baby get too hot or too cold.
- Don't smoke; and keep your baby in a smoke-free atmosphere.
- Never hang toys over the crib within easy reach of your baby.

Crib death Each year, a few babies die unexpectedly in their cribs. There is no explanation for crib death, or Sudden Infant Death Syndrome (SIDS), but doctors have suggested some safety precautions (see left) that can help to minimize the risk of crib death occurring. If you always put your baby to sleep on her back, make sure that she is not exposed to cigarette smoke, and be careful to see that she does not become overheated – you can greatly reduce the risk of crib death.

If you think your baby is unwell, consult your doctor immediately.

Putting your baby in the "feet-to-foot" position

Place your baby's feet at the foot of the crib, so that she cannot wriggle her way under the covers, and tuck in the covers securely so they reach no higher than her shoulders and cannot ride up and cover her head. Babies whose heads are accidentally covered with bedding get too hot and run a greater risk of crib death.

Lay your baby *with her feet at the foot of the crib*

Drop-side cribs
It is possible that drop-side cribs will be banned in Canada because of multiple reports of infants suffocating or being injured when the drop side becomes detached. Cribs with sides that have movable upper sections would still be allowed.

Temperature regulation
Babies regulate their body temperature by losing heat from their face and head. If a baby slips beneath the bedclothes so that her face and head are covered, heat can't be lost as easily. Make sure the bedding is arranged so that this can't happen. Unless the room is very cold, babies should not wear hats indoors for sleeping.

Settling for sleep

There will be times when your baby won't settle down to sleep after a feed. Gentle rocking or a quiet period in your arms may help to relax him and send him off to sleep. Make sure you keep the following soothing methods for times when he is really irritable, so he does not develop incorrect sleep associations and become too dependent on them.

Sucking
Your baby will be soothed by sucking, either at the breast or on your clean little finger. He may suck his own fist. If you don't mind him having a pacifier, use a natural-shaped one.

Soothing contact
Rubbing your baby's back rhythmically may soothe him enough to send him to sleep. Don't alter the rhythm or you will disturb him, and don't stop until his eyelids have closed.

An infant carrier
If your baby wakes every time you put him down, try carrying him around in a carrier: the motion of your body will keep him asleep (see page 85).

Ensure there is adequate support for his head

Gentle rocking soothes your baby

Rocking
Rock your baby to and fro in your arms to lull him to sleep. You may have to keep it up for some time, and he may wake every time you stop to put him in his crib, but it's still a tried and tested way to send him to sleep.

Your older baby's bedtime routine

From about six months, your baby will settle down to sleep more happily if the whole process of going to bed takes place in exactly the same way every day – babies love routine and rituals. From now on, he won't be quite so ready to go to sleep in strange surroundings, and his sleep patterns will be easily upset by a change in daily life, so try to impose the normal routine even if you're away from home.

What time is bedtime?
It's up to you and your partner to choose a time that fits in with your own routine, and one that you can stick to more or less every day. Make sure it's late enough that you're both home, and not so late that the routine takes up all your evening. Any time between 6pm and 8pm is perhaps the most suitable.

The bedtime routine
1 Start the routine in the same way every evening. A bath is ideal, because it's both fun and relaxing. If he doesn't like being bathed, 20 minutes spent playing a gentle game together might help him unwind.

2 If your baby still has a bedtime feeding, give it to him in his room, so he understands this to be a friendly, familiar place, not somewhere he is banished to at night while family life continues elsewhere.

3 Put your baby into his crib. If he is over one year old, you can give him a favourite teddy or a soft toy.

4 Now perhaps your partner could take over, so that you're both involved in the bedtime routine. This last half hour or so should always be the same, to mark it as the end of the day. You may want to sing a lullaby to help your baby drop off.

A car ride
If you get desperate, you can always try putting your baby in his car seat and going for a short drive round the block: the motion will probably put him to sleep automatically. When you return home again, leave him undisturbed in his car seat, and carry both indoors. Cover him with a blanket to keep him warm. Many parents find that this is an effective way to soothe an irritable but otherwise tired baby.

Other methods
Lullabies are an age-old method of soothing your baby to sleep. Your baby won't mind if you can't sing in tune, as long as you rock him to and fro. Playing music softly in his room may also help your baby to drop off to sleep. For difficult sleepers, a soother CD of the rhythmic swishing sounds he would have heard in the womb may work.

Sleeping bag
A sleeping bag will keep your baby comfortably warm all night. It is more practical than a blanket or quilt, and can make your night easier, too. Sleep sacks also reduce the risk of SIDS (see page 123) and suffocation. Your baby will soon learn to associate sleep with being put in his bag. Choose one without a hood, and make sure it is the right size around the neck so your baby won't slip down inside it. Sleeping bags come in different weights appropriate to the season – heavier for winter and lighter for summer. You can also adjust the amount of clothing you baby wears underneath the sleeping bag.

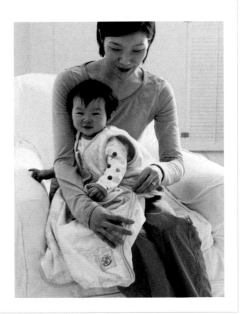

Rhythmic movements
Pushing your baby to and fro in his carriage or stroller will often soothe him to sleep, although he may keep trying to look at you. If this doesn't work, you can try taking your baby out in his carriage for a walk in the open air. Make sure he is adequately dressed and covered for the weather. Use this soothing method only when your baby is particularly unsettled.

5 Read a story with your baby to relax him and help him wind down. Don't give up if you think he isn't paying attention: he will be tired, and won't respond to the pictures with his usual lively interest, but that doesn't mean he isn't listening or learning for that matter.

6 Tuck your baby up, making sure that his feet are at the foot of the crib if he is under one year old. Turn the light down, or switch a nightlight on. Spend a moment or two lingering in the room before you go, so that he is still aware of your presence, as he drops off to sleep.

Sharing a bed with your baby

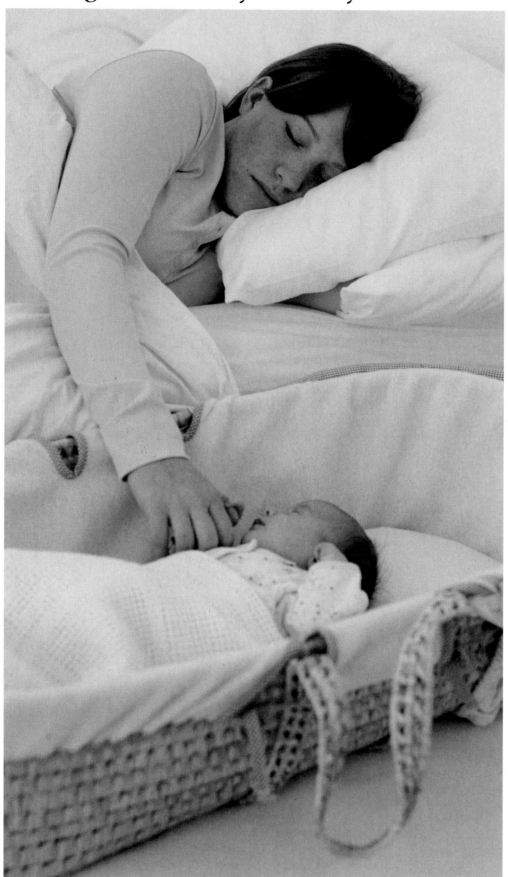

For the first six months, the safest place for your baby to sleep – night and day – is in an approved bassinet or crib in a room with you. But if your baby won't settle, it is very tempting to bring him into your bed. Snuggled close to you, he will fall asleep more easily. In fact, this is the most common sleeping arrangement among many cultures around the world. Bed-sharing has been shown to encourage and sustain breastfeeding. However, bed-sharing can increase the risk of crib death unless you take proper safety precautions. It may also become a habit that is difficult to break when it is time to move your baby to his own crib.

Co-sleeping safely

- Don't sleep with your baby if you or your partner smoke, drink, or take drugs or medication that make you drowsy.
- Don't place your bed directly against furniture or a wall. Your baby could become trapped between the bed and the wall.
- Be careful your baby doesn't get too hot. Your own body heat will keep him warm, so he will only need light coverings.
- Never co-sleep in an unsafe environment such as on a couch or waterbed.
- Co-sleeping products are not recommended.

Overcoming sleeping problems

Establishing a routine

By three or four months, most babies start to sleep 15 hours a day (10 hours at night, and the remainder divided among three daytime naps). You may still be getting up once or twice a night for feeds at the beginning of this stage, but by the time your baby is six months old, she'll be physically capable of sleeping through the night. Whether she actually will depends on whether she's learning sleep habits and patterns that will encourage this. She will still need about 14 hours of sleep a day, and may sleep for as long as seven hours at a stretch, with two one-and-a-half to two hour naps a day. She no longer needs a feed during the night. By nine months to a year, your baby will probably be sleeping for about 10–12 hours at night, and napping twice a day for an hour and a half to two hours at a time.

You can prevent a lot of future sleeping problems if you try to establish a consistent bedtime routine as early as possible (see page 124–5). The goal is to develop appropriate sleep associations so that she is able to soothe herself back to sleep during the night. From the time your baby is three months old try to:
● keep bedtime and nap times as regular as you can
● put her down to sleep at night before she nods off, so that she doesn't become dependent on you to fall asleep
● help her to learn how to settle and soothe herself – by sucking her thumb, or cuddling a favourite blanket or toy, which is always put in her crib with her (only after she is 1 year old). Most babies discover such a "comfort object" for themselves, and it works wonders, but once the favourite is established, make sure that you always have a duplicate handy for the inevitable night when it can't be found at bedtime
● give her a massage between bath and bedtime. This should make her feel relaxed and prepare her for sleep.

Night waking

Lots of babies, especially newborns, are night owls. During the day, they sleep, wake to feed, then after a little while, go happily back to sleep. At night, however, they seem much more unsettled, stay awake for longer, and often cry much more. Things usually get better when your baby is a few weeks old, but if they don't you can try to reset her biological clock by helping her differentiate the night from the day.
● Try to wake her at the same time each morning, however tempting it is to let her sleep longer, so you get some rest for a few more minutes.
● Try waking her when she has slept for about four hours during the day, and even if she doesn't seem to want to feed, play with her and talk to her. When she wakes at night, keep the lights dim and be as quiet and soothing as possible.
● Don't panic and change her bedtime routine. Night waking is usually a temporary issue, and resolves itself in most cases.

Daytime sleep
During the day, don't close her curtains when you put her to sleep and don't try to keep the house unnaturally quiet.

Unsettled babies

How do you deal with a baby who either refuses to go to sleep, or who wakes and won't settle easily during the night? This depends on the baby's age. A newborn needs cuddling, while a toddler needs a consistent routine. If by the time your baby is six months she is still waking frequently, or refusing to settle to sleep, there are two basic approaches you can use (see below) – try them both, and see which works best for you and your baby. If all else fails, and you resort (as many parents do) to bringing your baby into bed with you, remember that this does increase the risk of crib death (see page 123). She will still have to learn new sleep associations when it is time to move back into her crib.

1. The checking routine
If your child is crying, go back into her room. Pat her on the back, and tell her that everything is OK, but that it is time to go to sleep. Don't pick her up or cuddle her; be gentle but firm. Leave. Wait about five minutes, then check again. Do this repeatedly until she falls asleep, extending the time between each visit, but never leave her crying for more than 15 minutes without going back in to reassure her.

2. The flexible routine
Don't let your baby cry it out. Instead, try to see if there's any obvious cause. Comfort her to sleep; rock her or lie down with her until she drops off. You can buy CDs of special sleep-inducing baby music, or sing special songs to her as part of her bedtime ritual.

By six months, she may be starting to suffer from separation anxiety, misses you, and needs to know you are still around. Giving her more daytime contact with you may help – for example, by breastfeeding, playing with her, carrying her in a sling. Or, as she becomes more physically active, she may simply be overtired. Try putting her to bed a half an hour or so earlier than her usual bedtime.

Clothes and dressing

In the early weeks, your baby may need clean clothes as often as she needs a clean diaper. But once she turns into an active toddler, she will need far fewer items of clothing – she will outgrow them long before they are outworn. Choose clothes that are machine-washable, comfortable and unrestricting, with easy-to-manage fastenings and elasticized waistbands to help her learn to dress and undress herself. She shouldn't have to worry about her clothes, and nor should you.

Buying clothes for your baby

Clothes for a young baby should be easy to put on, and if possible made from natural fibres, which allow your baby to regulate her own temperature as well as she can. Don't use harsh detergents or fabric conditioners to wash your baby's clothes, as they may irritate her skin. The basic item of clothing now and throughout the first six months is the all-in-one sleeper.

Sleeper

Undershirt with snaps

Envelope neck

Undershirt

Mittens

Hat
On a cold day, your baby needs a hat to stop him losing heat through his head. In hot weather, he needs a sun hat for protection.

Sweater
Avoid mohair or fluffy wool and any knit with large holes that could catch fingers.

Clothes with snaps
Look for clothes with snaps up the front and around the crotch – these will be easy to put on over diapers, which can be bulky. Envelope necks make it easy to put clothes over your baby's head.

Socks
These should be soft and roomy, so that toes are not restricted.

Clothing basics

For babies of any age, clothing should be easy to put on and take off and should allow plenty of room for movement. Practical, easy-to-wash fabrics are essential as clothes will become dirty quickly.

Basic items for your new baby

Start with the following (size determined by weight), then add other items as needed. Buy extras, or you will be washing all the time. You need:
- eight sleepers, minimum
- six undershirts
- two sweaters
- two nighties
- two pairs of socks
- fabric booties
- tie-on mittens
- sun hat or warm hat
- outdoor clothes (winter).

Denim jeans *look good and are hardwearing*

Rolled-up pants

Larger pants can be rolled up when your baby is small and rolled down as she grows.

Snaps *at the crotch make diaper changing easier*

Sleepers

This perennially popular style is practical and hardwearing for when your baby starts to crawl.

Cotton *is breathable*

Cuffs and sleeves *should not restrict movement*

Dresses

Most dresses for baby girls come with matching underwear to go underneath. Tights keep a baby's legs warm.

Easy-care fabric *is important*

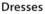

Elasticized fabric booties

These are useful in cold weather before she is walking; they must be very roomy inside.

Outdoor clothes

Your baby should be adequately dressed in colder weather as she loses heat easily.

How to dress your baby

Dressing and undressing your baby is a lovely opportunity to let him learn about his own body as you stroke and caress his soft skin. He may hate being dressed, but you can make it pleasurable with lots of nuzzling, cuddles, kisses, and chat; be especially gentle, too. Gather up the clothes you need, and undo all the snaps. Lay your baby on his changing mat.

Putting on an undershirt

1 Hold the undershirt with the front facing you, and gather it up. Put the back edge at your baby's crown.

Position the back edge at the top of his head

2 With one swift, gentle movement, bring the front edge of the undershirt down to your baby's chin. Hold the fabric gathered up together, and stretch it as wide as you can, so that none of it drags on his face.

3 Gently lift your baby's head and upper body, and pull the back of the undershirt down so it is round his neck and lying behind his shoulders. Lower him to the mat without jolting or letting his head flop.

4 If your baby's undershirt has sleeves, put the fingers of one hand down through the first sleeve, and stretch it wide, then with the other hand, guide his fist into your fingers.

5 Hold your baby's hand with your first hand, and ease the sleeve over his arm with the other. Pull the undershirt down below his arm. Do the same with the other sleeve, pulling the undershirt, not your baby.

6 Pull the shirt over his stomach. Lift his lower body by his ankles, and pull the back down. Do up the snaps at the crotch.

Lay the sleeper out flat

Putting on a sleeper

1 Pick your baby up while you lay the clean sleeper out flat on the changing mat, the front upward, and all the snaps undone. Lay your baby on top, his neck in line with the sleeper's neck opening.

An undershirt *underneath the sleeper is usually necessary in anything but the hottest weather*

Pull the suit, *not your baby*

Guide your baby's fist *into the sleeve*

2 Gather up the fabric of one sleeper leg into your hands, to open out the foot part. Ease your baby's foot in, getting his toes right into the toe of the suit, and pull the leg of the suit up. Do the same with his other foot.

3 Push the thumb and fingers of one hand up through one sleeve from the wrist end, gathering up the fabric of the sleeve over your hand. Stretch the opening as wide as you can. With your other hand, guide your baby's fist into your first hand.

Check that *his toes are not cramped*

4 Holding your baby's hand between your thumb and fingers, ease the sleeve over your hand and up his arm, drawing it up to his shoulder. This way your baby's fingers and nails can't get caught.

5 If the sleeper is on the large side, turn back the cuffs, so he can explore with his hands, and learn about his body.

6 Fasten all the snaps, starting with the ones around his thighs and crotch, and working up to his neck.

Undressing your baby

Lay your baby on his changing mat. Your baby may be unnerved by the feel of cold air against his skin as you undress him, so nuzzle his bare stomach, and make the most of this opportunity for skin-to-skin contact. Have a towel on hand to wrap your baby in when you've undressed him, or dress him again quickly.

Taking off a sleeper

1 Undo the sleeper snaps. Hold one ankle inside the suit, and pull the suit leg off. Do the same with the other.

Hold his ankle *while you pull the leg of the suit off*

2 Undo the snaps on his undershirt, then lift his lower body by his ankles, and slide the undershirt and sleeper up underneath him as far as you can.

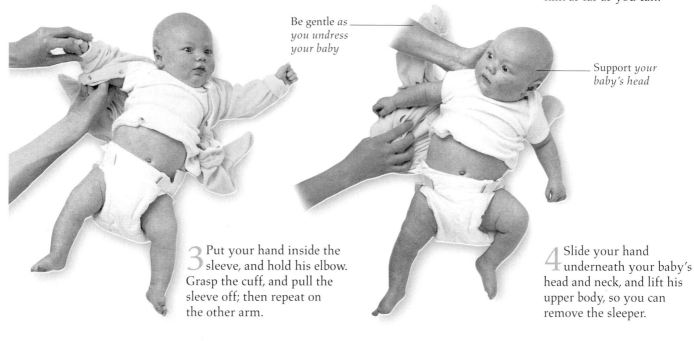

Be gentle *as you undress your baby*

Support *your baby's head*

3 Put your hand inside the sleeve, and hold his elbow. Grasp the cuff, and pull the sleeve off; then repeat on the other arm.

4 Slide your hand underneath your baby's head and neck, and lift his upper body, so you can remove the sleeper.

Taking off an undershirt

1 Hold his elbow inside the undershirt with one hand, bunch up the undershirt, and ease all the fabric over his fist. Do the same on the other side.

2 Gather up all the undershirt in your hands, so there is no spare fabric that might drag over your baby's face as you take it off.

3 Stretch the opening as wide as you can, then with one swift movement take it up and over your baby's face to his crown.

4 Slide your hand underneath your baby's head and neck, and lift his upper body, so you can slide out the undershirt.

How your child learns to dress himself

By about two years of age, your child will probably manage to pull off his own socks or T-shirt, and the majority of children will begin to dress themselves by the age of about three. You can encourage this new independence by buying clothes that are easy for your child to manage, and by letting him dress and undress himself as much as he can.

Ways to help

● Allow plenty of time – if you're not in a rush, you won't get too irritated by his slowness.
● Lay out his clothes in the order he needs to put them on.
● Buy pants or skirts with elasticized waistbands. Always avoid zip flies for a pre-school boy in case he gets any part of his penis caught.
● Look for clothes with large buttons, snaps, or Velcro fastenings.
● Teach him to start doing buttons up from the bottom upward.
● Let him choose his "favourite" foot, then mark his shoe, so he can get it on the correct foot.
● Avoid jackets with difficult zippers.
● When you have to help, make a game of getting dressed, playing "peek-a-boo" as you pop garments over his head.
● Once he's dressed, let him stay dressed, even if he gets dirty.

Choosing shoes

Bare feet are best for babies who are learning to walk. They make it easier to balance, and walking barefoot makes for healthy feet. Once your child is ready to walk outdoors, he will need shoes, but even then let him go barefoot as much as possible. Shoes are necessary only to protect feet, not to "support" them – the muscles give all the support the foot needs. Buy shoes from a store where they will measure the length and the width of the foot. Have the fit checked every three months. Buy new socks at the same time as new shoes: too small socks can be just as deforming as too small shoes.

What sort of shoes should I buy?

Any leather or canvas shoe is suitable, provided your child's feet have been properly measured so that the shoes fit in length and width. In practice, you may find that cheaper shoes, such as canvas sneakers, aren't available in half sizes and different width fittings. Rubber boots aren't usually available in half sizes, but they're still essential for wet weather walks. Buy them on the large side, and fit an insole.

Avoid all plastic shoes: plastic doesn't mould itself to the shape of your child's foot like leather or canvas. Only use second-hand shoes if the fit has been properly checked.

What to look for in your child's shoes

The space between *your child's big toe and the end of the shoe should be 0.5–1.25cm (¼–½in)*

Wide toes *are important to give your child's toes room to splay out inside*

T-bar with buckle

Open-toed sandal

The fastening *should hold your child's foot snugly: buckles or Velcro are easiest for your child to manage*

The seams *must be smoothly finished, so nothing can rub your child's skin*

Undressing himself
Your two year old will enjoy the challenge of undressing himself, given lots of time.

Bathing and washing your baby

A large part of taking care of your new baby day-to-day will be keeping her clean. A newborn baby's skin is delicate and easily irritated by sweating, urinating, or dribbling. As your baby grows and starts to feed herself and explore the world around her, she will generally get more dirty, too. Sponge bathing is quite enough to keep her clean, but most babies love being bathed, and bathtime will quickly become an important part of your daily routine together.

Equipment for bathing and washing

There are plenty of products available designed to make bathtime easier for you, but make sure that you only buy products intended for use on babies.

Adult shampoos, soaps, lotions, and creams contain too many additives and chemicals to be safe for your baby's delicate skin.

Equipment for bathing

Baby bath
Until your baby is ready to go into an adult bath (between three and six months), a proper baby bath will make bathtime easy for you. Place it at a convenient height on a worktop, or put it on the floor. If you buy a special bath stand, make sure it puts the bath at the right height for you.

Small bowl of clean warm water   **Cotton balls**

You will need clean warm water and plenty of cotton balls to wash your baby's eyes, ears, and face.

Waterproof apron
A cotton fabric with waterproof backing will feel softer to your baby than PVC.

A rubber bath mat *stops your baby from slipping down*

Rubber bath mat
Once your baby moves into the big bath, a suctioned rubber bath mat is essential to stop her from sliding on the bottom of the tub.

Baby toiletries

Bath liquid   **Lotion**   **Oil**   **Moisturizer**   **Shampoo**   **Soap**   **Cotton swabs**

Baby bath liquid makes an excellent alternative to both soap and shampoo. **Baby lotion** is useful for cleaning your baby's diaper area if his skin is very dry. **Baby oil** moisturizes your baby's skin when it is dry or scaly.
Baby moisturizer can be used instead of baby oil.
Baby shampoo may be needed once a week.
Baby soap need only be used if you don't use bath liquid.

With a young baby, place her on your lap, and soap her all over, then rinse the soap off in the baby bath. Remember to hold her firmly. Use soap sparingly and rinse it off thoroughly – for the first few weeks water alone is quite enough to keep your baby clean.
Cotton swabs are useful for cleaning between your baby's fingers and toes and behind his ears, but never push them into his ears, nose, eyes, or bottom.

Hair and nails

Hairbrush This should have soft bristles, and be small enough for your child to brush his own hair from about 18 months.

Baby nail scissors These have rounded ends and short blades, so there's no danger of hurting your baby by accidentally jabbing her.

Baby hairbrush

Nail scissors

Towel

Keep a large, very soft towel for your baby's use only. Warm it on a radiator if you have one. Some towels have a corner piece that makes a hood.

Washcloth   **Natural sponge**

Keep a new washcloth or sponge for your baby's use only, and wash the washcloth regularly. Don't let an older baby put the sponge into her mouth.

Tips for washing your young baby

● Until your baby is six months old, always use a bowl of clean warm water to wash her eyes, ears, mouth, and face.

● Only clean the parts you can see; do not try to clean right inside your baby's nose or ears, just wipe away any visible mucus or wax with a damp cotton ball. Otherwise you may push the dirt back up into the nose or ear.

● With a baby girl, never try to separate her vaginal lips to clean inside them. You will hinder the natural flow of mucus that washes bacteria out. Be very gentle.

● With a baby boy, never try to push back his foreskin to clean under it: you may hurt him, or tear or damage the foreskin.

● Always wipe from front to back when you are cleaning a baby girl's diaper area. This prevents germs from spreading from the anus into the vagina and causing infection.

● When wiping your baby's eyes and ears, use a fresh cotton ball for each one, or you may spread infections.

● Always leave cleaning your baby's bottom until last, and use a fresh cotton ball for each wipe. Dip the cotton ball in warm tap water.

Sponge bathing a young baby

Sponge bathing simply means cleaning only the parts of your baby that really need cleaning – her hands, face, neck, and diaper area – without undressing her completely. Sponge bathe your baby as part of your morning or bedtime routine – it's an excellent alternative to a bath, particularly during the first six weeks when your baby may not feel very comfortable about bathing in the baby bath. Make sure the room is warm and that you have all the supplies that you need. Wash your hands. Pour some clean warm water into a small bowl and check the temperature. Lay your baby on her changing mat and undress her down to her undershirt.

You will need

- Warm room
- Baby changing mat
- Bowl of warm tap water
- Cotton balls
- Tissues
- Warm towel
- Clean diaper
- Clean clothes

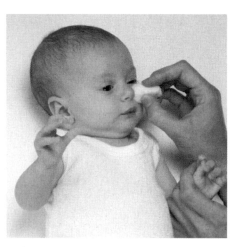

1 Wipe each eye from the nose outward with a cotton ball dipped in the warm water. Use a fresh piece for each wipe, and for each eye. Dry gently with a tissue.

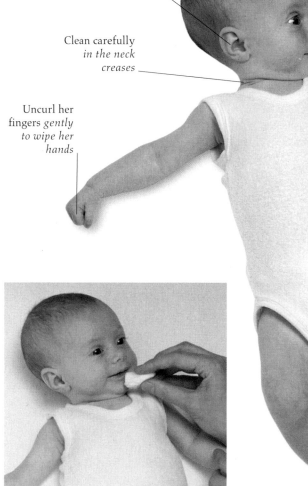

Never poke *a cotton swab into your baby's ears*

Clean carefully *in the neck creases*

Uncurl her fingers *gently to wipe her hands*

Wipe each eye *with a fresh cotton ball*

Remove all traces *of milk and dribble*

Pull up her undershirt *to clean her tummy and diaper area*

2 With a fresh moist cotton ball, wipe each ear. Don't try to wipe inside: just wipe over and behind it. Use a fresh piece for each ear, and dry with the towel. Wipe away dirt behind her ears.

3 Clean your baby's face of milk and dribble by wiping around her mouth and nose, then wipe over her cheeks and forehead. Dry with the towel.

4 Wipe under her chin and in her neck creases with a fresh moist cotton ball, as sweat here can irritate her skin. Dry well.

5 Wipe under her arms with a fresh moist cotton ball, gently pulling her arms up to flatten out the creases. Clean between her fingers. Dry well.

Cleaning your baby's cord stump

The shrivelled-up stump of your baby's umbilical cord will probably have dropped off by the time she is just over a week old. Careful cleaning makes sure infection cannot set in, and helps the cord separate.

Once the stump of cord has dropped off, you will need to clean the navel daily until it is fully healed.

Consult your doctor as soon as possible if the navel looks red, swollen, inflamed, or pus starts to weep at the base of the stump. A small amount of bleeding is normal, and usually nothing to worry about.

Clean the *stump with a cotton ball*

It is essential to wash your hands before you start. Gently clean the cord stump with cotton balls and clean water. If it is soiled use soapy water. Dry thoroughly and leave it exposed to the air as much as possible. Fold the front of your baby's diaper down so it is clear of the cord and avoid getting any urine on it.

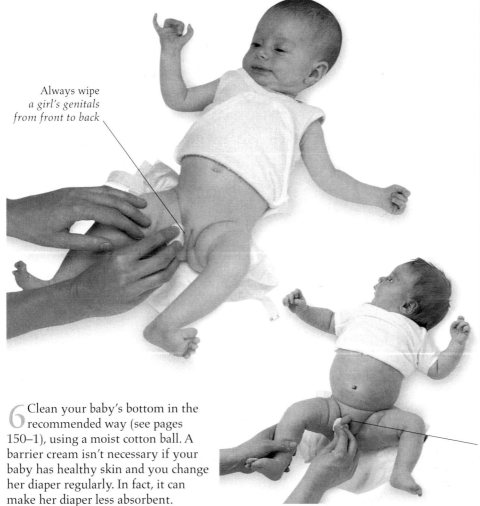

Always wipe a girl's genitals from front to back

6 Clean your baby's bottom in the recommended way (see pages 150–1), using a moist cotton ball. A barrier cream isn't necessary if your baby has healthy skin and you change her diaper regularly. In fact, it can make her diaper less absorbent.

Never pull back a boy's foreskin

Bathing your young baby

Most babies come to love the sensation of being bathed, but a new baby often dislikes the feeling of being "unwrapped," and you may feel nervous about holding your baby's small, slippery body. In the first weeks, you can simply sponge bathe your baby to keep her clean, but practise with a full bath once a week, and a hair wash every two weeks. Make sure the room is warm. You can kneel, sit, or stand to bathe her, but make sure your back doesn't start to ache.

You will need

- Baby bath
- Changing mat
- Your baby's bath towel
- Hairwashing towel
- Waterproof apron
- Bowl of clean warm water to wash her face
- Cotton balls and washcloth
- Baby bath liquid (optional)
- Clean diaper
- Baby oil (optional)
- Clean clothes

Getting ready for the bath

1 Test the water temperature with your elbow: it should feel just warm, and be 10cm (4in) deep. Add bath liquid, if used.

2 Lay the bath towel on the changing mat, place your baby on it, and undress her down to her diaper.

3 Wrap her up snugly in a towel and wipe her eyes and face with a cotton ball dipped in the bowl of clean water.

Cleaning her bottom
Lay her on her mat. Take off her diaper, and clean her bottom, wiping from front to back to prevent germs from the anus entering the vagina (see pages 150–1).

Washing your young baby's hair
Cradle her head in one hand, her back along your forearm, and tuck her legs under your elbow. Gently pour water from the bath over her head with a cupped hand. With most brands of bath liquid, you don't need to rinse her hair in fresh water. Bring your baby on to your lap to pat her head dry with a second towel.

Q&A

"My four-week-old baby has crusty patches on his scalp. What can I do about them?"
This is a harmless form of dandruff known as cradle cap. Rub your baby's scalp with baby oil, and leave overnight. Then wash the crusts off, and gently brush the scalp with a soft brush. If the cradle cap doesn't improve, ask your doctor or nurse practitioner for advice.

Putting your baby in the bath

1 Unwrap the towel while she is on your lap. Support her head and neck on your forearm, your hand holding her firmly around her far shoulder and upper arm. Put your other hand under her bottom and thighs and lower her in.

One wrist supports her head, the other her thigh

2 Smile and talk to your baby all the time as you use your free hand to splash water gently over her body. Take it very slowly if she doesn't seem relaxed.

Hold her far shoulder all the time

Lifting her out and drying her

1 Two or three minutes in the water is enough for a very young baby. Lift her out of the water by sliding your free hand under her bottom: she will be slippery, so hold her firmly.

Support her head so it can't flop

2 Wrap her in the towel on your lap, and cuddle her dry. Put her on her mat, and dry all her skin creases. Put on a clean diaper.

Bathing in the big bath

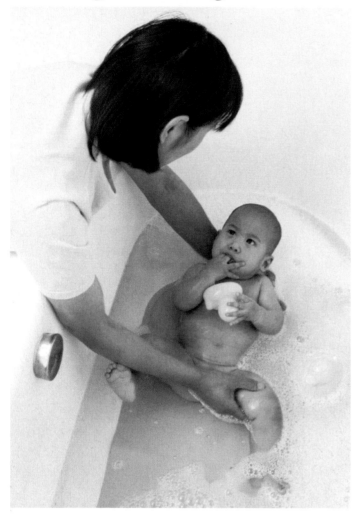

Your baby will probably be ready for the big bath at the age of six to seven months – and some babies are ready for the experience even earlier. If your baby hasn't yet learnt to enjoy bathtime, give him a few more weeks of being bathed in his baby bath, until he really is too big for it or is more confident. To bathe your six-month-old baby, arrange everything you will need beside the bath. Make sure the room is warm. Put your baby on his changing mat to wash his face, eyes, and ears, using clean warm water. Then undress him carefully, and clean his bottom thoroughly before placing him gently in the bath.

Washing your baby

1 Put the rubber mat on the floor of the bath and run in cold water, then hot, so that the water is just warm. Lay your baby on the rubber mat. Keep his head and shoulders supported on your arm, his ears clear of the water.

2 If you are using soap, roll the bar in your free hand then run your hand over his body. If you've put bath liquid in the water, just splash the water over him.

3 Rinse the soap off by splashing water gently over him. It may not be necessary to rinse off the bath liquid. Make sure to support his head when you lift him out. Take care, he will be slippery.

You will need

- Rubber bath mat
- Waterproof apron
- Baby bath liquid, or baby soap, and baby shampoo (shampoo not needed every time)
- Large soft towel
- Baby's own sponge or facecloth
- Cotton balls or a soft facecloth for washing your baby's face
- Clean diaper
- Pouring and other toys for an older baby
- Toothbrush for an older child
- Clean clothes

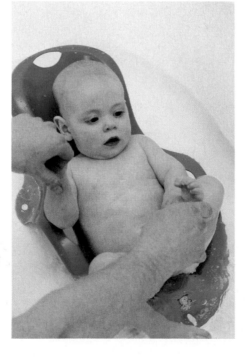

Bath seat

Once your baby can sit up by himself, you can put a bathtub seat or bath ring into the bath to make him more stable and leave your hands free. Choose one with strong suction cups to help keep the seat in place, and put it well out of reach of the taps. Remember though that this doesn't mean that you can leave him alone in the tub even for a minute. He can still wriggle himself off the seat and slide into the water.

Drying your baby

Wrap him in his towel and cuddle him dry. Make sure that you dry him thoroughly, especially in the creases under his armpits, at the top of his thighs, and around the neck region. The area between the fingers and toes also need careful attention.

Making bathtime fun

Once your baby can sit steadily, bathtime becomes a wonderful playtime – not just a way of getting him clean. Search out some bath toys: things that pour, such as plastic jugs and funnels, sandcastle buckets with holes, even plastic colanders, will fascinate him, and floating toys, such as boats or ducks, are ideal, too. About once a week, use a pouring toy to wash your baby's hair, but don't let water run over his face – he will probably hate it.

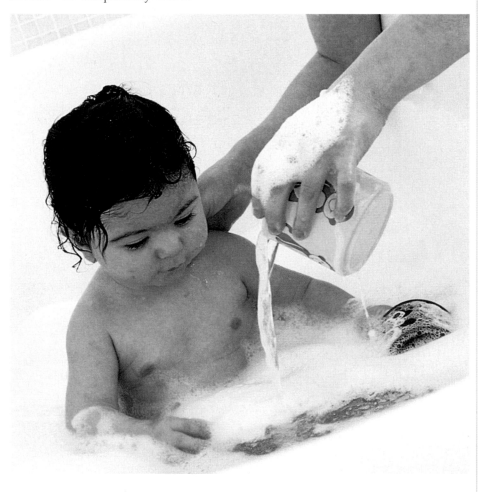

Washing your baby's hair

It is only necessary to wash your baby's hair about once a week. Wet the hair first. If using a baby shampoo, slide your supporting hand forwards and pour a small amount into the palm.

Support your baby's head with your free hand. Rub shampoo gently over his hair. Be careful not to get shampoo in his eyes. If you have bath liquid in the water, just wash the water over his hair.

Swap hands again and rinse the shampoo off with a wet, well-squeezed-out sponge or washcloth. You may want to turn this into a game to make it more enjoyable for him.

Applying shampoo
Use the tiniest drop of baby shampoo – apply it to your baby's wet hair and lather gently.

Using a sponge
Rinsing with a sponge or facecloth can prevent shampoo and water from running down his face.

Bathtime safety tips

● Never leave a baby or small child alone in the bath or move out of easy reach, even for a second. It takes no time for a child to slip and drown, even in very shallow water.
● Always test the water temperature with a sensitive part of your body.
● Even when your baby can sit steadily, keep a hand ready to support him if he slips.
● Never top up with hot water while your child is in the bath. If any topping up is necessary, mix hot and cold water in a jug so it's just warm, then pour it in.
● A rubber mat in the bottom of the bath is essential.
● Never let your child pull himself to standing in the bath even when he can stand steadily.
● Make sure the thermostat on your water heater is not too high.
● If the tap gets hot, tie a facecloth around it so your child can't burn himself on it.
● If you bathe with your baby, have the water cooler than you would usually have it.

Babies who hate water and washing

Bathing

Some babies are frightened by bathtime – and often a baby or toddler may suddenly take a dislike to bathing. If this happens, give up baths altogether for a short time: daily sponge bathing will keep a small baby clean, although a mobile baby will need an all-over sponge bath on your lap (see below). After two or three weeks, try having a bath with your baby to help him overcome his fear of the water. If your baby is particularly anxious, being held close to you will be comforting for him. Introduce some toys to make the experience fun for your baby. You can also use a jug to pour water over him, which can help to stop water going into his eyes.

Hairwashing

Babies and young children often particularly dislike having their hair washed, even if they love bathtime. If your child doesn't like having his hair washed, abandon it for a couple of weeks. Respect his dislike, but help him to be more reasonable about it: for example, go out together in the rain and show him how pleasurable raindrops feel on his face.

Reintroduce hairwashing at bathtime gradually. It may help to give him a facecloth to hold over his eyes and face: often it's the feel of water on their faces that children dislike most. If your child will wear one, you could try putting a plastic "halo" round his hairline to keep the water off his face.

Handwashing

Even if your child dislikes having his hands washed, it's very important to do this before and after every meal. Make the experience more fun by washing his hands between your own wet and soapy ones.

Playing with water
Sit your baby beside a bowl of water on the kitchen floor and let him splash and play. Pouring jugs and floating toys can often persuade a child that water can be fun.

Sponging her hair
You can keep your child's hair clean by sponging out any bits of food and dirt that she may have in her hair with a damp facecloth or a sponge.

Giving your baby a sponge bath

If your baby doesn't like water, there is no need to bathe him: once he can hold his head up, a daily sponge bath on your lap is enough. First, lay him on his mat and wipe his eyes, face, and ears with clean cotton balls. Sit him on your lap and keep everything you need within reach.

Wear an apron *that covers your upper body*

You will need

- Large bowl of warm water, with a little baby bath liquid added
- Small bowl of warm water and cotton balls for your baby's face
- Waterproof apron
- Your baby's own sponge or facecloth
- Warm towel
- Clean diaper

Top half

1 Take off the top half of your baby's clothing. Wet the sponge, squeeze it out well, and wash his neck. Dry well with the towel. Remember to dry thoroughly in all the creases, because leaving excessive moisture in them can lead to skin irritation.

Put the towel *over your lap before you begin*

2 Dip the sponge in the water again, squeeze it out so it doesn't dribble, then wash all over his chest and tummy. Dry him well with the towel.

3 Hold your baby's arms up to wash and dry his underarms where sweat and fluff can accumulate. Wash and dry his forearms, then let him dip his hands in the bowl of water if he wants to. Make sure you dry them well with the towel.

Hold your baby's *arms up to flatten out his skin creases*

Hold your baby *firmly all the time: he will wriggle*

4 Lean him forwards over your arm to wash and dry his back and shoulders. He won't like water trickling down his back, so squeeze the sponge out.

Bottom half

1 Put a clean undershirt on your baby, and take off his pants and socks. Wash his feet and legs next. Gently pat him dry, particularly between his toes.

2 Finally, take off your baby's diaper and clean his tummy, genitals, and bottom in your usual way (see pages 150–1). Lay him on your lap if you feel confident, or put him on his mat. Put on a clean diaper and dress him in his nightclothes.

Caring for your child's teeth

It's never too early to start looking after your child's teeth. It is recommended that you use a toothbrush as soon as a tooth appears. However, if you are nervous about using a brush, you can wipe his teeth and gums with a wet handkerchief. As soon as you feel comfortable, introduce him to a baby-size toothbrush: clean his teeth for him (see below) after breakfast and at bedtime. Taking care of the first, or "milk," teeth helps to ensure that the permanent teeth coming through at around six years are correctly positioned and in healthy gums – and you will be establishing good, lifelong habits in your child.

The more teeth cleaning seems like a game, the more your child will co-operate. Playing dentist, cleaning your own teeth with him, and spitting out messily into the sink will all help.

Cleaning your baby's teeth

1 Wet a clean washcloth, piece of gauze, or small soft toothbrush. Sit your baby on your lap. Toothpaste is not necessary at this age. However, if you choose to use it, only apply a pea-sized helping of toothpaste that doesn't contain fluoride. At this age, babies tend to eat toothpaste rather than spit it out.

2 Rub your wrapped finger over your baby's gums and teeth. Let her spit into the sink if she wants to copy you.

Why do teeth decay?

Teeth decay because bacteria in the mouth react with sugar to form acid, which eats through the hard enamel covering the teeth. Candy and sugary foods and drinks increase the risk of tooth decay, particularly if they're eaten between meals because the teeth are bathed in sugar most of the time.

You can minimize the chance that your child will have cavities by: not allowing him to sleep with a bottle of milk or juice in his mouth (even repeated breastfeeding at night can cause a constant drip of sugar-containing fluids that decays the teeth); avoiding fruit juices for as long as possible; never sweetening his pacifier; providing healthy snacks; brushing his teeth after sweet treats.

Fluoride

Fluoride is a chemical that hardens tooth enamel. Brushing twice daily with fluoride-containing toothpaste will help protect your child's teeth from decay. Many communities have fluoride in the water supply. After six months, your baby will need extra fluoride if the water supply has less than 0.3ppm (micrograms per litre). Speak to your doctor or dentist about the need for extra fluoride.

Too much fluoride?

You needn't worry if your child swallows a little toothpaste as you brush his teeth, but he might love the taste so much that he wants to eat it from the tube. Don't let him. Too much fluoride can cause staining of the teeth, called fluorosis. This is why it is recommended that you give your child only a pea-sized amount of child appropriate (lower dose fluoride) toothpaste when you brush his teeth twice a day.

Visiting the dentist

It's sensible to get your child used to seeing the dentist before he is likely to need any treatment. He can go to the dentist even before he has a full set of teeth. This will allow him to get used to the noises, smells, and surroundings, and prepare him for future visits. If he seems frightened, sit him on your lap in the chair and show him what the equipment does. By the time he is about two and a half he should have dental check-ups every six months. Your dentist will advise you on helping your child to care for his teeth – so see him even if you are sure your child's teeth are healthy. If there are cavities, it's vital that they are spotted in good time.

How the teeth come in

Your baby might cut his first tooth at any time during the first year, and he will be teething into his third year. Babies' teeth usually appear in the same order.

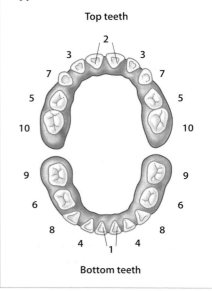

Teaching your child how to clean his teeth

As soon as the teeth come through, start cleaning your child's teeth for him with a wet toothbrush and a pea-sized helping of fluoride toothpaste. Brush them for him for as long as he will let you; he will probably want to brush his teeth himself from about the age of two. Always supervise your child – he needs to brush his teeth correctly. Teach him by standing behind him in front of a mirror, and, holding his hand, showing him the correct movements.

Top teeth: *brush downwards, away from the gums*

All biting surfaces: *brush back and forth along the flat tops of the teeth all around the mouth*

Get the brush *right to the back of your child's mouth*

Brush the gums *with a circular motion, both on the outside and inside by the tongue*

Bottom teeth: *brush upwards, away from the gums*

Making a game of teeth cleaning
Play games at bathtime to encourage your child to copy you; clean his teeth properly afterwards.

Cleaning your child's teeth
Stand your child on a step at the washbasin, with you behind her and to one side. Hold her head back so you can see into her mouth as you brush. Let her rinse and spit out – that's most of the fun.

Cutting nails

Your newborn baby
Keep your newborn baby's fingernails short so that there's no chance of him injuring himself by scratching his skin.

A young baby's nails are so soft that you may be tempted to peel the ends off with your fingers or teeth. However, it is preferable to use a pair of baby scissors or nail clippers with specially rounded ends. Hold his hand firmly, and press the finger pad away from the nail to avoid nicking the skin as you cut or clip.

Make sure that you always cut the fingernails straight across, otherwise the side edges might grow into the skin. Check for any sharp points when you finish.

If your baby wriggles while you are trying to cut his fingernails, don't try to fight him. Instead, trim them while he is sleeping peacefully.

Your older baby
Sit your baby on your lap, with him facing forwards. Hold one finger at a time and cut his nails with special baby scissors. It is best to follow the shape of his fingertips.

Cutting toenails
Lay a young baby on his mat; sit an older baby on your lap. Hold his foot firmly as he may try to kick you. Most children dislike having their toenails cut, so it might be a good idea to do it while your child is asleep.

Diapers and diaper changing

The first few weeks of your newborn's life may seem like a constant round of diaper changing. Her bladder is small, and she wets frequently. By changing her whenever her diaper is wet or soiled, you keep her comfortable and prevent diaper rash. As the months go by, you will notice that her diaper needs changing less frequently. By around two years, your child will start to recognize the feeling of a full bladder, and may be ready for potty training.

The contents of your baby's diaper

One way of knowing that your baby is feeding well is by checking the contents of her diaper. Listed below are the common sights on a baby's diaper during the first few weeks of his life:

● **greenish-black, sticky tar (first two or three days only):** this is meconium, which fills the bowels before birth, and passes out in the first two or three days
● **greenish-brown or bright green semi-fluid stools, full of curds (first week only):** "changing stools" show that your baby is adapting to feeding through her digestive system
● **orange-yellow, mustard-like stools, watery with bits of milk curd in them, often very copious:** the settled stools of a breastfed baby
● **pale brown, solid, formed, and smelly stools:** the settled stools of a bottle-fed baby
● **green, or green-streaked, stools:** quite normal, but small green stools over several days may be a sign of under-feeding.

Consult your doctor if:

● your baby's stools are very watery and smelly, and your baby is vomiting and off food: diarrhea is life-threatening in a young baby (see page 223)
● you see blood on the diaper
● anything at all worries you.

Types of diapers

Your baby won't much mind whether you use disposable or cloth diapers, provided the diaper fits snugly, and she's not left in a wet or dirty one. Disposables give your baby a neat, slim-line appearance. Cloth diapers are bulkier, and so the clothes you buy your baby may need to be a size larger to accommodate the diaper.

Reusable diapers have developed a lot since the time terry diapers were the only choice available. Because they are much easier to use, they are becoming more and more popular among parents. They are cheaper than disposables, and can be environmentally friendly, too. See pages 149 for more on types of diapers.

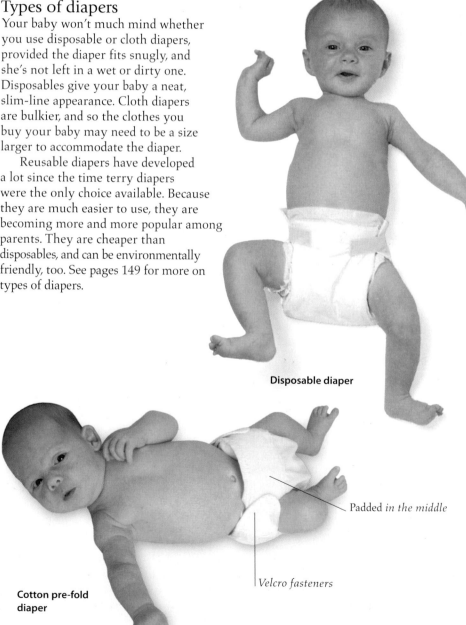

Disposable diaper

Padded *in the middle*

Velcro *fasteners*

Cotton pre-fold diaper

Changing your baby's diaper

Make sure you have everything you are going to need and choose a warm place to change your baby's diaper. Since you will be changing her diaper frequently, make your changing area a pleasant place for both of you – a mobile above your baby's head, a teddy nearby, bright decals stuck to the walls or furniture will all amuse your baby and encourage her to lie still for you. A changing mat is cheap and convenient, and your baby will be safe if you put the mat on a clean and dry floor. A specially designed changing table may be useful for storing clean diapers and toiletries, but your baby can fall off a table. If you do put the mat on a raised surface, never turn your back on your baby even for a second.

Changing time
Changing your baby's diaper is the perfect opportunity for you or your partner to talk to and play with her: incorporate lots of games and tickles, to make changing time fun.

The raised edge *on the mat won't stop your baby from rolling off*

A game *or two before you put a clean diaper on her will get some air to her bottom*

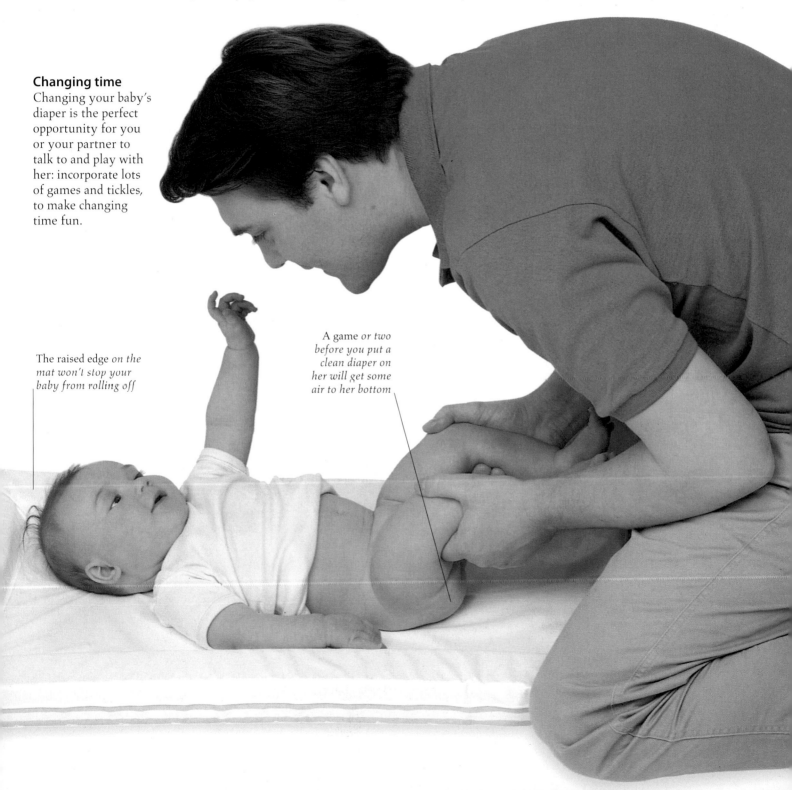

Equipment for changing your baby's diaper

Although it may seem to be a daunting array of equipment at first, keeping a full set of everything you will need together in one place will make diaper-changing seem that much easier. You can flush used tissues and diaper liners down the toilet, but put cotton balls, wipes, and disposable diapers, folded up and sealed, in a bin lined with a plastic bag. Drop reusable diapers into the appropriate bucket, before washing and rinsing them thoroughly (see page 153).

Equipment for cleaning your baby's bottom

Changing mat
A padded, wipe-clean mat with raised edges is invaluable. In warm weather, put a cloth diaper under your baby's head: the plastic may make her sweaty.

Baby wipes
These are useful for cleaning your baby's bottom. You can also use towelettes moistened with water.

Clean the mat with a baby wipe

Washcloths
Use some wet washcloths, then some dry ones, to clean her bottom.

Tissues
These are needed to wipe away feces and to dry your baby's bottom.

Cotton balls
Put out a handful of cotton balls before you start the diaper change so you don't have to put a dirty hand into the bag.

Barrier cream
Use barrier cream sparingly, and only if your baby's bottom is sore. Be careful not to get any cream on disposable diapers as the tapes will not stick.

Changing your baby's diaper
Keep everything you need to change your baby's diaper nearby, in a place where you won't need to turn your back to her.

Baby bath liquid and lotion
A few drops of baby bath liquid added to the bowl of warm water is a good alternative to water alone for cleaning your baby's bottom. A little baby lotion on a cotton ball is also effective.

Baby bath liquid   **Baby lotion**

What kind of diapers should you use?

In a few months' time you will have gained enough experience to change a diaper in a matter of seconds, and almost in your sleep, but to begin with diapers and diaper-changing may seem to take up a disproportionate amount of your day. When you are deciding whether to use reusable or disposable diapers, you will be thinking about cost, convenience, comfort for your baby, and the environment. You really have three choices when it comes to diapering your baby: use disposables, use a diaper service, or buy and wash your own cloth diapers. Disposable diapers are convenient and, being more absorbent, they are less likely to cause diaper rash than cloth diapers. However, they are expensive and environmentally unfriendly.

Reusable diapers, as well as being cheaper than disposables, have become much more convenient than the old-fashioned terry or cloth squares. Most are shaped like a disposable diaper and fasten with Velcro, snaps, or plastic clips. Disposable biodegradable liners, which catch the feces but allow moisture to seep through, make dealing with a dirty diaper easier. You can also choose from a variety of shapes and sizes to suit your baby. You will need about 15–20 diapers in each size. Don't forget to account for the time and expense of washing them when making your decision.

Disposable diapers are more expensive – especially when you consider that you will be using about 70 diapers a week. However, there are times, when you are travelling or on holiday for example, when you will really need the convenience of disposables. Consider choosing biodegradable diapers that can be composted. Many are also made from recycled materials that are free from chemicals and unbleached.

Reusable diapers

All-in-one reusable diaper

All-in-one reusable diapers offer the convenience and all the features of a disposable diaper. They combine an absorbent diaper and diaper liner and an outer waterproof shell that prevents leakage. They fasten around the baby's hips with Velcro tabs and look similar to disposable diapers. They are less difficult to use than conventional cloth diapers and avoid the need for diaper pins, but are harder to wash and dry because the integral waterproof shell usually can't be put in the tumble drier.

Terries

The traditional terry-towelling squares are the cheapest and most basic reusable diapers available. These must be folded into a triangular shape, fastened with diaper pins and used with a waterproof outer wrap – you can use plastic pants with snap fasteners to give a good fit. They dry quickly, but aren't as absorbent as some of the modern reusable diapers.

Pre-fold

These are basic cotton non-terry diapers that are folded into a rectangular shape

All-in-one reusable diaper

with a padded bit in the middle, and a waterproof outer diaper wrap, all secured with snaps or Velcro. These take less time to dry but may not be as absorbent as shaped diapers.

Shaped diapers

A shaped diaper is a cloth diaper shaped like a disposable diaper, which you use with a waterproof outer wrap. They fasten either with Velcro tabs or snaps.

Disposable diapers

Disposable diapers are sized according to your baby's weight. When you are happy with a brand, buy in bulk. "Ultra" or "High Performance" diapers are very absorbent, and will effectively keep the wetness away from your baby's skin. Some disposables have an outer cover that is breathable, allowing air to circulate next to the skin. "Standard" diapers are cheaper and bulkier, and you will have to change your baby more often. Diapers for boys have more padding at the front, while those for girls have more padding underneath.

Elastic around the legs protects against leaks

Always buy non-chlorine-bleached diapers if you can

Disposable diaper

Experiment until you find a brand with reliable adhesive tapes and good absorbency

Cleaning a girl

Clean your baby girl's bottom thoroughly at every diaper change. Otherwise she will soon get red and sore. Put your baby on her mat and undo her clothing and diaper. If she's wearing a fabric diaper, use a clean corner to wipe off the feces. With a disposable diaper, open it out, wipe off the feces with tissues and drop them into the diaper. Then lift your baby's legs and fold the diaper.

Fold underneath

1 Wipe away feces with tissues, then wipe all over her tummy up to her navel with a clean moist washcloth or baby wipe.

2 Using a fresh washcloth or wipe, clean inside all the creases at the top of your baby's legs, wiping downwards towards her bottom.

Dry the skin creases thoroughly

3 Lift her legs up with a finger between her ankles, and clean her genitals next. Always wipe from front to back to prevent germs from the anus entering the vagina. Do not try to clean inside the vaginal lips.

4 With a fresh baby wipe, clean her anus, then her buttocks and thighs, working inwards towards the anus. When she's clean, remove the disposable diaper, seal the tapes over the front, and drop it in the bin.

5 Dry her diaper area with tissues, then let her kick for a while without a diaper, so that her bottom is open to the air.

6 If using, apply barrier cream above and around the genitals, on the vaginal lips and anus, and over the buttocks. Wash your hands.

Diaper rash

All babies get a red or sore bottom from time to time. Consult your doctor if the rash won't clear up.

To avoid diaper rash:
- change your baby's diaper frequently
- clean and dry her bottom and skin creases thoroughly, using warm water and tissues
- leave your baby without a diaper as often as possible so that her bottom is open to the air
- if using cloth diapers, buy tie-on or snap-on plastic pants, as these allow air to circulate

- wash and rinse all cloth diapers thoroughly.

At the first signs of redness:
- change diapers more frequently
- use a healing diaper rash cream
- leave your baby without a diaper on for as much of the day as possible
- if using cloth diapers, try a more absorbent type of liner
- stop using plastic pants: they make diaper rash worse because they help keep urine close to the skin. If you don't like the leaks, switch to disposables for a while.

Cleaning a boy

Your baby boy's urine will go everywhere so you need to clean his bottom very thoroughly at every diaper change to guard against a sore bottom. Put your baby on his mat, and undo his clothing and his diaper. If he's wearing a cloth diaper, wipe off the worst of any feces with a clean corner. With a disposable, undo the tapes, then pause (see right).

1 Your baby boy will often urinate just as you take his diaper off, so wait a couple of seconds with the diaper held over his penis to avoid urine going everywhere.

2 Open the diaper out. Wipe off the feces with tissues, and drop them into the diaper, then fold it down under him. Start by wiping his tummy up to his navel with a moist washcloth or baby wipe.

Clean carefully under his testicles

3 With a fresh washcloth or wipe, clean in the creases at the top of his legs and at the base of his genitals, wiping away from his body. Hold his testicles out of the way while you wipe underneath them.

4 With a fresh washcloth, wipe all over your baby's testicles, including under his penis, as there may be traces of urine or feces here. Hold his penis out of the way, but take care not to drag the skin.

5 Clean his penis, wiping away from the body: do not pull the foreskin back to clean underneath, this will keep itself clean.

Put barrier cream *over his lower tummy to protect against diaper rash*

6 Lift your baby's legs to clean his anus and buttocks, keeping a finger between his ankles. Wipe over the back of his thighs, too. When he is clean, remove the diaper.

7 Wipe your hands clean, and then dry his diaper area with tissues. Let him kick for a while if he has a sore bottom. Always keep tissues at hand, just in case he urinates.

8 If using, apply barrier cream sparingly above the penis (but not on it), around the testicles and anus, and over the buttocks. Wash your hands afterwards.

Putting on a disposable diaper

Before you put on a new diaper, make sure that you clean your baby's bottom thoroughly and, if using, apply a barrier cream to help prevent diaper rash. Wipe your hands well on a tissue, as the diaper's adhesive tapes won't stick very well if you get grease on them or on the front of the diaper.

Bring the diaper *straight up: don't twist it to one side*

Spread the diaper *taut over your baby's tummy*

2 Bring the front up, pointing the boy's penis toward his feet (or he may urinate into the waistband).

1 Open up the diaper with the tapes at the top. Lift your baby by her ankles with one finger between them, and slide the diaper under her, until the top edge lines up with her waist.

3 Hold one corner in position and, with the other hand, peel the tape, and pull it forwards to stick to the front, parallel with the top edge of the diaper.

4 Do the same with the other side, making sure the diaper is snug round your baby's legs, and not twisted round to one side.

Diaper bins

There are many options for discarding disposable diapers. The bin pictured here seals each diaper into a plastic wrapper. The bin only needs to be emptied when all the wrappers are used. This type of bin controls odours better than traditional diaper pails, and makes it easier to dispose of the contents quickly and hygienically. However, it is expensive and costly to the environment.

Plastic wrappers *effectively seal in germs and odours*

Fold the waistband *over if it is too high: it could chafe your baby's navel*

5 The diaper should fit snugly round your baby's waist allowing room enough for one of your fingers. Check the fit, and if it's too loose, peel the tapes, and reposition them.

Putting on a reusable diaper

Shaped diapers

These reusable diapers come in two parts: an absorbent inner diaper, sometimes used with a liner, and an outer wrapper. The inner diaper square is folded and placed inside the outer wrapper (as shown here), or sometimes a shaped or ready-folded inner diaper is used inside the wrapper. The inner diaper catches feces and absorbs urine, while the wrapper holds everything in place, and prevents wetness from leaking through to the baby's clothes. If you use squares, it is a good idea to have them folded ready for use. Like a disposable, a reusable diaper should be changed when your baby soils it.

1 Lay the outer wrapper out flat, with the inside facing you and the tabs at the top.

2 Take one of the absorbent diapers and fold it into thirds along its length, forming a long rectangle.

3 Fold the liner over the diaper, and then fold the diaper and liner again to form a long rectangle.

4 Place the absorbent diaper (with the liner on top) down the centre of the outer wrapper.

5 Put the baby down on the diaper, bringing the front up and fastening the tabs snugly around her hips.

Washing reusable diapers

Diaper rash is caused by bacteria. You can help prevent diaper rash by keeping your diapers as germ-free as possible. Rinse all diapers, no matter how lightly soiled, before putting them in the diaper pail. A solution of borax and water in the pail will help remove stains and make washing easier. Machine wash at 60°C, which is hot enough to kill any bacteria. Use laundry detergent and bleach if you wish, but do not add any fabric softener, as this reduces the absorbency of the diapers and can cause skin irritation. Run the diapers through a second wash cycle using just water, adding white vinegar to the last rinse cycle. This gets rid of soap residue and acts as a natural whitener and clothes softener.

Hang the diapers outside to dry as it helps to bleach and disinfect them. Although the reusable diapers can be tumble-dried, constant tumble-drying may eventually affect their absorbency, and reduce the amount of use you get out of them. In addition, tumble-drying uses up a lot of energy, and will negate the environmental benefit of using reusable diapers. Avoid putting plastic pants or outer wrappers in the dryer.

Diaper pail safety
Make sure that your baby cannot get into the diaper pail.

Giving up diapers

When it comes to toilet training, each child is different. The process will be much easier if you wait until she is ready for this big step. Once she is capable of recognizing the signs of a full bladder or bowel (which happens after age two), and is interested in using the potty, your job is to provide the setting and the encouragement. Progress may be uneven as bowel and bladder control may not happen at the same time. Be patient!

Tips to help

● Choose a time for potty training when your child's life is relatively free of new situations and when you can approach it with a relaxed attitude.
● Set the situation up so she is more likely to succeed than fail – if she thinks she always fails, she will stop trying.
● When she's successful, show that you're pleased with her.
● When she has an accident, be sympathetic about it.
● Allow her to learn at her own pace.

Training pants
Padding and a waterproof backing make these more absorbent than underwear. Disposable training pants are also available.

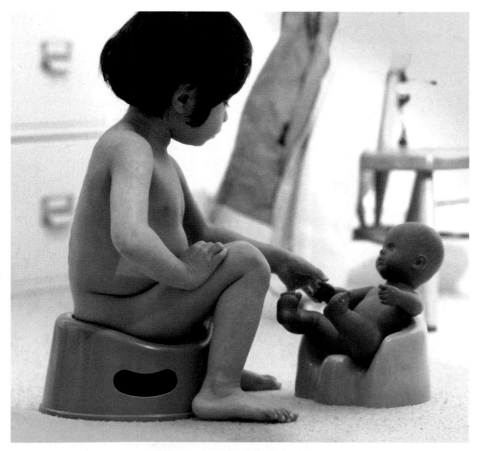

Your child's potty
Your child will soon understand what it's for, and will be proud of herself for learning a new skill. Always be encouraging and complimentary.

Achieving daytime control

1
Wait until your child is ready
Most children are ready for potty training between the ages of 2 and 3 years. Your child is ready to learn to use the potty if she:
● shows an interest in the potty
● recognizes that she's done something in her diaper, perhaps by pointing and shouting
● is often dry after a nap.

2
Introduce the potty
Show her a potty and tell her what it's for. Put it in the bathroom for a few days before doing anything further, so she gets used to it. Show her how to sit on it, but with her diaper on for now.

3
Set aside a suitable time
You might want to set aside two weeks during the summer for potty training, when your child can wear training pants while playing outside in the yard. She won't have to worry about outer clothing, and a few accidents won't disrupt the household. *Don't* start when your routines are already upset: a holiday away from home, for example, is not a good time.

4
Put her in underwear, reminding her often to use the potty
For these two weeks, let your child wear underwear or training pants, which will absorb at least a little of the urine. Have the potty nearby, and suggest she sits on it after a meal, a drink, a snack, or a nap, or whenever she shows any signs of needing it.

5
Help her to use the potty
Encourage her to sit on the potty, but do not pressure her. Pull down her underwear and help her to sit down on it (tuck a boy's penis in). If she's managed to tell you she needs it, thank her.

If your child jumps up too soon
Suggest she sits there a little longer – about five minutes – and distract her with a toy or a book. If nothing happens, let her get up and carry on playing.

When she does go in the potty
When she does use the potty, always praise her. Wipe and clean her quickly, from front to back. Hold the potty steady as she stands up, and pull up her underwear for her. Don't show disgust at the contents of the potty, just flush them down the toilet, wipe the potty clean, then rinse it with disinfectant. Wash your hands.

6
When your child has an accident, don't scold her
You can't expect her to remember to use the potty at this stage. If she wets or dirties her underwear, don't scold her – it's really your fault for not reminding her to sit on the potty often enough. Clean her bottom with a sympathetic air and put fresh underwear on her. If after two weeks your child shows no signs of understanding, and is not telling you she needs the potty on at least some occasions, she's not ready to give up diapers yet. Put her back in them for a few more weeks, then try again – you may have several two-week training stints before she gets herself to the potty on most occasions when she needs to.

7
Leave a diaper off during naps
Once your child is using the potty fairly reliably during the daytime, and her diaper has been dry after a nap for about a week, you can leave her diaper off. Suggest she sits on the potty after she wakes from her nap. Napping without diapers will help her towards staying dry at night.

8
When you go out
Until your child is fairly reliable, put a diaper on her when you go out, but try to make sure, without forcing her, that she uses her potty beforehand. If you're going on a car journey, put her in a diaper. Take a potty, spare clothes, and an old towel, in case of accidents.

9
Suggest using the toilet
After a few weeks of using the potty during the day, suggest that she try being like you and use the toilet. Help her pull her underwear down and sit her on the seat for the first few times, until she gets the hang of it. For a boy, lift the seat and lid, and show him how to aim his penis, otherwise help him pull his underwear down and climb up to sit on the seat. You can use a clip-on toilet seat to make the hole smaller and less daunting for her. Stay nearby until she's finished, wipe her bottom, and help her down; she won't be able to wipe her own bottom until she is at least four. Wash her hands and yours.

Achieving night-time control

1
Wait until she is dry at night
If you have taken a dry diaper off your child in the morning for about a week, you can start leaving her diaper off at night.

2
Let her sleep without anything on her bottom at all
For the first week, put her to bed without a diaper or underwear; protect the mattress with a waterproof sheet if you want to. Make sure she uses the toilet before bedtime. She should sleep through without any problems. If she doesn't, and she wets the bed, she's simply not ready to give up night-time diapers yet.

3
If she lapses into bedwetting
If your child starts to wet her bed after being dry at night for weeks or months, it may be because she has suffered some sort of stress in her life. If she seems ill or has a fever, take her to the doctor to rule out an infection. Never scold or punish her for bedwetting. If she wakes up wet in the night, be sympathetic as you clean her up. If it happens more than once, put her back in diapers until she's more settled and you have taken off a dry one for seven consecutive mornings. She may not be dry at night until she is five or six, but this is not unusual. Withholding a bedtime drink won't help her.

Reaching the toilet
Put a step out so your child can climb up. She will probably want to flush the toilet when she finishes – that's part of the fun.

Getting out and about

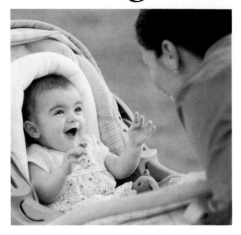

As she grows older your baby will love going out and about. She'll find everything fascinating and new – dogs, people, even supermarket shelves. To facilitate this, some form of stroller and a car seat are essential items. Other useful items are a baby carrier for a young baby, or a backpack carrier if your baby is older. A diaper bag with a detachable changing mat is convenient for outings. Pack it with diaper-changing equipment, spare clothes, and other useful items for your excursion.

Methods of transport

Choosing a method of transporting your baby can be bewildering. Consider how many months of the year you'll be using your purchase, how old your baby is, and where you'll be walking. A convertible carriage stroller with a removable bassinet might be ideal. However, other strollers allow you to clamp the car seat onto the frame of the stroller.

A waterproof hood *will protect your baby from the rain*

Folding stroller
from three months
- 👍 Your baby can face you, or forwards.
- 👍 Rigid seat-back gives your baby good support.
- 👍 Can be free-standing when folded flat.
- 👍 Light, and easy to manoeuvre.
- 👎 Your young baby cannot lie flat.
- 👎 Your baby is not protected from the elements.
- 👎 A plastic hood for wet weather protection is often an extra.

The folding mechanism *should be easy to use*

Carriage with removable bassinet
from birth
- 👍 Your young baby can face you.
- 👍 Your young baby can sleep in it day and night.
- 👍 Your baby can be snug under a weatherproof cover for outdoor use.
- 👍 Some types convert to take a stroller seat.
- 👍 Chassis folds flat.
- 👎 Can be awkward to take on public transport.
- 👎 Some types are too wide to fit through a small door.

A large tray *is useful for shopping and changing equipment*

Car seat adaptable stroller
from birth

- 👍 Gives your baby a comfortable ride.
- 👍 Can be used up to about one year.
- 👎 Hard to use on public transport.
- 👎 You need ample storage.

The car seat *fixes easily onto the chassis*

The stroller seat *can lie flat for a newborn baby*

The stroller can *be moved to a seated position as your baby grows*

Umbrella-style stroller
from about six months

- 👍 Folds up neatly, so it is good on public transport, and also when storage space is limited.
- 👍 The cheapest option; also the lightest.
- 👎 Soft seat-back gives poor support, so not suitable for babies under six months.
- 👎 Often no shopping tray.

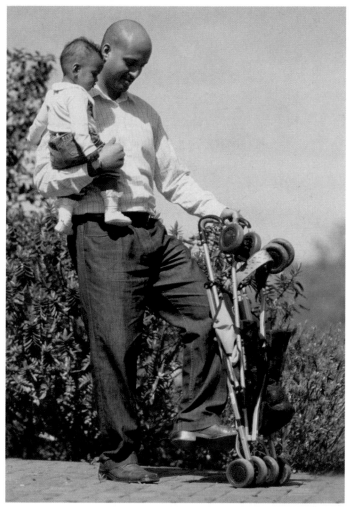

When your child is walking
Once she is up and about, she will be eager to explore her surroundings. This enthusiasm may tire her out at times, so be ready to pick her up, or take a stroller with you. If you are worried about her safety when you take her outside, a harness is an ideal way to keep your child from wandering off, while giving her more freedom than when she's holding your hand. It will also provide additional safety when she starts to walk.

Carriage and stroller safety
- Always lock the stroller before putting your baby in.
- Always fit and use the harness.
- Put the brake on as soon as you stop.
- Never let your child pull herself up or try to stand.
- Never hang heavy bags on the handles: it may tip.
- Never let your child play with a folded stroller.
- Make sure the carriage or stroller you buy conforms to Canadian safety standards.
- Stroller hinge mechanisms can injure (and even amputate) little fingers. Always follow instructions and keep your child away when you open or close the stroller.

Car travel

There is excellent evidence that infants and children are safest in cars when they are secured in special car seats. The seat must suit your child's age and weight and be installed properly in your car. The safest place for babies and children 12 years of age and under is in the back seat. Children aged 12 and under must not be in a seating position that has an airbag. It is important for parents to stay up-to-date with the latest information and to do everything they can to keep children as safe as possible while on the road.

Being extra safe

New legislation concerning car seat safety came into effect on January 1, 2011, so any car seats sold after this time will comply with the new safety guidelines. However, if you have a car seat purchased before this time, it is fine to use as long as it has not passed its expiry date and is properly installed. All car seats are different, so ensure that your child fits within the weight and height range. Weight is more important than age or height in determining the appropriate seat for your child. Do not be in a hurry to move up to the next stage, particularly from the rear-facing position.

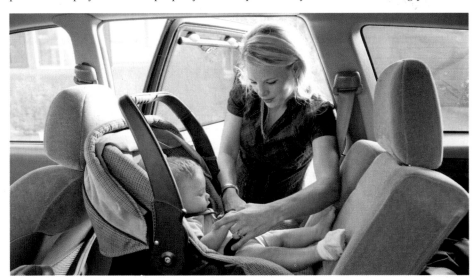

Children should always be in the back seat – the middle of the back seat is the safest place for a single car seat. The internal seat belt or harness should be installed using the slot positions that are at or slightly below your baby's shoulders. The chest clip should be at your baby's underarms, and the harness straps should be fastened tightly. Only one finger should fit between the harness strap and your baby's collarbones. Items not provided by the car seat manufacturers, such as liners, trays, or comfort straps, may interfere with the safety of the seat.

In-car entertainment

Make long car journeys as enjoyable as possible:
- play CDs of stories and songs
- sing songs and recite rhymes
- point out interesting objects
- take toys such as finger puppets or an activity centre
- take snacks and drinks
- stop frequently.

Car seat installation

As car designs vary so much, it is virtually impossible to make a child car seat that can be fitted correctly into all cars. For this reason, it is critical to follow the manufacturer's instructions carefully. However, newer cars have a Universal Anchorage System (UAS) that allows the car seat to be directly attached to the car's frame. You may also see the term LUAS, which stands for Lower Universal Anchorage System, or LATCH, which stands for Lower Anchors and Tethers for Children. These are now standard for child car seat installation, intending to make fitting quick and easy. Because universal anchorage systems create a rigid link between the child seat and the car, it makes them extra secure. These systems have linkage points built into them to enable the child seat or seat base to be simply plugged into the clips in the car's frame. A forward facing seat still requires a tether strap attached to a tether anchor for additional safety. In many larger centres, there are professionals who can check the car seat installation for you.

Stage 1: Rear-facing infant seat
(from birth until she outgrows the seat's weight/height limit)

Newborns and young infants have weak neck and back muscles so they require a seat that is relatively inclined. Use a rear facing infant seat on the back seat from birth until she outgrows the seat's weight/height limit. Do not be in a hurry to move to the next stage, since research has shown that this is a safer position for the weak neck muscles of young children. Secure the seat directly to the car using the Universal Anchorage System (UAS) or the car seat belt as instructed by the manufacturer. Strap your baby in with the harness.

Safety in the car

● Use only car seats that conform to Canadian motor vehicle standards (seats certified to US standards do not meet Canadian standards).

● Make sure the car seat installation conforms to LUAS (see facing page).

● Never let any child travel unrestrained. **Always** strap your child into her seat with the safety harness.

● Never travel with your baby in your lap or your arms.

● If your car has air bags, do not put the baby seat in the front passenger seat. Children are always safer in the back seat.

● If you have an accident, replace your seat belts, your child's car seat, and the seat's anchorage kit: they may have been damaged.

● Never buy second-hand car seats, harnesses, or anchorage kits for the same reason.

● Install a mirror on your windshield so that you can see your child without turning around.

● Use booster seats in the back seats for older children.

● Never leave your baby or child unattended in a car.

Stage 2: Forward-facing child seat
(from 10kg/22lbs until she outgrows the seat's weight/height limit)

A forward-facing child seat should be used until your child outgrows the seat's weight/height limit. This type of seat has improved side impact protection and a head support pad that increases the length of the backrest, and as such increases the usable height for the child in the seat. The harness straps are narrower than a vehicle seat belt and fit children's small shoulders. Do not hurry to move to the next stage. Your child is safer in a car seat than a booster as long as she fits the car seat's height/weight limit. Some car seats have a recline feature and can be used in the rear-facing position from birth. Make sure to install the seat as instructed by the manufacturer on the back seat of your car.

Stage 3: Booster seat
(from 20kg/45lbs until she outgrows the seat's weight/height limit)

A booster seat should be used when your child is over the maximum weight and height for his car seat, but no sooner than this. It should be placed in the back seat with the shoulder strap over the child's shoulder and across the chest, with the lap belt low and snug across the hips. Buckle up an empty booster seat so that it won't move around.

Stage 4: Seat belt
(over 37kg/80lbs)

The back seat is still the safest place for your child. The belt should be placed over the shoulder and across the chest, with the lap belt low and snug across the hips.

When you have to leave your child

The first time that you leave your baby is a real milestone for you, even if it is just for an hour or two of shopping, a trip to the gym, or a visit to the cinema. Leaving your precious new baby in the care of even the most trusted friend, grandparent, or babysitter can be painful. You may feel a bit guilty because it suddenly seems such a relief to be free, albeit briefly, from the feeling of total responsibility that you have for your tiny infant.

Getting your child used to other people

Babysitters

Nothing is more important during your baby's early months than your ever-loving presence, but eventually he has to learn to lead a separate existence. His eventual transition to school will be easier and his confidence will grow if he has opportunities to explore the world outside his immediate family, and learns to be independent of you, and to make close relationships with other people – grandparents, babysitters, and friends.

It isn't frivolous or selfish to get your baby used to a regular babysitter when he is young. And if you plan to go back to work within a year or so, then it is essential that he gets used to the idea that someone else can be relied on to love and care for him. There are several things you can do to make babysitting easier both for the sitter and your baby.

● Tell your baby what's going to happen, even if he is too young to understand. He will sense your reassurance.

● If you go out in the evening, make sure he knows the babysitter, so that if he wakes he won't be terrified at seeing a stranger.

● Don't introduce any new babysitting arrangement when your baby is tired, hungry, or sick. Pick a time of the day when you think he'll be at his most alert and happiest.

● If you have a new babysitter, don't rush to go out even if you are in a hurry. Spend some time holding him and letting him size up this new person. Let your baby see that you like the babysitter.

● Show the babysitter which toys are his favourites and how to play the games he likes best.

● If the babysitter has to put your child to bed, make sure she knows every detail of his bedtime routine, so that your child will go to bed happily.

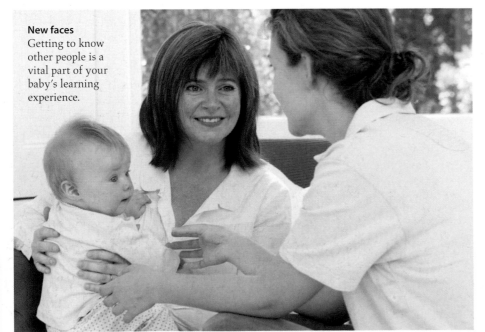

New faces
Getting to know other people is a vital part of your baby's learning experience.

Separation anxiety

At some time, usually between seven months and a year, your baby may start to seem reluctant even to let you out of his sight for a second. He'll cling when you try to put him down, or cry if he is left with anyone else. Don't worry about such behaviour. This "separation anxiety" is normal and means that he recognizes you as separate from him, and realizes how essential you are to him. Even the most clingy baby will eventually become independent. But, meanwhile, patiently accept his dependence on you. If you have to go out, always tell him. Say goodbye confidently, even if you're feeling nervous – your child is sensitive to your emotions and if he senses your anxiety, he may be even more upset. Tell him where you are going, and reassure him that you will be coming back.

Cuddlies and security blankets

By eight or nine months, most children form a strong attachment to a favourite soft toy, blanket, or a special object. This powerful need for something cuddly grows even stronger after the first birthday. The child may carry it around continually during the day, take it to bed at night, cuddling or sucking it for comfort. Eventually, it becomes a kind of talisman, something the child turns to for comfort whenever he is frustrated, frightened, or sad. Your child's cuddly will become grubby, shabby, and eventually probably unsanitary, because your child will be reluctant to let you wash it, as its familiar smell is part of its comforting charm. Don't try to persuade him to give it up. It fulfils a real need. Keep it handy, make sure babysitters know about it, and try to forestall the disaster of losing it by keeping a duplicate somewhere safe.

Comfort objects
Attachment to an object often helps your child to adapt to new situations.

Childcare options

Going back to work

Whether you are going back to work because you love your job or whether it is a matter of financial necessity, it is bound to be stressful at first. How smoothly it goes depends almost entirely on the childcare arrangements you make. It will take a little while for everything to settle down, so don't worry too much if the first few days are difficult. Children are pretty adaptable, and most settle down quickly under a new routine. But keep a careful eye on your child during the first few weeks you are back at work. If his behaviour deteriorates or if he seems generally unhappy, you may need to re-think your childcare plans.

Grandparent care

This may be an ideal arrangement provided that the grandparent is willing. It is important that they know and respect your views on childcare – and vice-versa. Problems may arise if you feel that the grandparents are "taking over."

Shared care with a friend or relative

If you intend to work part-time and have a good friend or close relative who also has small children, this may provide a workable solution. It's important to formalize the arrangement and stick to it, so that neither party feels they are being taken advantage of.

Caregiver

Regulations concerning caregivers vary among provinces. Licensed childcare programs have to meet and maintain certain provincial standards to ensure that the health, safety, and developmental needs of the children are being met. Unlicensed caregivers may look after small numbers (up to five) of children in their home. Talk to the caregiver yourself, to make sure that she is the kind of person you want to care for your child. It may be difficult to find a place for a very young baby.

Day care centre

Private day care centres offer full day care, usually from around 7:30am to 6pm, and often stay open during holiday periods. Although day care is expensive, there is a fairly high ratio of staff to children and a stimulating environment. Staff may have a diploma in Early Childhood Education. Most day care centres have a separate baby area for children under the age of two.

Nanny care

Although this is the most expensive option, having a nanny means that your child has one-to-one care in his or her own home. A qualified nanny will have a childcare qualification such as an Early Childhood Development diploma. In many cases, new immigrants to Canada are given visas that enable them to work as live-in childcare providers. These women come with varied backgrounds, education, and skills. When hiring a nanny, always ask to see her registration documents and childcare qualifications, and always check references.
N.B. An au pair is a mother-helper, not a caregiver. Au pairs are untrained and will have little or no childcare experience. He or she may babysit but is not a suitable person to take sole charge of a baby or young child.

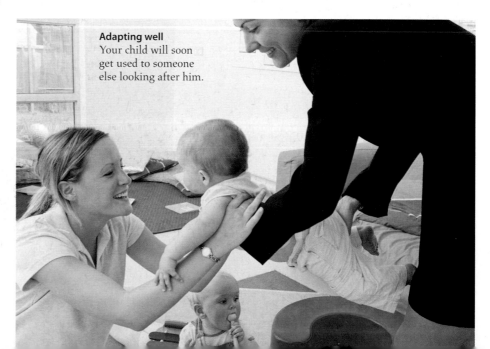

Adapting well
Your child will soon get used to someone else looking after him.

Growing and learning

Watching your child grow and learn is a rewarding experience. Every stage brings something new: at first it's rolling over, sitting, crawling, walking. Once he's mastered those, he will learn to talk, and will refine his co-ordination and dexterity. Although there's nothing so thrilling as watching him take his first steps, the next year will bring some subtler achievements that will fill you with pride. Throughout these pre-school years, your child needs your attention and stimulation.

The first six months

During these months you will see your baby develop a real personality, and he will reward you with plenty of enchanting smiles and gurgles. Although there are a lot of toys aimed at this age group, he needs – and loves – your company most of all. When he's wakeful, talk and smile with him. Plenty of stimulation in the form of things to look at, sounds to hear, and textures to explore is vital, too. You don't need expensive toys: old photographs, rattles, and non-glass mirrors will all do just as well.

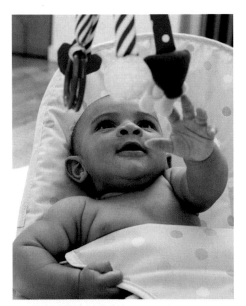

Using her body
Give your baby the chance to explore what she can do with her limbs and body. Lying on her tummy, she will push up on her arms and kick her legs out behind her; she may even balance on her tummy. Massaging her gently with baby oil will teach her about her body, too.

Objects and noises
At around six weeks, let your baby spend some of his wakeful times in a bouncing chair on the floor. (Before this, he will enjoy lying on the floor on a blanket.) If you show him something colourful that makes a noise, he'll show his interest by wriggling around. He may be able to hold something light if you put it in his hand, and soon he'll reach out clumsily to grab things.

Learning about each other

During the first couple of months of life your baby can't focus beyond about 25cm (10in), so bring your face close when you talk to her, and exaggerate your expressions and smiles. It's this eye contact that helps your baby become a person, and shows her what building a loving relationship is all about.

Rolling

Sometime during these six months, your baby will learn to roll over, from front to back first, then from back to front. It will give him a great sense of achievement: he's beginning to make his body move for him. Remember that even before he's learnt to roll he can fall off things, so never leave him unattended on a high surface, not even the bed.

Learning to sit

As your baby gets more control over his body, help him learn to sit by surrounding him with cushions. They will help him balance, and protect him if he topples over.

Premature babies

Your premature baby will probably reach all his developmental milestones later than other babies. Remember that in reality he has two "birthdays": one is the day he was born, but the more important one for the first few months is the date on which he was expected to be born. If you take those missing weeks in the womb into account, you will almost certainly find that his progress is not slow at all. Take him to the doctor for regular monitoring; he should have caught up with other children born at the same time by the age of two.

Stepping stones chart

Babies don't all develop at the same rate, or learn a particular skill at a particular time. But because everything they learn acts as a "stepping stone" to the next stage of development, they do acquire skills in the same order. The chart below shows the "stepping stones" in various areas of your child's development – physical skills, manual dexterity, sight, hearing and language, and social development and play. Your child may learn to do something either earlier or later than the average age given in the chart.

Stepping stones in child development

Age	Gross motor skills (physical movements)	Fine motor skills (manual dexterity)	Hearing, vision, and language	Social development and play
One month	Lies on back with head to one side. When held sitting his head falls forwards with back curved. Held standing on hard surface presses down feet, straightens body, and makes reflex "stepping" movements.	Hands normally closed, but if open will grasp a finger if it touches his palm.	Startled by loud noises. Turns head and eyes towards light. Eyes will follow a dangling toy held 15–20cm (6–8in) away and moved slowly from side to side. Cries and coos.	Stops crying when picked up and spoken to. Looks at mother's face intently when she feeds or talks to him.
Three months	Lies on back with head in mid-line. Kicks vigorously. Held sitting can hold head erect and steady. Placed face down lifts head up briefly. Held standing with feet on hard surface sags at knees.	Watches movements of own hands, and begins to clasp and unclasp hands. Holds rattle placed in his hand for a few moments, but can't look at it at the same time.	Alert, and interested in people's faces. Moves head to look around. Eyes converge as a toy held above his face is moved nearer. Smiles at mother's voice. Vocalizes when spoken to. Turns head and eyes towards a sound.	Smiles at 5–6 weeks. Recognizes and begins to react to preparations for bath, feeds, etc. by smiles, coos, and excited movements. Responds with obvious pleasure to friendly handling, tickling, being talked or sung to.
Six months	Raises head when lying on back. Sits with support. When hands are grasped can pull himself up. Rolls over, front to back. Placed face down lifts head and chest up. Held standing takes his weight and bounces.	Stretches out both hands to grasp interesting objects. Begins to transfer objects from one hand to the other. Shakes rattle, and looks at it at the same time. Takes everything to mouth.	"Sings" and chats to himself using single and double syllables, such as ka, muh. Turns to mother's voice at once. Screams if annoyed. Recognizes and responds to various emotional tones of mother's voice.	Laughs, chuckles, and squeals aloud in play. Still friendly with strangers, but sometimes shows some anxiety, especially if mother is out of sight. When he drops a toy, he forgets about it.
Nine months	Sits alone for 10–15 minutes on floor. Progresses on floor by rolling or squirming. Tries to crawl on all fours. Pulls self to standing with support, but can't lower himself. Held standing steps purposefully on alternate feet.	Examines objects by passing them from one hand to the other. Stretches out one hand to grasp small objects. Will hold out toy to adult, but can't yet let go unless pressing against hard surface. Grasps spoon while being fed.	Shouts to attract attention, listens, and shouts again. Babbles tunefully, using long strings of syllables, e.g. dad-dad. Understands "no" and "bye-bye." Imitates adult noises, like cough, brrr, etc. Watches people and activities with interest.	Looks at toys falling over edge of carriage or table. Can find partially hidden toy. Plays "peek-a-boo." May be wary of strangers, clinging to known adult and hiding face.

Age	Gross motor skills (physical movements)	Fine motor skills (manual dexterity)	Hearing, vision, and language	Social development and play
12 months	Sits well. Crawls rapidly. Pulls self to standing. Walks around furniture. Walks with one or both hands held. Stands or walks alone for some time.	Picks up small objects with thumb and index finger. Points at things he wants. Holds spoon but cannot use it alone. Drinks from cup with little assistance.	Responds to own name. Babbles loudly. Understands familiar words and commands. First words with meaning (usually "mama" or "dada"). Imitates speech.	Shows affection to familiar people. Tries to help with dressing. Throws toys, watches them fall. Waves and claps hands. Puts cubes in and out of box.
15 months	Walks with feet apart. Goes from standing to sitting by collapsing backwards, or falling forwards on hands. Crawls upstairs. Bends over to pick up toys.	Builds tower of two cubes after being shown. Grasps crayon and imitates scribble. Brings spoon to mouth to lick. Holds cup when given, and gives it back.	Speaks 2–6 familiar words, and understands more. Obeys simple commands, e.g. shut the door. Looks with interest at pictures in a book, and pats pages.	Helps more constructively with dressing. Easily upset. Depends on mother's reassuring presence. Can push big-wheeled toy on level ground.
18 months	Walks well. Runs stiffly, can't run round obstacles. Carries toys. Walks upstairs with helping hand. Creeps backwards downstairs. Sits on stairs, bumps down a few steps.	Picks up tiny objects with pincer grasp. Preference for one hand obvious. Scribbles with crayon with preferred hand. Builds tower of three cubes after being shown.	Jabbers, uses 6–20 words, and understands more. Sings and tries to join in rhymes. Enjoys picture books, points at and recognizes coloured items. Turns two pages at a time.	Takes off shoes, socks, and hat. Does not take toys to mouth. Plays contentedly alone, but likes to be near adult. Emotionally depends on familiar adults, especially mother.
Two years	Runs safely. Walks backwards. Pulls wheeled toy. Climbs on and off furniture. Goes up and down stairs holding rail, two feet to a step. Sits on wheeled toy and moves forward with feet.	Builds tower of four or five cubes. Draws circles and dots. Can imitate vertical line. Identifies familiar adults in a photograph after being shown once.	Turns pages one by one. Uses 50 plus words. Puts two or more words together to make sentences. Refers to himself by name. Asks names of objects. Joins in rhymes and songs.	Follows mother around, and copies what she does. Plays simple make-believe games. Plays near other children, but not with them. Has tantrums when frustrated, but easily distracted.
Two and a half years	Walks upstairs alone, and downstairs holding rail, two feet to a step. Climbs easy climbing frame. Jumps with two feet together. Kicks a large ball. Sits on tricycle and steers, but can't yet pedal.	Can build tower of seven or more cubes, and line up blocks to form a "train." Can draw a horizontal line and circle when shown how. Eats skilfully with spoon, and may use a fork.	Uses 200 plus words. Knows full name. Uses "I," "me," and "you." Always asks questions beginning "what?" and "how?" Can say a few nursery rhymes. Recognizes self in a photo, once shown.	Rebellious and throws tantrums if frustrated. Less easily distracted. Enjoys make-believe play. Likes to watch other children play, and may join in for a few minutes. Has little idea of sharing toys.
Three years	Walks alone upstairs with alternating feet, downstairs with two feet to a step. Climbs with agility. Rides tricycle. May walk on tiptoes. Sits with feet crossed at ankle.	Eats well with fork and spoon. Washes hands. Pulls pants up. Builds tower of nine cubes or more. Draws man with head and some features. Paints with large brush. Uses scissors.	Can give full name, sex, and often age. Holds simple conversation and relays past experiences. Listens to stories, and demands favourites. Can match 2–3 primary colours.	Less prone to tantrums. Helps adults in activities. Enjoys floor play with bricks etc. Plays with other children. Understands taking turns. Friendly with younger siblings.

The second six months

Your baby will cram a great deal into these months. He will sit up unsupported, may crawl, and even stand or walk by his first birthday. It won't be steady progress, and not every child goes through each stage. This is the age when he learns to explore every new thing by putting it in his mouth. From now until around three years old, make sure your child never gets hold of any small, dangerous objects.

Exploring boxes
Don't be surprised if your baby finds the boxes his toys arrive in just as fascinating as the toys. Check for and remove any staples, and make sure there aren't any sharp edges.

Making noises
A wooden spoon and a saucepan make a perfect drum – your baby will love banging away and listening to the loud noise he creates.

Sitting up
Your baby will lean forwards and splay his legs out wide and straight, when he first learns to balance sitting up. (Put a cushion behind him until he's steady.) Now he has both hands free to explore.

"Pat-a-cake"
Sing the rhyme and clap your hands together as he claps his. He will enjoy this little play.

Crawling
Getting about on all fours is a great achievement. He may not use each leg in the same way: a lop-sided shuffle with one knee and the other foot is quite normal.

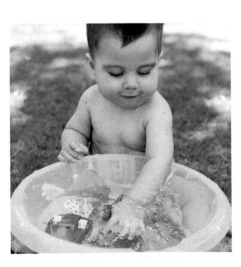

Water play
Show your baby how water feels on his hands. Sieves and plastic jugs make good substitutes for toy buckets.

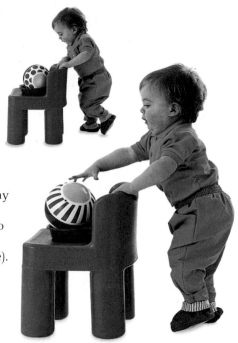

Boxes and objects
Give your older baby a box
and some empty cotton spools
or brightly coloured blocks,
and he will happily take
them out one by one, then
put them back in again.

Introducing a ball
At seven months, your baby
may be fascinated to see a ball
rolling around but surprised
when he accidentally makes
it move. By a year, he may be
able to pick it up and throw it.

Pulling up and cruising
At 10 months, your child may
be able to co-ordinate his
arms and legs well enough to
pull himself up on furniture
(clear away anything unstable).
The next stage is to start
shuffling sideways holding
on – known as cruising. He
will probably sit down with
a heavy bump.

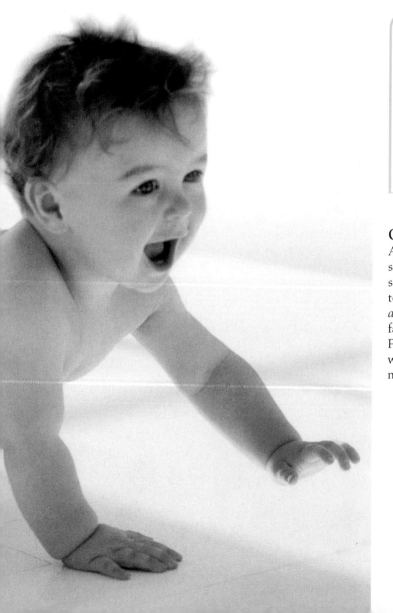

Playpens and babywalkers
A **playpen** can be a useful safe place if you have to leave
your mobile child alone for a few moments – to answer
the door, for example. Never leave him in it for more
than a few minutes as he will get bored and frustrated. A
babywalker is a chair on wheels that your baby can propel
with his feet. The sale of baby walkers has been banned in
Canada since 2007 because of serious injuries. If you have
a baby walker, discard it, removing the wheels first so that
another baby is not injured.

Climbing stairs
As soon as your child
shows interest in the
stairs, for his own safety
teach him how to go up
and down on all fours,
facing into the stairs.
Fit a baby gate for
when you're
not watching.

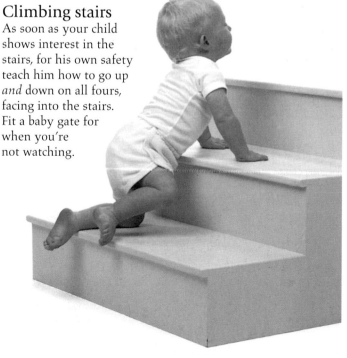

The second year

First steps and first words will probably be your child's most exciting and significant achievements during his second year. Handedness becomes apparent around the middle of this year: he will show a preference for one hand, and once he starts to draw and paint, this will become more marked. Although he'll amuse himself for short periods, you're still his essential and most valued playmate, and his most effective teacher, too.

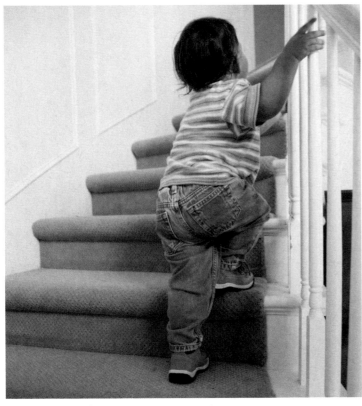

Using stairs

Towards the end of this year, your child may grow confident and skilful enough to go up and down the stairs upright and facing forwards.

Learning to walk

Once your child has taken her first hesitant steps unsupported, it will only be a few days before she's waddling about enthusiastically, though unsteadily. She'll keep her feet wide apart, and her arms out for balance. Let her go barefoot as often as possible: she only needs shoes for walking about outdoors.

First steps will be unsteady

Building a tower
From about 18 months, your child will be able to build a tower of four or even five blocks.

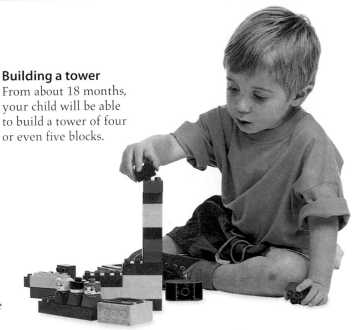

Walking skills
A pull-along toy improves his sense of balance.

Imitating you
Copying you is how your child learns – and "helping" is always a favourite game. Toy tools make it easy for him to join in.

Greater mobility
At around two years, a stable ride-on toy will improve his co-ordination and confidence, and provide a new challenge.

Using crayons
Introduce non-toxic crayons from about 18 months. He'll scribble now; soon he'll make up and down strokes.

Learning shapes
Sorting shapes into their correct holes is a challenging lesson. Give plenty of praise, when he gets it right.

Practising speech
A telephone and doll are two invaluable toys for practising the art of communication by copying what you do.

Learning about himself
Teach your child to point to his eyes, nose, and ears, and see if he can point to yours. It expands his vocabulary, and helps him learn to see himself as a person in his own right.

Learning to talk
Your child will say his first word – probably "dada" or "mama" – sometime around his first birthday, and from then on he may learn roughly two or three new words a month. By the age of two, he may be able to string two words together – "me go," for example – and will have about 200 words in all. You can help him to improve his vocabulary by:
- talking to him
- continuing to include picture books and rhymes in your playtimes
- listening to him, being interested in what he's saying, and trying to understand
- not interrupting him to make him repeat things "properly" – he won't get the pronunciation right at first
- using adult language when you talk back to him, so he can hear the words spoken correctly
- being clear and direct: "Put the brick on the top" is less muddling than "Let's see if we can get this nice red brick on top of the other."

The third year

This year, your child may surprise you with a burgeoning imagination that can make an absorbing game out of anything. Don't waste money on expensive kits and toys that can only stifle his creativity. A big cardboard box makes a house, a car, a boat, a spaceship – then when it gets battered, you can throw it away and get another one (remove any staples). A sheet draped over two chairs is a haven, a tent, a house – anything he can think of. Towards the end of this year, your child might join a playgroup, and start to play with other children in a constructive way. You'll notice that he's becoming open to suggestion and reason when you want him to do things.

Dressing up
The "let's pretend" game is fun at any age. Your old clothes, shoes, handbags, and hats are all ideal items for a dressing-up box, and much more fun to play with than the special child-size outfits available in the toy stores.

Irregular shapes
Jigsaws demand concentration, dexterity, and visual understanding. If he gives up quickly, try giving him a simpler one.

Colour and paint
Painting is a good way to learn about colour and texture. Give him thick brushes and non-spill pots, and protect his clothes.

Imaginary friends
Dolls and teddies will become friends to your girl or boy, and she will want to control their lives in the way you control hers.

Jumping and running
Learning to jump, run, and balance are new physical challenges. Jump with him to show him how to bend his knees as he lands.

Using her hands
Help your child refine her hand movements. She can screw and unscrew small objects now, and will enjoy using pastry cutters to make shapes out of play dough or your pastry.

Playing together
A sandbox is always fun. Show your child how to use buckets and shovels, and teach her not to throw sand. She will soon find her own level of creativity. Cover the box when not in use to stop dogs and cats fouling it.

Sharing and playing
It takes time for children to learn to take turns and share toys. Set your child a good example – it's easiest if he learns to share with you first. Sometime around the age of two and a half to three, your child will start to play *with* other children for the first time, sharing his toys amicably and joining in a common project. This is the ideal age to introduce him to a playgroup: the more your child is with others of his own age, the more quickly and easily he will learn to join in – and to fit in.

You can provide plenty of good play opportunities yourself: a sandbox, a wading pool, interlocking plastic bricks, dressing up, making Christmas decorations – all these are great ways for children to learn to play together constructively. Your supervision is vital throughout the pre-school years, to keep a check on safety or to step in if tempers start to fray.

Games to play with your baby

Most parents realize how important it is to talk to their baby, but not everyone finds it easy to do this without feeling embarrassed or self-conscious. That's one reason why the games that parents traditionally play with their babies are so important. They provide a natural way for you to interact with your baby. Many of them involve simple repetitive rhymes and songs that even a baby quickly learns to recognize and that will help to stimulate his own language development. Here are some favourite games to play with your young child.

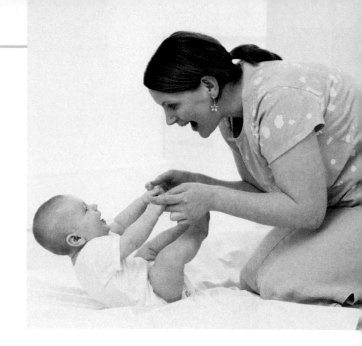

Tickling and touching games

Games that involve you lovingly handling his body are fun for your baby, and you will be surprised at how soon he will learn to understand and respond when you start to play one of them. When you sing "The wheels on the bus," you can involve his whole body, his legs becoming the wheels, his arms the opening and closing doors, and the wipers. He will enjoy having his toes wiggled in "This little piggy," and having you lightly run your fingers from his toes to his head for "All the way home." In games such as "Round and round the garden," and "There was a little mouse that lived just there," he will be overcome with excitement at anticipation of the tickly ending.

Hiding and finding games

Search-and-find games can be fascinating from babyhood right through to primary school age. A baby's first "treasure hunt" is to see you hide one of his toys under a blanket or towel right in front of him, and then, when you say "Where did the toy go?" make the discovery that the hidden toy is actually still there, under the blanket. You can step up the excitement by using three towels – which one is the toy under? To find it, your baby has to follow rudimentary rules – the toy is under a towel, not somewhere else quite different – and to remember under which towel his toy has gone.

"Peek-a-boo" is an immensely popular variation on this. The surprise of seeing your face dip out of sight and then come back into view can send your little one squealing with pleasure. You can try playing it with your baby in a "jolly jumper": as he twirls around you'll disappear, then he'll shout delightedly as he bounces around to face you again. And even if your baby loved it when he was only six months old, he will still enjoy variations on this search-and-find game later on. As he grows older, he'll imitate you and may "hide" from you behind his hands or under a towel. He'll pass through a stage where he thinks you can't see him simply because he can't see you. This is normal and can be fun when you turn it into a game.

Activity games

Games that involve bouncing on a parent's knee, such as "Yankee Doodle went to town" and "This is the way the ladies ride," can be as boisterous or as gentle as the baby's age and temperament dictate. Your baby will very quickly learn to indicate when she wants to do it again – and when she has had enough. Remember to give her some time to relax after a boisterous game by cuddling her quietly.

Singing and language games

Nursery rhymes and songs are part of your child's heritage. A few of the many excellent CDs of music and songs for small children are invaluable on car journeys. Best of all though is to sing to your baby yourself. All babies seem to love being sung to. Singing lullabies to your baby, such as "Twinkle, twinkle little star" and "Rock-a-bye baby," can help soothe her. She will enjoy the rhythm and rhymes of these and other lullabies. In finger play songs, such as "Eensy Weensy Spider," the action of your hands can reinforce the meaning of the songs and help your baby to remember them.

Songs are one of the best ways to encourage your baby's language development and help her to understand and identify the world around her. "This little piggy" for example, explores the concepts of going and coming, and opposites ("went to market," "stayed at home," "had roast beef," "had none"). "Old McDonald had a farm" will teach her about animals and animal noises.

In her third and fourth years, your child will start to appreciate rhyming and nonsense rhymes. You can reduce her to helpless laughter with your own nonsense variation on a song she knows well ("Hickory dickory dee, The mouse ran up the tree...") and you will find she will very soon start imitating you and making up her own versions.

Playing catch

All children seem to love a game of simple catch. Sit down on the floor, with your baby directly opposite to you, and gently roll a soft ball or wheeled toy towards him. He may pick the toy up and want to return it to you. Alternatively, he may simply want to hold the toy and examine, or even chew it. He may puzzle you by holding out the toy for you to take and then pull it back again. This is quite common – although he's learned to grasp something, he may not yet have learnt to let it go. Don't try to pull the toy away from him. Just tell him what a nice toy it is, and keep on chatting to him.

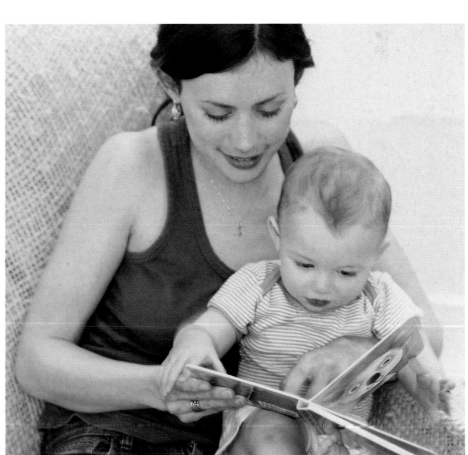

Reading

Your baby will like to have you read to him long before he has any idea of what reading is all about. He will enjoy the physical closeness as he sits on your knee, and is cuddled. Your baby will like the sound of your voice as you talk to him about the pictures in the book. He will like the bright colours of the pictures themselves. To begin with, reading is just another opportunity for you to spend time with your baby and talk to him. But eventually, he will understand what it is you are talking about.

Becoming a person

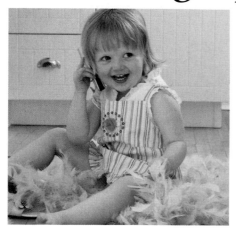

Your baby soon shows her own particular temperament, but her personality is also shaped by your responsiveness. Showing her how special she is to you, and treating her as an individual with her own wishes will help her become confident. Toddlers are easily frustrated, and at times you will need all your tact to help her without making her feel that you're taking over. Watching as she explores and discovers the world around her should make these pre-school years enormously rewarding for you.

Getting along together

Learning to get along well together in pre-school years is a process of adjustment for both of you. Your child has to learn the boundaries of acceptable behaviour, while you may have to adapt your own natural style as a parent, which may not always make you tolerant, consistent, and fair. Your child needs you to show her, not just tell her, how to behave well. Thoughtfulness, politeness, and kindness – all this she will only learn by copying you, when you show the same behaviour to her.

How to handle your child

Your child will respond best to you and do as you say more willingly if you can be both affectionate and firm. It isn't easy to get the balance right.

● Be consistent in what you say and do. If your child is spanked when she is naughty, she will hit other children when she is cross with them.

● "Dos" work better than "Don'ts." "Hang your coat up so no one will step on it," elicits a more positive response than "Don't drop your coat on the floor."

● Say please and thank you, when you ask her to do something.

● Agree with your partner about what you will allow, and back each other up.

● Try to persuade rather than coerce. If she's in the middle of some absorbing activity, try telling her "Let's finish this, and then it'll be time to go to bed," rather than "Clear away those toys, now it's bedtime."

● Don't be too restrictive. Try listening to the way you talk to your child. Do you find you're nearly always issuing orders: "Stop that," "Do as you're told," "Don't touch"?

● If you were unreasonable over something, say so, and apologize.

● Don't assert your authority unnecessarily – avoid a clash of wills.

● Always explain *why* she mustn't do something as well as *what* she mustn't do, even if she's too young to understand.

Learning for herself
Give your child help when she needs it, but don't take over – it's her toy, and she needs to feel she can succeed.

Rules to keep your child safe

Until your child has reached at least two and a half, you can't expect her to understand reasons for not doing things, nor to remember what she mustn't do. It's your responsibility to make sure her curiosity can't lead her into much danger, and that the important rules are enforced.

For example, "You must never go out of the yard on your own" is an abstract rule that your toddler cannot comprehend, much less remember when she's busy playing or absorbed in her toys. You can only keep an eye on her, and make sure that she doesn't stray out by putting a secure latch on the garden gate.

According to research, fire, falls, poisoning, and strangulation pose the biggest risk to children. Childproof your home to minimize any dangers. Make sure smoke and carbon monoxide detectors are installed and regularly tested. Remove toys from the stairway, and install a baby gate and a handrail by the stairs. Never hang toys on your baby's stroller or crib where she can reach them, don't let electrical cords trail, and put covers over electrical sockets. A baby gate across the kitchen door may be the best way to keep her safe when you're cooking.

Loving and spoiling

You may worry that the normal affection you give your child will spoil him. It won't. He needs your love, combined with plenty of attention. But you can spoil him by being over-lenient when he misbehaves. Letting him get his own way through tears and tantrums will not help him in his relations with friends and adults.

If you go out to work, you may find yourself "making it up" to your child for not being there by lavishing toys on him. Toys can't take your place, and you may be giving him unrealistic expectations of what you can afford. Instead, when you can be around, give him your time, your love, and plenty of attention.

Showing your love
Your child will prefer your love and attention to any toys. Don't worry about spoiling him with love – you can't.

Developing a sense of identity

At around the age of 18 months or so, your child begins to realize that he is a separate person. He will start to refer to himself by name, and he will enjoy looking at photos of himself, too. From now on, he will want to take charge of his life more and more, and assert his own wishes and personality. You can help him foster this determination to do things for himself and nurture his burgeoning sense of identity.

Encouraging independence

● Make things easy. From age two onwards, organize his possessions, so that he can do as much as possible for himself. Buy clothes that are easy to manage, so he can dress and undress himself as much as possible; put a step by the sink so he can wash his hands without your help; and install a low peg so he can hang up his own coat.
● Encourage him to help you. "Helping" is a game at the moment, not a chore. Simple jobs, like unpacking the shopping or setting the table, make your child feel he's achieved something, and show him that helping is part of family life.
● Let him make his own decisions. The opportunity to make simple decisions gives your child the feeling that he has some control over his own life. So let him choose which T-shirt he wants to wear, or how his room is arranged, or where he'd like to go for a walk.

Helping your child to feel special

Your child, just like every child, needs to feel that he's special – that you love him and that he is worth loving. It's this message that helps to make him emotionally strong and able to cope away from the security of home. There are plenty of little ways you can show how special he is to you:
● Don't forget to say you love him, or be too busy to give a hug or a cuddle when he wants one.
● Respect his feelings and respond to his needs. When he's miserable, he needs to cry and be comforted. Saying "Don't be a crybaby" is denying him the right to feel sad.
● Praise him and be enthusiastic about each fresh achievement.
● Listen and show interest when he talks to you.

Becoming a person
Try to appreciate your toddler for the lively, fascinating, and independent individual he is fast becoming.

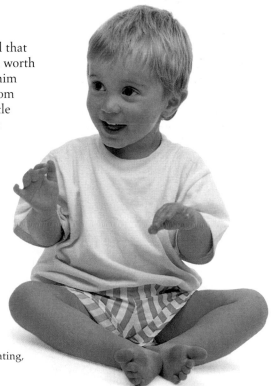

Good and bad behaviour

When they are well and happy, children usually behave acceptably. But every child has off-days, and every child wants to test her limits – and yours – by seeing how far she can go. Bad behaviour is often an effective way of gaining your attention, too. The time of greatest conflict will probably come at some stage during her third year: tears and tantrums often go hand in hand with being two years old.

Dealing with bad behaviour

Act quickly, pick your child up and remove her from the source of the trouble with a firm "NO." At the same time, distract her attention with some other activity or toy.

Most types of bad behaviour, tantrums, fussing, and whining for example, are simply best ignored. If your child never manages to elicit a response from you, and is never allowed to win any arguments by such behaviour, she will soon stop. Just be calm, and carry on as normal. If necessary, put her outside the room until she calms down.

Rewards for good behaviour

It's very easy to give your child more attention when she behaves badly, and less when she behaves well and you feel you can relax. But rewarding your child with praise, affection, or a story on your lap when she behaves well is much more effective. You will encourage the behaviour you want, and teach her a very useful lesson in life – that being nice to people works much better than being nasty.

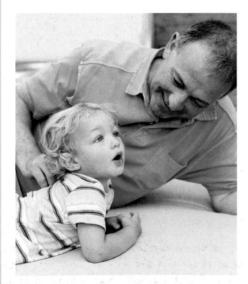

Appreciate good behaviour
Make sure you recognize and praise your child's good behaviour.

Consequences for bad behaviour

Whatever consequence you decide upon, it has to be immediate if it is to have any effect on your toddler. Threats of future action, perhaps the withdrawal of treats and privileges, are useless and unfair for young children. Your child will not be able to understand why she is having this delayed consequence. You and your partner also need to be unanimous in carrying out the consequence – it will confuse your toddler if you contradict each other.

An immediate consequence that your child *will* understand is to be isolated for a short time to cool off. A quarter of an hour spent somewhere safe but alone – the hall is often suitable – will be long enough for her to forget whatever it was that she wanted to do, and give you time to cool down as well.

Should I spank my child?

Do not spank or hit your child. It's not a good way to deal with bad behaviour. What is more, you are teaching her that physical force is an acceptable way to make people do what you want. You must learn other ways to discipline your child.

How to avoid getting to the end of your rope

However clever you become at managing your child, there will always be days when her behaviour seems completely unbearable, and you know you are close to losing control.

The solution is simple: take your child out. Whatever the weather, a trip to the park, the shops, or a friend's house will distract both of you from your respective moods, and help you recover your sanity and sense of humour.

Being firm

You needn't be angry or upset when you discipline your child, just consistent, so your child gets the clear message that she's not allowed to behave in that way.

Dealing with aggressive children

All small children fight occasionally, especially when they are bored or tired. When the fights get out of hand, step in quickly:
● separate the fighting children immediately
● distract them by introducing some other game or a change of scene
● don't take sides – it's nearly always impossible to work out the rights and wrongs of any situation.

If your child bites another child:
● give all your attention and concern to the bitten child
● remove the biter immediately, and put her somewhere else, safe but alone, for a few minutes.

Your child is bound to snatch and grab when she first starts to play with other children, but with help from you she will soon learn to share. It helps to get your child used to being with other children from an early age, so ask your doctor or other parents about local toddler groups, where your child can meet and interact with other children of her age. A few children will continue to be very rough and aggressive, and their behaviour will eventually make them unpopular. For your child's sake, help her to be gentle with others:
● give her a good model to follow by always trying to be gentle, patient, and loving towards her
● make it clear through the way you act that it's your child's behaviour you dislike, not her
● always step in and stop your child immediately if she starts to hit another child; be firm, but don't shout or be aggressive yourself
● never let her get her own way by behaving aggressively or unpleasantly.

If your child's behaviour continues to worry you, and you can't seem to find a way to deal with it, seek advice from your doctor or nurse.

Childhood habits

Many small children develop habits such as thumb-sucking, head-banging, breath-holding, hair-twirling and pulling, nose-picking, and nail-biting, which they resort to usually when they are angry, frustrated, bored, or simply in need of comfort. These habits are common and harmless, but they often worry parents. Although children usually grow out of them by the time they are four, sometimes they can be hard to break.

Thumb-sucking and pacifiers

About half of three year olds suck their thumbs, and a few still do so when they are six or seven. Persistent thumb-suckers may gradually push their front teeth forwards. However, unless the habit continues after the age of six, when the second set of teeth come in, the distortion won't be permanent. Sucking on a pacifiers is less likely to distort the teeth, so if your baby shows signs of being a habitual thumb-sucker, it might be worth offering her a pacifier as an alternative.

Head-banging, rolling, and rocking

Some time in their first year, many children develop a habit of rocking rhythmically on all fours in their crib, rolling their heads from side to side, or banging their heads on the head-board. Usually they'll do this as they are going off to sleep or as they wake up, and often the rocking is violent enough to move the crib across the floor. Although this is alarming to watch, and to listen to, you really do not need to worry about it. Infants and young toddlers who do this seldom hurt themselves, although they may damage the furniture. These rhythmic behaviours nearly always disappear by the time the child is three or four.

Some toddlers develop an equally worrying habit of banging their head on a hard surface during the day, usually to express frustration or boredom. Again, the child won't hurt herself, apart from the odd bruise. It's usually best to take no notice, although you may want to offer the child a pillow to soften the impact. If you ignore the habit, it will eventually disappear.

Head-banging or rocking that starts in older children, or persists after the age of four, needs to be taken more seriously. Discuss with your doctor; it may mean that your child has some emotional problem.

Breath-holding attacks

A few young children deal with pain or frustration by holding their breath. They may do this for up to half a minute, and sometimes they will even pass out. Immediately when this happens, the child automatically starts to breathe again, and no harm is done; but the child quickly discovers this is a splendid way to gain attention. Ignore the attacks as much as possible, and they will probably have stopped by the time your child is four.

Hold on to his security blanket

Even when your child seems to have outgrown his security blanket, hold on to it – he may be happy to have it back when he is stressed or ill.

Sucking a thumb or cuddly blanket can be a source of comfort

Thumb-sucking
Many toddlers suck their thumbs. Try to discourage the habit once the second set of teeth have come through.

"Bad dreams" and night terrors

Even a child as young as one year old may have nightmares about something that has frightened her during the day, even though she doesn't yet understand what a dream is, and certainly couldn't tell you about it. If a very young child wakes from a nightmare, simply cuddle and comfort her until she calms down.

By the time she is two years old she may try to tell you about it, and you can reassure her that it was "only a dream," although she won't yet really understand this concept. By three or four, she will have a much better idea of what is "real" and "not real." But she will still need you to soothe her fears and make it clear that you won't let anything bad happen to her. It may reassure her to have a night-light in her room, and for the door to be left ajar.

A few children, however, have night terrors, which are quite different from nightmares. Nightmares usually occur in the second half of the night when the child is sleeping lightly, and dreams are at their most plentiful. A night terror will start much earlier, usually between one and four hours after the child has gone to sleep, when she is sleeping very deeply. You will hear your child screaming or moaning as if in terror, but when you rush in to her, she won't seem to recognize you, may push you away, and scream even more if you try to hold her. This is because she is not properly awake, and if left alone will quite quickly go back to sleep. So don't try to wake her or even hold her. Simply wait beside her so that you're there if she does wake. In the morning, she will have no memory of what happened, and be none the worse for it.

your **child's health**

Everything you need to know to recognize and treat common childhood illnesses, plus a guide to first aid.

The first three months

Babies are born with natural immunity which protects them against many infections for about six months. But for the first three months, it's best to seek medical help immediately if you think your baby is ill. The symptoms listed here relate to the most common health problems that affect babies under three months, and will guide you to the relevant section (see pages 182–5). Pages 186–7 cover illnesses for children of all ages. Remember, however, that only a doctor can give you a definite diagnosis.

Emergency

Call for an ambulance or go to the nearest hospital emergency department if your baby:
- brings up green vomit
- has a body temperature higher than 39°C (102.2°F) for more than half an hour
- vomits AND cries uncontrollably as if in great pain
- is breathing very noisily or rapidly
- has a taut, bulging fontanelle when he isn't crying

Fontanelle

- has purple spots on his skin that don't fade if glass is pressed against it
- passes stools containing blood and mucus, which resemble redcurrant jelly.

Loss of appetite

If your baby does not want to feed, but seems generally contented and well, there is no need to worry. If he refuses two feeds in succession, or does not demand a feed for six hours, **call your doctor now.**

☎ Seek medical help

Call your doctor now if your baby seems unwell or shows one of these symptoms:
- cries more than usual, or his crying sounds different from usual over a period of about an hour
- seems abnormally listless, quiet, or drowsy
- refuses two successive feeds, or does not demand a feed for more than six hours
- seems particularly irritable or restless.

Crying

If you fail to calm your baby after an hour or so, or if his crying sounds unusual, **call your doctor.** If your baby cries inconsolably for two or three hours at about the same time each day, but shows no other signs of illness, he might have colic (see page 118). This may continue for several weeks, but will resolve itself without any treatment.

Slow weight gain

If your baby does not seem to be gaining weight at the normal rate (see charts on pages 254–7), consult your doctor or nurse practitioner. Occasionally an underlying illness can make a baby grow more slowly than normal.

Premature babies

Babies who were very small at birth, or who were born a month or more before their due date, are more vulnerable to infections during their first weeks. Until your baby is older and has put on weight, try to keep him away from anyone who has a cough or cold, and, if possible, don't take him into public places for the first two or three months.

Cold hands and feet, *see Chilling (page 184)*

Areas of dry, flaking skin *mean that your baby's skin needs moisturizing, so avoid soap and rub a little baby moisturizer into the dry areas*

Tears from one or both eyes *even when your baby isn't crying: this happens when the tear duct has not opened completely, so his tears can't drain away. It is quite common, and usually corrects itself by the time the baby is a year old. Consult your doctor if it continues beyond this age*

Vomiting, see page 185

Red blotches with a tiny red centre, *see Spots and rashes (page 182)*

Brown, scaly patches on the head, *see Cradle cap (page 183)*

Pus *in the inner corner of the eye, or eyelashes gummed together after sleep, see* Sticky eye *(page 183)*

Tiny white spots, *usually on the nose or cheeks: these are called milk spots or milia. Many babies develop them during the first few weeks of life. They need no treatment, although they may last for several weeks*

Hot, flushed, damp skin, *especially on the neck or chest, see* Overheating *(page 184)*

Hiccups, *particularly after feeding: these are nothing to worry about, and will go without any treatment*

Painless bulge around the navel *that increases in size when your baby coughs, sneezes, or cries: this is a hernia, and is caused by a weakness in the abdominal wall. It will probably disappear without any treatment within a year*

Diarrhea, see page 185

Redness or rash *around the genitals, see* Diaper rash *(page 182)*

Spots and rashes

What are they?

Many newborn babies go through a spotty stage in the first few weeks, so don't worry unnecessarily if your baby develops a few spots – they don't usually mean that she is ill in any way. One of the most common rashes in young babies is called newborn urticaria (erythema toxicum). Newborn urticaria usually appears during the first week of your baby's life, and will generally disappear without any treatment.

What can I do?

If your baby has newborn urticaria (see symptoms box), simply ignore the spots. Unlike urticaria in older children, which may require treatment, newborn urticaria will disappear on its own within two weeks, so it is not necessary to put any lotions or creams on the spots. Don't be tempted to alter your baby's feeds in any way – the spots are not due to milk disagreeing with her.

Symptoms

- Red blotches with a tiny red centre, which come and go on different parts of the baby's body, and last only a few hours.

☎ Seek medical help

Call your doctor now if the spots are flat, pink, dark red, or purplish (a petechial rash). Consult your doctor as soon as possible if:
- a spot has developed a pus-filled centre
- you think a spot has become infected.

Diaper rash

What is it?

Diaper rash is an inflammation of the skin on a baby's bottom. It may occur if your baby has been left in a dirty diaper for too long, because as urine and feces are broken down ammonia is released, which burns and irritates her skin. It can also be due to an allergy to detergent used when washing cloth diapers. A similar-looking rash may be caused by a yeast infection, which can affect the mouth (see Thrush, page 213), as well as the diaper area. Yeast rashes usually start in the creases at the top of the legs.

Symptoms

- Red, spotty, sore-looking skin in the diaper area
- smell of ammonia.

What can I do?

1 Change your baby's diaper frequently, and clean and dry her bottom thoroughly at each change (see pages 150–1). Inside cloth diapers, use an extra-absorbent type of liner.

2 Whenever possible, let your baby lie on a diaper with her bottom exposed to the air. Don't use plastic pants or wraps over cloth diapers until the rash subsides, because these prevent air circulating to her bottom.

3 Look for white patches inside your baby's mouth. If you see any, she may have an oral yeast infection called thrush (see page 213).

4 Don't use harsh detergents or fabric softener to wash her diapers, as they can trigger an allergy. Rinse her diapers thoroughly.

5 Use a diaper rash cream (available at the pharmacy), and apply it when you change your baby's diaper, to soothe and heal the skin.

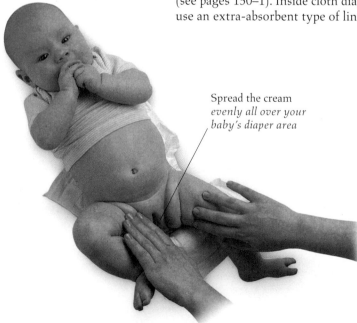

Spread the cream *evenly all over your baby's diaper area*

☎ Seek medical help

Consult your doctor as soon as possible if:
- the rash lasts several days
- you think your baby has yeast.

What might the doctor do?

The doctor may prescribe an antibiotic cream if the rash is infected, or an anti-fungal cream if your baby has a yeast infection.

Cradle cap

What is it?
Thick, brownish, crusty patches on a baby's scalp are known as cradle cap. Sometimes it may spread to the baby's face, body, or diaper area, producing a red scaly rash. Although it looks unsightly, cradle cap is harmless and doesn't seem to distress the baby. It generally clears up by the age of about two years.

Symptoms

- Brownish, scaly patches on the scalp.

☎ Seek medical help
Consult your doctor as soon as possible if the rash spreads and:
- seems to irritate your baby
- looks infected or begins to ooze
- does not clear up after five days.

What can I do?

1 Rub the cradle cap scales on your baby's head with baby or olive oil to soften them. Leave the oil on for 12 to 24 hours, then brush your baby's hair gently to loosen the scales. Finally, wash her hair – most of the scales should simply wash away.

2 If the rash spreads, keep the affected areas clean and dry. Don't use soap, baby lotion, or baby bath liquid.

What might the doctor do?
If the condition persists, or if the rash looks infected or starts to ooze, your doctor may prescribe an ointment to be rubbed gently on the area.

Sticky eye

What is it?
This is a very common mild eye infection. If your baby develops any of these symptoms after she is two days old, she may have conjunctivitis (see page 209) or a blocked tear duct.

Symptoms

- Eyelashes gummed after sleep
- pus in the corner of the eye.

☎ Seek medical help
Call your doctor now if your baby has a bad discharge of yellow pus. **Consult your doctor as soon as possible** if:
- your baby develops symptoms of sticky eye after first two days of life
- it does not clear up after three days.

What can I do?
Clean your baby's eyes twice a day with a cotton ball dipped in warm boiled water. Wipe outwards from the inner corner of her eye, and use a fresh cotton ball for each eye.

What might the doctor do?
If the doctor thinks your baby has conjunctivitis, he may, in some cases, prescribe antibiotic eye drops.

To administer eye drops
Swaddle your baby in a blanket with her arms inside and hold her on your lap in the crook of your arm, or ask someone to hold her for you. Apply the drops to the inner corner of her eye. You can also place the drops in the inner corner of her eyes, with her head held central, and wait for her to open her eyes spontaneously. The drops will then roll into her eyes.

Chilling

Why are babies at risk?
For the first few weeks of his life, your baby will be unable to regulate his body temperature very efficiently. If he becomes too cold, his body temperature will drop and he may become dangerously chilled quite quickly. Babies who were born prematurely are particularly vulnerable to this.

Symptoms
First signs
- Crying and restless behaviour
- cold hands and feet.

Signs of serious chilling
- Quiet and listless behaviour as the baby gets colder
- cool skin on chest and stomach
- pink and flushed face, hands, and feet.

☎ Seek medical help
Call your doctor now if your baby:
- shows signs of serious chilling
- has a body temperature below 35°C (95°F).

What can I do?

1 Warm your baby up by taking him into a heated room and feeding him. Once he has become chilled, it doesn't help just to pile on extra clothes or blankets.

2 Take your baby's temperature (see page 193). If it is below 35°C (95°F), he is dangerously chilled, so **call for an ambulance immediately**.

How can I prevent chilling?
Keep the room your baby sleeps in at about 16–20°C (65–68°F). When you undress and bathe him, the room should be warmer still. Be sensible about taking your child out in cold weather – wrap him up well, and don't stay out for too long. Make sure his head, hands, and feet are well covered; particularly his head, as a lot of body heat is lost through the head. Never leave him to sleep outside in his carriage on a cold day. Dress your baby according to the temperature of the environment, and adjust his clothes as the temperature changes.

Put a hat under the hood to keep his head warm

In cold weather
Dress your baby in an all-in-one outdoor suit, or wrap a shawl over his other clothes, and use mittens and booties. Keep an eye on him to make sure he's not getting too hot.

Overheating

Why are babies at risk?
Overheating is as dangerous for young babies as chilling, especially if they are feverish or unwell. Overwrapping of babies at night is thought to be one of the factors that contributes to crib death (see page 123).

What can I do?

1 Take your baby to a cooler place and remove a layer of clothing.

2 Take your baby's temperature (see page 193) and, if it is raised, offer him plenty of fluids to prevent dehydration.

Symptoms
- Restless behaviour
- hot, sweaty skin
- raised temperature.

How can I prevent overheating?
Dress your baby according to the weather. On very hot days, he can sleep in just a diaper and an undershirt, but always remember the danger of chilling (see above). Never leave him to sleep in the sun; his skin will burn easily. Provide shade, and check him frequently as the sun moves around.

☎ Seek medical help
Call your doctor if your baby's temperature does not return to normal within one hour.

Vomiting

Why do babies vomit?
All babies regurgitate a small amount of milk during or just after a feed, usually due to gas. This regurgitation is perfectly normal, and does not mean that your baby is ill, but until you are used to it, you may think that he is vomiting. If your baby vomits, he will bring up most of his feed. This is less likely to happen in a breastfed baby.

Frequent vomiting, especially if your baby also has diarrhea, may be caused by gastroenteritis (see page 222). This is extremely serious in a young baby because the loss of fluids can make him dehydrated very quickly.

Forceful vomiting
Sometimes a baby vomits with great force, so that the vomit shoots across the room. If your baby does this at two successive feeds, **consult your doctor as soon as possible.** The most likely reason is that he has brought back part of his feed with a large burp of gas. However, if it happens after every feed, especially if he is hungry all the time, he may have a condition called pyloric stenosis, in which the outlet from the stomach becomes blocked – if your baby has this, he will need a simple operation to treat the problem.

What can I do?
Continue to feed your baby as usual, but to replace fluids lost through vomiting, start by giving him small, frequent drinks of cooled, boiled water. A preferable fluid replacement is an oral rehydration solution (ORS) that is suitable for babies. This can be obtained at the pharmacy and must be mixed precisely according to the manufacturer's instructions. Do not make it up any stronger or weaker. Don't attempt to make your own rehydration solution from salt and sugar at home. Your baby may initially refuse the water or oral rehydration solution, so be persistent.

If your baby is vomiting, and is not keeping fluids down, see your doctor urgently. Although vomiting and diarrhea are not often dangerous in adults and older children, they can cause a young baby to become dehydrated very quickly and so require prompt attention. Don't give your baby any anti-nausea medications, or change your baby's formula unless your doctor has advised it. Breastfed babies should continue to be breastfed.

☎ Seek medical help
Call your doctor now if:
● your baby vomits and shows any other signs of illness
● your baby vomits the whole of two successive feedings.

Emergency
Call for emergency help immediately if your baby:
● vomits all his feeds in an eight-hour period
● has a dry mouth and lips
● has a dry diaper for more than six hours
● brings up green vomit
● has sunken eyes or a sunken fontanelle
● is abnormally drowsy.

What might the doctor do?
The doctor may prescribe a powder to be mixed with water for your baby to drink. If your baby has lost a lot of body fluid, the doctor might send him to hospital, where he may be given liquid intravenously.

How can I prevent an upset stomach?
If you are bottle-feeding your baby, sterilize all the feeding equipment, and throw away any unfinished feeds. When making up feeds, cool them quickly under cold running water and store in the fridge. Never keep a feed warm for a long period.

Diarrhea

What is it?
Until babies start eating solid food, they will usually pass fairly runny stools a few times a day. If your baby passes watery, and possibly greenish, stools frequently, he has diarrhea. This is a serious condition in a young baby, since there is an increased danger that he may become dehydrated quite quickly.

What can I do?
It is important to prevent your baby from becoming dehydrated, so make sure that he has plenty to drink. Offer your baby cooled, boiled water between his normal feeds.

If you are concerned that your baby is becoming dehydrated despite your efforts to get him to drink, contact your doctor immediately.

☎ Seek medical help
Call your doctor now if your baby has fever or is passing blood in the stool, or has had diarrhea for six hours **and** other symptoms, or if diarrhea lasts more than 24 hours, or if he may be dehydrated (see emergency box, above).

Diagnosis guide

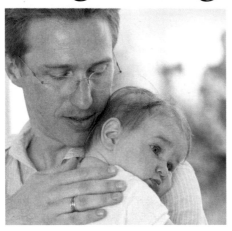

If your child is unwell, try to identify her symptoms by referring to the guide below. If she has more than one symptom, look up the most severe one. This gives you a possible diagnosis and refers you to a section covering the complaint, which contains a brief explanation of the nature of the illness, with information about how you can help your child, and advice on whether you need to call a doctor. Bear in mind that only a doctor can give an accurate diagnosis.

General symptoms of illnesses

All children suffer from minor illnesses at some stage. The following are the most common symptoms babies and young children develop when they are ill.

Fever (see page 192)
A raised temperature (fever) may mean that your child has an infection, so you should check for other signs of illness. However, healthy children may get a slight fever during energetic play or in very hot weather, so check your child's temperature again after she has rested for about half an hour. If it is still over 38°C (100.4°F), she may have an infection.

Changed behaviour
If your child is less lively than usual, more irritable, whiny, or simply unhappy, she may be ill.

Unusual paleness
If your child looks much paler than usual, she may be ill.

Hot, flushed face
This may be a sign of a fever.

Loss of appetite
Although a child's appetite varies from meal to meal, a sudden loss of appetite may be a sign of illness. If your baby is under six months old and has refused two successive feeds, **call your doctor now.** If your older child goes off her food for more than 24 hours, look for other signs of illness (see chart).

Part of body	Symptoms	Page reference
Eyes and ears	• Eyes looking in different directions	See "Strabismus" p.210
	• Red, sore, or sticky eyes or eyelids	See "Eye problems" pp.209–10
	• Itchy eyes, especially if accompanied by runny nose or sneezing	See "Colds and flu" pp.200–1
	• Aversion to bright light, especially if accompanied by fever, headache, and stiff neck	See "Meningitis" p.208
	• Earache, partial deafness, discharge from ears, itchy ears	See "Ear problems" pp.211–12

Part of body	Symptoms	Page reference
Skin, hair, and teeth	● Sore mouth ● Itchy head or tiny white grains in the hair ● Red lump, perhaps with pus-filled centre ● Red raw skin ● Spots or rash ● Spots or rash accompanied by sore throat or fever ● White or brown lump on sole of foot/dry, painless lump anywhere on the body ● Red, tender skin ● Areas of very itchy, dry, red, scaly skin ● Sore around the mouth	See "Thrush" p.213 See "Head lice" p.232 See "Spots and boils" p.226 See "Chapped skin" p.229 See "Skin problems" pp.226–32 or "Insect stings" p.252 See "Infectious illnesses" pp.203–8 See "Warts" p.230 See "Sunburn" p.229 or "Burns and scalds" p.245 See "Eczema" p.228 See "Cold sores" p.230 or "Impetigo" p.231
Brain and nerves	● Momentary lapses of attention ● Loss of consciousness, combined with stiffness and twitching movements	See "Epilepsy" p.233 See "Epilepsy" p.233
Bones, muscles, and joints	● Puffy face, swollen glands at the angle of the jaw-bone and on the side of the neck ● Stiff neck accompanied by fever and headache	See "Mumps" p.206 See "Meningitis" p.208
Lungs and airways	● Runny or blocked nose, sneezing ● Swollen glands accompanied by sore throat ● Sore throat ● Sore throat accompanied by fever and general illness ● Sore throat accompanied by a rash ● Sore throat accompanied by puffy face ● Breathing difficulty, wheezing, rapid breathing ● Whooping cough	See "Colds and flu" pp.200–1 See "Tonsillitis" p.214 or "German measles" p.203 See "Throat infections" p.214 See "Colds and flu" pp.200–1 See "German measles" p.203 See "Mumps" p.206 See "Coughs and chest infections" pp.215–9 See "Whooping cough" p.207
Digestive organs	● Stomach pain ● Stomach pain accompanied by nausea, vomiting, or diarrhea ● Abnormal-looking stools ● Diarrhea ● Constipation ● Intense itching around the anus ● Vomiting or nausea ● Vomiting with great force	See "Dealing with a stomach ache" p.220 See "Gastroenteritis" p.222 See "Diarrhea" p.223 See "Diarrhea" p.223 See "Constipation" p.221 See "Pinworms" p.232 See "Vomiting" p.222 See "Forceful vomiting" p.185
Urinary organs	● Pain when urinating, odd-coloured urine, frequent urination ● Sore tip of penis/painless bulge in the groin or scrotum ● Intense itching around the vagina ● Soreness, itching, or redness around the vagina, vaginal discharge	See "Urinary system infections" p.224 See "Genital problems in boys" p.225 See "Pinworms" p.232 See "Genital problems in girls" p.225

First signs of illness

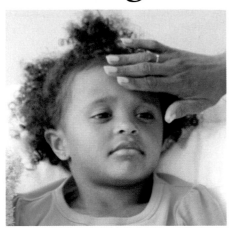

Even if your child has no definite symptoms, you will probably know when she is not feeling her best. She may look pale, be more clingy than usual, cry or whine, or seem very irritable. She may be off her food. When your baby is teething, don't assume that the symptoms are due to this. All symptoms should be taken seriously in a baby under a year old – babies can become ill very quickly. If your child is over a year old, keep a check on how her symptoms progress over the next few hours.

Calling the doctor

If you think you know what is wrong with your child, read the relevant section among complaints covered on pages 200–33. This advises you whether you need to call the doctor. As a general rule, the younger the child, the more quickly she should be seen by a doctor. If you are unsure what to do, phone your doctor and describe your child's symptoms to him, and tell him her age. The doctor will tell you what to do, and will know whether your child needs medical attention.

Don't ever hesitate to call your doctor, even if you are not absolutely sure that something is wrong. Trust your instincts and get advice when you need it.

Degree of urgency

Whenever you are instructed to call the doctor, you will be told how quickly your child needs medical help.
- **Call for emergency help immediately:** this is a life-threatening emergency. So call 911 for an ambulance, or go to the nearest hospital emergency department.
- **Call your doctor now:** your child needs medical help now, so contact your doctor immediately, even if it is the middle of the night. If you can't reach him, call for emergency help.
- **Consult your doctor as soon as possible:** your child needs to be seen by a doctor within the next 24 hours.
- **Consult your doctor:** your child should be seen by a doctor within the next few days.

Feeling unwell
Your child may become more clingy, and demand extra attention when she is ill.

Symptoms

The most common early symptoms of illness in children are:
- raised temperature – 38°C (100.4°F) or more
- crying and irritability
- vomiting or diarrhea
- refusal to eat or drink
- sore or red throat
- rash
- swollen glands in the neck or behind the jaw.

Emergency

Call for emergency help immediately if your child:
- is breathing very noisily, rapidly, or with difficulty
- has a convulsion
- loses consciousness after a fall
- is in severe, persistent pain
- has a fever and is unusually irritable or drowsy
- has a rash of flat, dark red or purplish blood-spots (petechial rash)
- screams with pain and turns pale when he screams.

Checking for symptoms

What can I do?

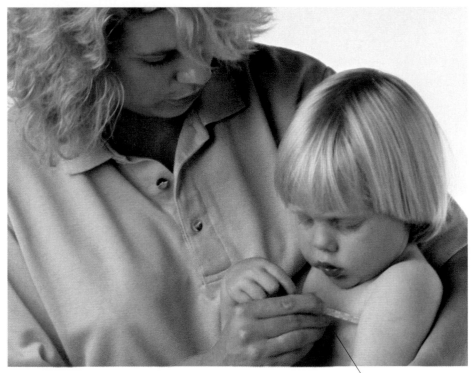

1 If you think your child is feeling unwell, or if he looks as though he has a fever, take his temperature with an aural or digital thermometer (see page 193). A temperature of 38°C (100.4°F) or above can be a symptom of illness.

Tuck the end *of the digital thermometer into your child's armpit*

"Is my child in pain?"

Q&A

If your baby is in pain, his crying may sound quite different from normal. When a baby or a small child cries or complains of pain, it can be difficult to discover where the pain is, and even more difficult to ascertain how bad it might be.

Serious pain will affect your child's behaviour, so watch him to find out how severe his pain is. Does it make him cry or stop him sleeping, eating, or playing? Does his face look drawn or has his colour changed? Would you know that he had a pain even if he didn't tell you? If not, his pain probably isn't too severe.

If your child is in pain, give him the recommended dose of acetaminophen syrup or ibuprofen suspension (not aspirin). Consult your doctor if the pain continues.

2 Check whether your child's throat is inflamed or infected, but don't try to examine the throat of a baby under a year old. Ask your child to face a strong light and open his mouth. If his throat looks red or has creamy spots, he has a sore throat (see Throat infections, page 214).

3 Feel gently along your child's jawbone and down either side of the back of his neck. If you can feel tiny lumps under the skin, or if any of these areas seem swollen or tender, your child has swollen glands, which is a common sign of illness.

4 Check to see whether your child has a rash, particularly on his chest and behind his ears – the most common areas for a rash to start. If he has a rash and a fever, he may have one of the common childhood infectious illnesses (see pages 203–8).

The doctor's examination

The doctor will ask you about any symptoms you have noticed in your child and how long he has had them, and will then examine your child. If your child is old enough to understand, explain what will happen when he visits the doctor. If the doctor suspects any particular illness, he may do other investigations as well as, or instead of, those shown below.

1 The doctor will feel the glands that lie along your child's jawbone, down the back of his neck, and in his armpits and groin. These may become swollen during an infectious illness.

2 He may feel your child's pulse to check if his heart is beating faster than usual. This is often a sign of a raised temperature. The doctor may also take your child's temperature.

3 By listening to your child's chest and back through a stethoscope, and asking your child to breathe deeply, the doctor will check the health of his heart and lungs.

4 If your child has a sore or inflamed throat, the doctor will examine his throat using a small light, pressing his tongue down with a tongue depressor.

5 The doctor may ask your child to lie on the examining couch so that he can gently feel his abdomen. He will check for swelling or tenderness in any of the internal organs.

Questions to ask the doctor

Don't hesitate to ask the doctor about anything that is worrying you. In particular, find out:
● how long your child may be ill, and what symptoms to expect
● whether he is infectious, and whether you should isolate him, particularly from small babies and pregnant women
● how you can make your child more comfortable while he is ill.

Going to hospital

It can be terrifying for a child to go to hospital, especially if she is separated from her parents. If your child is under two, all she really needs at this age is your presence. If your child is over two, playing with a favourite toy may help. Explain that teddy goes to the hospital to be made better by helpful people and soon teddy comes home again. Keep your explanations simple but truthful; your child will feel let down and mistrustful if you promise something won't hurt, and then it does.

Visiting your child

Hospital staff know how important it is for a parent to be with a child to comfort and reassure her, and should make it easy for you to visit her at any time. Many provide accommodation so that you can stay with your child – find out about this before her admission. She won't find the hospital so frightening if you continue to care for her as you would at home, so ask the nurses whether you can still bathe and feed her.

If you can't stay in hospital with your child, visit her as often as you can, and bring brothers and sisters to see her. Even if she cries when you leave, don't feel that she might settle better without your visits. It would only make her feel even more anxious, unhappy, and abandoned. Make a special effort to be with her for the first day or two, and when she has any unpleasant procedures such as injections, or is having stitches removed.

What to pack

Your child will need the items pictured here while she is in the hospital. Pack diaper changing equipment as well, if necessary. Label everything, particularly her toys, so that they don't get misplaced. Pack soap, a facecloth, a sponge, her toothbrush and toothpaste, her brush, comb, and a towel. Pack your own bag if you are staying overnight in the hospital with your child.

Dressing gown

Three pairs of pyjamas or three nighties

Slippers

Favourite toys

Washing equipment

Having an operation

If your child is old enough to understand, it will help to explain what will happen on the day of her operation. Ask the doctor how the anaesthetic will be given (it may be injected or inhaled through a mask). If inhaled through a mask, you will be allowed to stay with your child while she is given the anaesthetic, and also be allowed in the recovery room after she wakes up. Try to be with her after the operation since she may be frightened.

1 Warn your child that she will not be allowed to eat or drink anything on the day of her operation.

2 Tell your child that she will be dressed up for the operation in a hospital gown, and will wear a bracelet with her name on it.

3 While she is still in the ward, your child may be given a "pre-medication" (pre-med) to make her sleepy.

4 Tell your child that she will walk or be wheeled in her bed to the anaesthetic room, where she will be given an anaesthetic. She will fall asleep.

5 Reassure her that she will see you soon after she wakes up.

6 If your child has stitches, discourage her from scratching them. It will hurt only momentarily when they are removed.

The child with a temperature

In children, body temperature above 37.5°C (99.5°F) may be a sign of illness. However, a slightly raised temperature is not a reliable guide to her health. Fluctuations in temperature are common and not a cause for concern, but if your child's high temperature persists she may be ill, so check for other signs of illness. Babies and children can be ill with a normal or below normal temperature between 36°C (96.8°F) and 37°C (98.6°F), and some children can have a slight fever without being ill.

Signs of fever

Your child may have a fever if she:
● complains of feeling unwell
● looks pale, and feels cold and shivery
● looks flushed and her forehead feels hot.

Feel your child's forehead with your cheek if you think he has a fever – don't use your hand because, if it is cold, your child's skin will feel warm by comparison. If his forehead feels hot, take his temperature.

☎ Seek medical help

Call the doctor now if your child:
● has a raised temperature, as well as other signs of illness
● is under six months old, and has a temperature of 38°C (100.4°F)
● has a fever over 39.4°C (103°F), or over 39°C (102°F) if she is under a year old, and you can't bring it down
● has a fever for over 24 hours
● has a fever and is excessively cranky, irritable, or lethargic.

Choosing a thermometer

The best thermometers for babies and young children are the digital thermometer and the ear thermometer.

Safe and easy to use, the digital and ear thermometers give an accurate reading. Although they are more expensive than other thermometers, they are ideal for young children as they read the temperature quickly. Always keep spare batteries.

Digital thermometer

Window *with temperature reading*

Window *with temperature reading*

Ear thermometer

Taking your child's temperature

When your child is unwell, take her temperature reading every few hours. The right method depends on the child's age. Rectal temperature measurement is the most accurate method for babies under two years. However, most parents prefer taking the temperature under the armpit with a digital thermometer. Ear thermometers are more expensive and must fit easily in the child's ear canal. By five years, a child can usually cooperate with oral temperature measurement with a digital thermometer. Never use the old-style mercury thermometers.

The definition of fever depends on where the temperature was taken. Fever is defined as a temperature over 38°C (100.4°F) measured in the rectum or ear, over 37.5°C (99.5°F) measured in the mouth, or over 37.2°C (99°F) measured under the arm.

Using a digital thermometer

Underarm

1 Sit your child on your knee and lift her arm. Switch the thermometer on and tuck the end of it into her armpit.

2 Bring your child's arm down, and fold it over her chest. Hold the thermometer firmly in place for the recommended time – usually between 10 seconds and two minutes. Then remove the thermometer from under your child's arm.

3 Read your child's temperature in the window of the thermometer. Switch the thermometer off, then wash it in cool water and dry it.

The number *in the window is your child's temperature*

By mouth

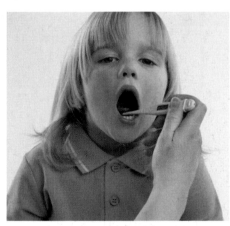

Switch the thermometer on, and ask your child to open her mouth. Place the thermometer under her tongue, and ask her to close her mouth. Wait for about three minutes.

Using an ear thermometer
Make sure a clean lens filter is in place. Pull the ear back gently, and insert the thermometer until the ear canal is sealed off. Press the button on top of the thermometer for one second, then remove the thermometer and read your child's temperature.

Hold the thermometer *firmly in place*

Bringing down a fever

Keeping him comfortable

1 If your child's temperature rises to 38°C (100.4°F), give him the recommended dose of acetaminophen or ibuprofen. Don't give ibuprofen to a baby under six months old. You should always call your doctor if your infant under three months develops a fever. Aspirin (ASA) should not be given to feverish children because of the risk of Reye's syndrome, a serious condition that can cause liver and brain damage.

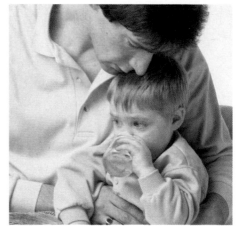

2 Your child may sweat profusely as his temperature falls, so give him plenty to drink to replace the lost fluid. If your child has a low-grade fever that isn't affecting his behaviour, don't give him any medication to lower his fever.

Keeping her cool

Do not overdress your child. In fact, if your child has a fever try to keep her cool, but not so much that she shivers. Do not give her a cold bath or sponge her with alcohol. Never try to "sweat" the fever out of her. When body temperature is rising, it's imperative to use light blankets and keep her in light clothing, so as not to increase the fever.

1 Keep your child cool by removing her top layer of clothing.

2 Change her bedding and pyjamas when her temperature is normal again, to make her comfortable.

3 Monitor your child's temperature at regular intervals. If it continues to rise and gets above 39.4°C (103°F), **call your doctor now.**

Monitor your child
Stay close to your child and make sure that she doesn't get too cold.

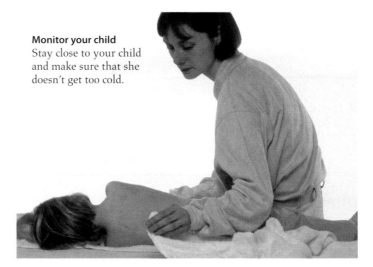

Febrile convulsions

Febrile convulsions are seizures caused by fever. You may see your child's body stiffen, her eyes roll, and her limbs twitch uncontrollably. Febrile convulsions happen in two to five percent of children between six months and five years of age, and while very frightening for parents, do not have any long-term effects.

What can I do?

Stay calm. Place your child carefully on a flat surface on her side in the recovery position (see page 241). Stay with her, but do not restrain her or put anything in her mouth. Call your doctor.

Preventing febrile convulsions

If a tendency to have febrile convulsions runs in your family, keep your child's temperature as low as you can when she is ill. Your doctor may instruct you to give her a dose of acetaminophen or ibuprofen when she shows the first signs of illness, to stop her getting a fever.

Delirious children

Some children become delirious when they have a high fever. If your child is delirious, she will be very agitated, and may even hallucinate and seem extremely frightened. This delirious state is alarming, but it isn't dangerous for your child. Stay with her to comfort her. When her body temperature drops, she will probably fall asleep, and will be back to normal when she wakes up.

All about medicines

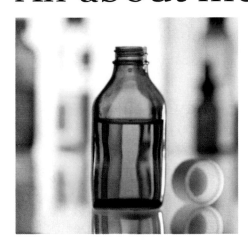

Most minor illnesses get better on their own, with or without treatment. If a medicine is necessary your doctor will tell you how often your child should take it, and for how long. Follow the directions carefully. Never mix a medicine into your baby's feed or your child's drink, since he may not finish it. If the doctor prescribes a course of antibiotics, your child must take the full course. Remember that viral illnesses such as colds do not respond to antibiotics. They simply have to run their course.

Giving medicine to babies

Always shake the bottle before pouring out the medicine and measure the dose exactly. If your baby cannot yet sit up, hold him as if you were going to feed him. If he can sit up, sit him on your lap, and tuck one of his arms behind your back. Put your hand firmly on his other arm to prevent him from struggling. If this doesn't work, ask another adult to hold him still while you give him medicine. You can prevent a baby from wriggling by swaddling him firmly. Keep some tissues handy.

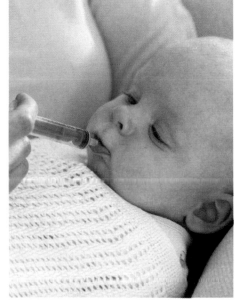

Medicine spoon
Measure your baby's dose, and pour half into another spoon. Keep both spoons nearby, then pick up your baby. Hold him so that he can't wriggle, then pick up one spoon, and rest it on his lower lip. Let him suck the medicine off, then repeat with the rest of the dose.

Medicine dropper
Measure the dose in a measuring spoon, then suck some of it into a plastic dropper. Put the dropper into your baby's mouth, and squeeze the medicine in. Give the rest of the dose. Don't use a dropper for a baby under four months old – he could choke. Don't use a glass dropper as it could break.

Syringe
Draw up the correct dose into the syringe, then pick up your baby, and rest the mouthpiece of the syringe on his lower lip. Tilt it slightly so that the medicine runs into your baby's cheek when you gently depress the end of the syringe (easiest method for babies).

Giving medicine to children

Most medicines for children are made to taste fairly pleasant, but if your child dislikes the taste, the following tips may help.

● Have your child's favourite drink ready to take away the taste of the medicine, and try bribery – a small treat or reward may help.

● Tell your child to hold her nose so that she can't taste the medicine, but never do this forcibly for her.

● If your child is old enough to understand, explain why she has to take the medicine – if she knows that it will make her feel better, she may be more inclined to take it.

● If you find it impossible to get medicine into your child, ask the doctor if he can prescribe it with a different flavour or in a different form.

Medicine and safety

Make sure that your child can't help herself to any medicines in your home.

● Keep all kinds of medications out of her reach, preferably in a locked cabinet.

● Always make sure that the medicines you buy have child-proof lids or packaging.

● Don't pretend to your child that her medicine is a soft drink.

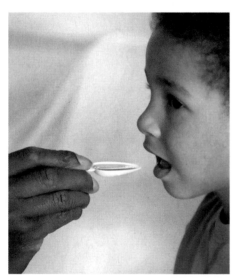

Medicine and tooth decay

Try to clean your child's teeth after giving her medicine. This is because many medicines for children contain sugar, and may cause tooth decay. If your child has to take medicine over a long period, ask your doctor or pharmacist whether a sugar-free alternative is available.

A taste tip
If your child does not like the taste of the medicine, pour it onto the back of her tongue – it won't taste so strong, because her taste buds are at the front.

Warning

Never give aspirin to your child unless advised to do so by your doctor; give her acetaminophen or ibuprofen syrup instead (see page 194). Buy the right strength and product that is appropriate for her age, and give the correct dose, which is calculated by weight. Don't give these medications for more than 48 hours, unless your doctor has advised this. If your child vomits suddenly and develops a high fever while she is recovering from an illness, **call for emergency help immediately.**

Giving nose drops

Children

1 Place a small pillow or cushion on a bed, and help your child to lie on his back with the pillow beneath his shoulders and his head dropped back. If your child is likely to wriggle as you give him drops, ask an adult to help you by holding his head.

2 Put the tip of the dropper just above your child's nostril, and squeeze out the prescribed number of drops. Don't let the dropper touch his nose – if it does, wash it before using it again. Keep your child lying down for about a minute.

Babies

Wrap your baby in a blanket, then lay her on her back across your knee, so that her upper back is supported. Keep your left hand beneath her head to support it, then give the drops as instructed for a child.

Giving ear drops

Children

1 Most children find ear drops too cold as they are squeezed into their ears, so ask your doctor whether you can warm them up (some medicines deteriorate if they are warmed). To warm the drops, place the bottle in a bowl of warm, **not hot,** water for a few minutes. Before giving to your child, check the temperature on the inside of your wrist.

2 Ask your child to lie on his side with the affected ear uppermost. Then place the dropper close to his ear, and gently squeeze the prescribed number of drops into the ear canal. Keep your child lying down for about a minute, and place a cotton ball very lightly in his ear to prevent excess liquid running out down his neck.

Babies

Wrap your baby and lay her on her side across your lap. Support her head with one hand, then give the ear drops as instructed for a child.

Giving eye drops

Children

1 Bathe your child's affected eye with a cotton ball dipped in warm, boiled water, then ask your child to lie on her back across your knee, or with her head in your lap. Put one arm around your child's head with your palm against her cheek, then tilt her head so that the affected eye is slightly lower than the other. Draw her lower eyelid gently down with your thumb.

2 Hold the dropper carefully over the gap between the lower lid and the eye, angling it so that it is out of your child's sight. If necessary, ask someone to hold her head steady. Gently squeeze out the prescribed number of drops, being careful not to touch the eye or the lid. Even if she cries, enough of the medicine is likely to stay in her eye.

Babies

The easiest method to give eye drops to a baby or child is to place the drops in the inner corner of the eyes, and with the head in a central position, wait for the baby to open his eyes. The eye drops will then roll in.

Eye ointment
If your child is prescribed an eye ointment, gently squeeze out a small amount into the outer corner of her eye.

Caring for a sick child

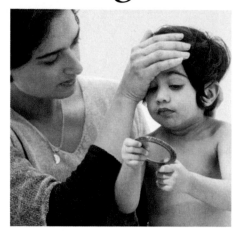

While your child is feeling ill, she may demand a great deal of attention, and may be irritable and easily bored. When ill, most children need a lot of extra cuddling and reassurance. Keep your baby with you during the day, so that you can check on her frequently. Let your child lie down in the living room, so that she is near you. At night, sleep in the same room as her if she is very unwell, so that you are nearby if she needs you. Many children vomit when they are ill, so keep a small bowl nearby.

Eating and drinking

Your child will probably have a smaller appetite than usual while she is ill. Don't worry if she doesn't want to eat much for a few days – it won't do her any harm. Allow her to choose her favourite food, and offer small helpings. Let her eat as much or as little as she wants: when she is feeling better, her appetite will return. Babies may demand feeds more frequently than usual, but take very little milk each time. Be patient if your baby behaves like this – she needs the comfort of feeling close to you as she feeds. Drink is much more important than food while your child is ill. Make sure that she has plenty to drink – about 1½ litres (3 pints) a day, especially if she has a raised temperature, or has been vomiting or has diarrhea – to make sure that she doesn't get dehydrated.

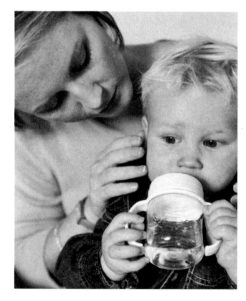

Giving your child a drink
Let your child choose her favourite drink – it doesn't matter whether it is a soda, fruit juice, milk, or water.

Encouraging your child to drink
If it is difficult to persuade your child to drink enough, make her drinks seem more appetizing by trying some of the ideas suggested below.

An unusually shaped straw *will appeal to her*

Small container
Offer frequent small drinks from a doll's cup or an egg cup, rather than giving large amounts.

Straws
Make drinks look appetizing and more fun by letting your child use a straw.

Training cup
Offer drinks in a training cup, which will help avoid spills while she is in bed.

Ice cubes
For a child over a year old, freeze diluted fruit juice into cubes, then let her suck the cubes.

Popsicle
Your child may prefer a popsicle – the "drink on a stick." Try to avoid ones with artificial colouring.

Sickness and vomiting

1 Hold your child while she is vomiting to comfort her. Sit her on your lap leaning over a bowl. When she begins to retch, support her head with one hand on her forehead, and put your other hand over her stomach, just below her rib cage.

2 After she has finished vomiting, do your best to reassure your child. Then sponge her face and wipe around her mouth. Give her a few sips of water, let her rinse her mouth out, or help her to clean her teeth, to take away any unpleasant taste that she may have.

3 Let your child rest after vomiting; she may want to lie down for a while. Wash out the container and put it within easy reach, in case she vomits again. If your child vomits frequently, she may have gastroenteritis (see page 222). Wash hands to prevent the spread of infection.

Comfort and entertainment

Staying in bed

There is no need to insist that your sick child stays in bed, although if she is feeling very ill she will probably prefer to stay there. If she wants to get up, make sure that she is dressed in cool, loose clothes, and that the room she is playing in is well ventilated, but not drafty. However, your child may want to lie down and go to sleep during the day, even if it isn't her usual naptime. If she doesn't want to be left alone, let her snuggle up with a pillow, a duvet, and her favourite cuddly toy on the sofa in the living room, or make up a bed for her wherever you are (a folding guestbed is ideal). In this way, your child still feels like she is a part of the family, and does not get too bored or lonely.

Playing in bed
If your child feels like staying in bed, but wants to sit, prop her up on her bed. Give her a picture book and read to her.

Entertaining your child

Try to keep your child occupied so that she doesn't get too bored, but remember that she will probably act younger than her age while she is feeling unwell. She won't be able to concentrate for very long, and she won't want to do anything too demanding. Bring out an old favourite toy that she hasn't played with for a while. If you give her small presents to keep her entertained and cheer her up don't be tempted to buy toys that are advanced for her age. Babies will enjoy a new mobile or a rattle that makes a new sound. Quiet activities such as interlocking building bricks, felt pictures, simple jigsaws, crayons or felt tip pens, a kaleidoscope, or Plasticine are ideal for sick toddlers and children. Protect the bedding with a towel if your child wants to play with something messy while she is in bed. She might enjoy a CD player

with her favourite songs or music, too. Remember that she will probably want more of your company than usual, so be prepared to spend some more time with her, looking at her books, and drawing pictures for her to colour in. She will be happier if you are within her sight, even if not actively playing with her.

Colds and flu

All children get colds and the flu. As soon as your child comes into contact with other children, she may get one cold after another – some children under six may have up to ten a year. As she grows older, your child develops resistance to many of these viruses.

Wiping your child's nose
If your child has a runny nose, dab it gently with a tissue to prevent it from becoming sore from frequent wiping. Throw the tissue away immediately and wash your hands, to avoid spreading infection.

Emergency

Call for emergency help immediately if your child develops a rash of dark, purplish-red spots (see page 208). Doctors refer to this as a petechial rash.

☎ Seek medical help

If your child has been feeling absolutely miserable, and especially if she is not yet one year old, **consult your doctor as soon as possible** if she has:

- a temperature over 38.5°C (101.3°F)
- wheezy, fast, or laboured breathing
- earache
- a throat so sore that swallowing is painful
- a severe cough
- not improved after three days.

Colds

What are they?

Perhaps the most common of all illnesses, a cold is a viral infection that irritates the nose and throat, so children don't catch a cold simply by being cold, by going out without wearing a coat, or by getting their feet wet. While it is not a severe illness, a cold should be taken more seriously in babies and children than in adults, because of the risk of a chest or ear infection developing. If your child develops a rash in addition to the symptoms of a normal cold, contact your doctor to determine what the rash could be.

Symptoms

- Runny or blocked nose and sneezing
- slightly raised temperature
- sore throat
- cough.

What might the doctor do?

If your baby cannot suck because her nose is blocked, and you can see the mucous, a suction bulb can be used to clear her nostrils. If the mucous is thick, your doctor may suggest saline nose drops or spray.

Over-the-counter cold medicines

These medicines (including medicated nose drops) should not be given to children under six as they do not help, and they can be dangerous. Unmedicated saline (salt water) nose spray or drops may help clear congested nasal passages.

What can I do?

1 Take your child's body temperature (see page 193), and give her a children's syrup containing acetaminophen to bring it down if necessary. Make sure she has plenty to drink, but don't force her to eat if she's not hungry. A drink before bedtime may help to keep her nose clear at night.

2 Spread a barrier cream, such as petroleum jelly, under your child's nose and around her nostrils if the area has become red and sore from a constantly runny nose or frequent wiping.

Flu

What is it?

The flu (also known as influenza) is a very infectious illness caused by hundreds of different viruses. It tends to occur in epidemics every two or three years, when a new strain of the virus appears to which people have not yet developed immunity. Flu season begins every year in late autumn and early winter. The peak season for the flu in the northern hemisphere is from November through March. If your child has caught the flu she will develop symptoms a day or two later, and will probably be sick for about three or four days. She may be sick enough to want to stay in bed, and could remain weak for several days after her temperature has gone down. A few children develop a chest infection, such as bronchitis or pneumonia (see pages 218–9), after having the flu.

Symptoms

- Raised temperature
- headache
- ache all over the body
- feeling shivery
- runny nose
- cough
- sore throat.

What can I do?

Take your child's temperature (see page 193), and if necessary, give her acetaminophen or ibuprofen suspension to reduce fever (see page 196). Offer her plenty of cool fluids – it's important that she has plenty to drink. See your doctor if the acetaminophen fails to bring her temperature down.

"Should I have my child vaccinated against the flu?" Q&A

The Canadian Paediatric Society recommends flu shots for all children between 6 and 23 months, and for older children with heart, kidney, or lung disease. The flu vaccine must be given every year because its composition is changed as new strains of the virus develop. The vaccine is also recommended for pregnant women so that their babies get antibodies against the flu through the placenta and breast milk. This protects young infants under 6 months for whom the flu shot does not work, and who are particularly vulnerable to severe influenza.

Put your baby *to sleep on her back*

3 A menthol rub may feel comforting but has not been shown to help coughing. Simply sitting upright in your lap may ease her cough.

4 She will be able to breathe more easily if you raise the head of the crib slightly. Place a book under the legs of the crib so that your baby's head and chest are slightly raised. Never prop up the mattress as this is considered unsafe practice.

5 Make sure that the air in your child's room isn't too dry. If you use a cool mist humidifier, it must be disinfected daily because of the risk of mould or bacteria. Hot water vapourizers are not recommended as they pose a risk for burns.

Sinusitis

The sinuses are air-filled cavities in the bones of the face. The lining of the nose extends into them, so they can easily become infected after a cold. This infection, sinusitis, often seems like a persistent cold, with nasal congestion, cough, and bad breath. Sinusitis is often misdiagnosed in children. At the first sign of nasal congestion or runny nose many parents (and doctors) think that the child is suffering from a sinus infection. Instead, these children often just have a common cold, and do not require treatment. True sinusitis may require antibiotics. However, yellow or green nasal discharge is common with colds and does not mean that antibiotics are needed.

Having your child immunized

At the two-month check-up, your baby will receive the first of many childhood immunizations. These vaccines contain harmless versions of the germs that cause the most severe infectious diseases. These make the body produce special proteins (antibodies) that will protect your child from that disease in the future.

Why should my baby be immunized?

Childhood immunization means protection against many serious diseases: polio, measles, mumps, rubella (German measles), pertussis (whooping cough), diphtheria, tetanus, meningococcus C (causes meningitis), rotavirus (causes diarrhea), varicella (chickenpox), *haemophilus influenzae* type b and pneumococcus (both can cause meningitis and other serious infections). By having your child immunized, not only do you protect her from these major childhood diseases, but you also help to eradicate the disease itself. The table shown on this page is an example of a typical immunization schedule. However, since immunization programs are provincial, you should check with your doctor or nurse for specific details. Occasionally your doctor may recommend an immunization that is not covered by the provincial program.

What are the risks and side effects of immunizations?

Immunizations may make your child mildly unwell or slightly feverish for a short time, but more serious side effects are extremely rare. Do not take her to be immunized if she has a feverish illness. However, there is no need to postpone immunization if she has a minor infection, such as a cold.

If your child develops a fever after her shots, give her the recommended dose of acetaminophen syrup. She may develop a small, hard lump at the injection site. This will go away in a few weeks and is nothing to worry about. If she becomes "floppy" and less responsive than usual, her crying sounds unusual, her fever lasts beyond 24 hours after the immunization, her temperature rises above 39°C (102.2°F), or she has a febrile convulsion, **call your doctor immediately.**

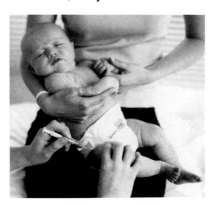

Having an injection
Hold your baby firmly on your lap while she has the injection, to comfort her and keep her as still as possible. To lessen the pain, you can give your baby sugar water (with a teaspoon or pacifier) just before the shot, or breastfeed your baby while she gets the needle.

Typical immunization program

Age	Vaccine	How given
6–32 weeks	Rotavirus	2 or 3 oral doses
2 months, 4 months, and 6 months	Diphtheria Tetanus Pertussis (whooping cough) Polio Hib*	1 injection
	Pneumococcal infection	1 injection
6–23 months	Influenza	2 injections
12 months	Measles Mumps Rubella	1 injection
	Meningococcus C	1 injection
15 months	Pneumococcal infection	1 injection
	Varicella (chickenpox)	1 injection
18 months	Diphtheria Tetanus Pertussis (whooping cough) Polio Hib*	1 injection
	Measles Mumps Rubella	1 injection
4–6 years	Diphtheria Tetanus Pertussis (whooping cough) Polio	1 injection
12 years	Hepatitis B (if not given in infancy)	2 or 3 injections
	Meningococcus C	1 injection
Girls aged 9–13 years	Human papillomavirus (HPV – can cause cervical cancer)	3 injections
14–16 years	Diphtheria Tetanus Pertussis (whooping cough)	1 injection

*Hib: *Haemophilis influenzae* type b, a bacterium that can cause one type of meningitis and other serious childhood diseases.

Infectious illnesses

Now that most children are immunized, many of these diseases have become much less common. If your child catches one of them, she will probably be immune for the rest of her life. Since most of these infectious diseases are caused by viruses, there are no medicines to cure them, but most children recover quickly and uneventfully. Many diseases are most infectious just before symptoms appear. It may be a good idea to notify the parents of your child's playmates, so they can watch for signs of illness in their own children.

Warning
If your child has a raised temperature while she is ill with one of these diseases, **do not** give her aspirin to bring the fever down, unless advised by the doctor, since it can cause a very serious disease called Reye's syndrome. You can give your child acetaminophen or ibuprofen suspension instead.

Emergency
Call for emergency help immediately if your child has an infectious disease and develops any of these signs:
- unusual and increasing drowsiness
- headache or stiff neck
- convulsions
- rash of flat, dark red or purplish blood-spots.

Rubella (German measles)

What is it?
Rubella was once common, but has become rare because of routine immunization (see opposite). It is a mild illness, so your child may feel perfectly well, and may not stay in bed. She will develop symptoms two to three weeks after she has been infected. Keep her away from others for seven days after the rash appears.

What can I do?

1 Take your child's temperature (see page 193) and, if necessary, give her acetaminophen syrup to reduce her fever.

2 Make sure that your child has plenty to drink, especially if she has a raised temperature.

Symptoms
Days 1 and 2
- Symptoms of a mild cold
- slightly sore throat
- swollen glands behind the ears, on the sides of the neck, and on the nape of the neck.

Day 2 or 3
- Blotchy rash of flat, pink spots appearing first on the face, then spreading down the body
- slightly raised temperature.

Day 4 or 5
- Fading rash, and general improvement.

Day 6
- Your child is back to normal.

Day 9 or 10
- Your child is no longer infectious.

☎ Seek medical help
Call for emergency help immediately if your child develops any of the emergency signs above. **Consult your doctor as soon as possible** if you think your child has rubella, but check first before taking your child to the doctor's office to avoid her coming into contact with pregnant women.

What might the doctor do?
Your doctor will confirm that your child has rubella, but there is no treatment for it.

Rubella and pregnancy
While your child is infectious, keep her away from any women who might be pregnant. Although rubella is a mild disease, it can cause defects in a developing baby if a pregnant woman catches it.

Measles

What is it?

Measles is a very infectious illness that causes a rash, fever, and a cough, and sometimes more serious complications, such as pneumonia and inflammation of the brain. It is a very rare disease in Canada due to widespread immunization.

What can I do?

1 Try to bring down her temperature (see page 194) and give plenty of fluids. She may feel very miserable and want to stay in bed.

2 If her eyes are sore, bathe them using a cotton ball dipped in cool water. Keep her room dark if this makes her more comfortable.

What might the doctor do?

Your doctor will confirm the diagnosis and keep a check on your child. He will treat any complications if they develop.

Symptoms

Symptoms develop 10–14 days after infection.

Days 1 and 2
- Runny nose, dry cough, and red watering eyes
- steadily rising temperature.

Day 3
- Tiny white spots, like grains of salt, in the mouth.

Days 4 and 5
- Dull red rash of slightly raised spots appears, first on forehead and behind the ears, gradually spreading to rest of the face and trunk. After two or three days, the rash fades and other symptoms disappear.

☎ Seek medical help

Call for emergency help immediately if your child develops any of the signs on page 203. **Consult the doctor as soon as possible** if you think your child has measles. Call him again if:
- your child is no better three days after the rash develops
- your child's temperature rises suddenly
- her condition worsens after she seemed to be improving
- she has earache or her breathing is noisy and difficult.

Roseola infantum

What is it?

Roseola is a mild illness that is very common in early childhood. It is characterized by a high fever that lasts for about three days, followed by a rash of pink spots. Most children will have had it by the time they are two.

What can I do?

1 Call your doctor if your child's temperature is 39°C (102.2°F) or above. In some cases, febrile seizures may follow the high temperature. Follow the protocols given on page 194.

2 Try to bring down the fever to make your child more comfortable (see page 194). Acetaminophen may bring his temperature down briefly.

3 Make sure your child has plenty to drink so that he is always adequately hydrated.

Symptoms

Symptoms appear 5–15 days after the incubation period.

Days 1 to 4
- High temperature
- sometimes a mild cold or cough.

Days 4 to 8
- Temperature returns to normal
- rash of pink, slightly raised spots appears over head and trunk
- rash fades, and the child is back to normal.

☎ Seek medical help

Call for emergency help immediately if your child develops any of the emergency signs listed on page 203.

Chickenpox

What is it?

Chickenpox is a very infectious illness, characterized by a rash of itchy spots that turn into fluid-filled blisters. It is usually accompanied by a slight fever. Your child may not feel very ill, but if he has a lot of spots he may itch all over. Symptoms appear two to three weeks after your child has been infected. It is a very common childhood illness. In later life, the chickenpox virus may be reactivated and cause shingles, so a child may catch chickenpox after contact with an adult who has shingles. Chickenpox can cause complications for a pregnant woman or her unborn baby. It is recommended that all children be vaccinated against chickenpox.

Symptoms

Days 1 to 4

● Groups of small, red, very itchy spots with fluid-filled centres, appearing in batches first on the child's chest, abdomen, and back, later elsewhere on the body
● fluid within the spots becomes white and cloudy
● slight temperature.

Days 5 to 9

● The spots burst, leaving small craters
● scabs form over the spots and drop off after a few days.

Day 10

● Your child is back to normal.

☎ Seek medical help

Call for emergency help immediately if your child develops any of the signs listed on page 203. Consult your doctor as soon as possible if you think your child has chickenpox, and call him again if he has any of the symptoms listed below:
● very severe itching
● redness or swelling around any spots, or pus oozing from the spots – this means they have become infected
● temperature of 39°C (102.2°F) or more
● severe cough or confusion
● infection persisting beyond nine days.

What can I do?

1 Take your child's temperature (see page 193), and give him the recommended dose of acetaminophen syrup to bring it down if it is raised. Give him plenty of fluids to drink if he has a fever. Although your child may not feel very ill, try to make sure that he has plenty of rest as this will aid his recovery.

2 Try to discourage your child from scratching the spots, since it can infect them, and also cause scarring when they heal. Cut your child's fingernails short and keep them clean, so that the spots are less likely to become infected if he does scratch them. Put scratch mitts on him.

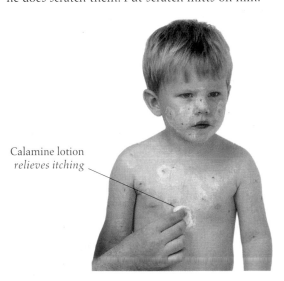

Calamine lotion *relieves itching*

3 Try to relieve your child's itchiness. Dab the spots gently with a cotton ball dipped in calamine lotion.

4 Give your child lukewarm baths with a handful of baking soda dissolved in the water to help reduce itching.

5 If your child is very itchy, he will probably find loose cotton clothes the most comfortable.

What might the doctor do?

Your doctor will confirm the diagnosis, and may prescribe an antihistamine cream or medicine to relieve your child's itching if it is very severe. If any of the spots have become infected, he may prescribe an antibiotic cream.

Mumps

What is it?

Mumps is an infection that was quite common among children until routine immunization was introduced. It causes swollen glands, particularly the glands just in front of and below the ears. Infrequently, mumps can cause deafness or inflammation of the testicles, but this is rare in a boy before puberty.

What can I do?

1 Give acetaminophen syrup to bring his temperature down, and hold a cold compress to his swollen glands.

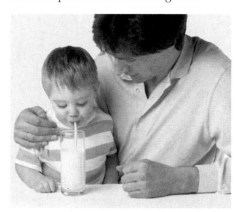

2 Give plenty of cold drinks, but avoid acidic drinks, such as fruit juice. Let your child drink through a straw, if it hurts him to open his mouth.

Symptoms

Symptoms appear 14–24 days after the infection.
● Raised temperature
● one or two days later, the child develops painful swelling on one or both sides of the face. This lasts for four to eight days.

Area of swelling

3 If it hurts your child to swallow, give him liquid or semi-liquid foods, such as ice cream and soup.

4 Keep him away from unimmunized teenagers and young adults, and from women in the first 16 weeks of pregnancy when mumps carries a slightly increased risk of miscarriage.

☎ Seek medical help

Call for emergency help immediately if your child develops any of the signs listed on page 203. **Consult your doctor as soon as possible** if you think your child has mumps, and call him again if your child develops bad stomach pain or a red testicle.

What might the doctor do?

Your doctor will confirm that your child has mumps, and treat any complications if they develop.

Erythema infectiosum (Fifth disease)

What is it?

Erythema infectiosum is a mild, and mildly infectious, illness that usually occurs in small outbreaks in the spring, and mostly affects children over the age of two years. The disease is characterized by a bright red rash that suddenly appears on both cheeks, hence its other name of "slapped cheek disease."

What can I do?

Give your child acetaminophen syrup if he has a fever. Offer him plenty of fluids to drink, and apply a cold compress on the site. If your child has a blood disorder (for example, sickle-cell anemia or thalassemia), consult your doctor. Erythema infectiosum can sometimes cause severe illnesses in such children. If your child has Erythema infectiosum, keep him away from any women who might be pregnant. Although once the rash appears he is unlikely to be infectious, the disease can, in rare circumstances, lead to miscarriage or problems in the fetus, if contracted during pregnancy.

Symptoms

Symptoms appear 4–14 days after the infection.

Day 1
● Bright red cheeks, with a contrasting pale area around the mouth
● mild fever
● joint pain.

Days 2 to 5
● Blotchy, lace-like rash spreading over trunk and limbs.

Days 7 to 10
● Rash fades. Your child is no longer infectious. The rash may recur over the next few weeks or months, particularly if your child is exposed to sunlight.

Whooping cough

What is it?

One of the most serious childhood diseases, whooping cough (also known as pertussis), is characterized by a severe and persistent cough. It is caused by a bacterial infection. It is highly infectious, so keep your child away from babies and children who have not been immunized. Immunized children can get a mild form of the illness. A few children with whooping cough develop a secondary infection, such as bronchitis or pneumonia (see pages 218–9).

Symptoms

Week 1
- Symptoms of a normal cough and cold
- slight temperature.

Week 2
- Worsening cough, with frequent coughing fits lasting up to a minute, after which your child has to fight for breath
- if your child is over 18 months, he may learn to force breath in with a "whooping" sound
- vomiting after a coughing fit.

Weeks 3 to 10
- Cough improves, but may worsen if your child gets a cold
- your child is unlikely to be infectious after the third week.

What can I do?

1 Stay with your child during any coughing fits, because he may become very distressed. Sit him on your lap, and support him gently as he leans slightly forwards. Keep a small bowl nearby so that he can spit out any phlegm that he coughs up, and in case he should vomit. Clean the bowl thoroughly with boiling water afterwards, to make sure that the infection doesn't spread to the rest of the family.

2 If your child often coughs and vomits after meals, offer him small meals at frequent intervals, just after a coughing fit if possible.

Emergency

Call for emergency help immediately if your child turns blue during a coughing fit.

☎ Seek medical help

Consult your doctor as soon as possible if you suspect that your child has whooping cough.

3 Keep your child entertained – he will have fewer coughing fits if his attention is distracted, but don't let him get too excited or overtired, as this may bring on a coughing fit.

4 Sleep in the same room as your child, so that you can be with him if he has a coughing fit at night.

5 Don't let anyone smoke near your child, and don't give him any cough medicines.

What might the doctor do?

The doctor may prescribe an antibiotic. Although it won't cure your child's cough, it may reduce its severity, and make your child less infectious. This is particularly important if you have a baby who is at risk of catching whooping cough from an older brother or sister who already has the disease. However, the antibiotic is only really effective if it is given right at the beginning of the infection.

Caring for a baby

Whooping cough is dangerous in babies, because they may not be able to draw breath properly after coughing. Your baby will need careful nursing, and may be admitted to the hospital. Your child may receive intravenous antibiotics to treat infection or reduce lung inflammation. He may find feeding difficult if he vomits frequently, so abandon your regular feeding schedule and offer a feed as soon as he has calmed down after coughing or vomiting.

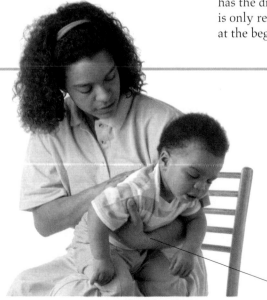

Coughing fits
When your baby has a coughing fit, sit him on your lap, and keep rubbing his back. Stay with him until he has stopped coughing and is breathing normally again. Then cuddle to comfort him, and put him down to sleep on his back as usual.

Rub his back *when he has a coughing fit*

Meningitis

What is it?
Meningitis is an inflammation of the tissues covering the brain, caused by an infection with bacteria or viruses. Viral meningitis is more common than bacterial meningitis, and is also less serious. It can be caused by several different viruses, and tends to occur in winter. Viral meningitis is more likely to affect children over five years old. Bacterial meningitis is quite rare, but it can be life-threatening. Even with timely antibiotic therapy, there may be permanent brain injury. Any bacteria can cause meningitis; however, vaccination against Hib has virtually eradicated one kind of meningitis. Unfortunately, other bacteria such as meningococcus (of which there are several strains) and pneumococcus can also cause meningitis. There are vaccines against meningococcus C and pneumococcus (see page 202), but it is impossible to prevent all cases of this serious disease. Children under five are particularly susceptible to bacterial meningitis.

The early symptoms of bacterial and viral meningitis are very similar, and can easily be mistaken for those of flu. However, the symptoms of bacterial meningitis are usually more severe. It can develop very rapidly, so that the child may become seriously ill within a few hours, with increasing drowsiness and sometimes loss of consciousness or convulsions.

Meningitis rash
Some children with meningitis develop a characteristic rash of tiny blood-spots under the skin, which can appear anywhere on the body. The spots are flat, pink, dark red, or purple. They look like pinpricks at first, but if untreated, grow bigger until they look like fresh bruises.

What can I do?
Call your doctor now, or take your child to the nearest emergency department if she seems abnormally drowsy or has any two of the symptoms listed in the emergency box below.

What might the doctor do?
The doctor may send your child to the hospital for a lumbar puncture test to confirm the diagnosis.

If viral meningitis is diagnosed no treatment is necessary except painkillers, and your child will recover completely within a week or two.

Bacterial meningitis will be treated with antibiotics and, if convulsions occur, with anticonvulsant drugs. If the disease is picked up early and treated promptly, most children recover completely. Rarely, the disease may be fatal, and in a few children it may cause some brain damage, especially if treatment is delayed.

The meninges
Three protective layers, known as the meninges, cover the brain and spinal cord. Meningitis occurs when the meninges become infected by viruses or bacteria.

Meninges · Brain · Skull · Venous space · Cerebrospinal fluid · Area shown in detail

Emergency
Call for emergency help immediately if your child has two or more of the following symptoms:
- vomiting and refusing feeds
- stiff neck
- restlessness and irritability, especially when picked up (this can be due to limb or muscle pain)
- tense or bulging fontanelle
- purple-red rash that does not fade when pressed
- fever with cold hands and feet – a temperature of 38°C (100.4°F) or more in babies under three months, and of 39°C (102.2°F) or more in babies between three and six months
- rapid or unusual breathing patterns
- skin that is extremely pale, blotchy, or turning blue
- a high-pitched moaning cry
- shivering
- floppiness and listlessness, or stiffness with jerky movements
- abnormal drowsiness, or your child being less responsive, vacant, or difficult to wake

Older children may also have:
- severe headache
- dislike of bright light and loud noise.

If your child has a dark, purplish rash, check to see whether it fades when pressed. To do this, press the side of a glass on to the rash. If the rash is still visible through the glass it may be a purpura rash, which requires immediate medical attention. Take your child to the nearest emergency department or call 911.

Purpura on light skin

Eye problems

Most eye disorders clear up quickly with or without treatment, but all problems affecting the eye should be taken seriously. Eye infections spread easily, so give your child her own facecloth and towel. Use a clean tissue to dry each eye. Keep your child's hands clean and try to stop her rubbing her eyes – this helps to prevent an infection, as well as stops it from spreading.

What might the doctor do?
The doctor may prescribe a cream to soothe your child's eyelids, or an antibiotic ointment.

☎ Seek medical help
Consult your doctor as soon as possible if:
- your child's eyes are sticky
- there is no improvement after about a week of home treatment.

Emergency
Call for emergency help immediately if your child has any injury that has damaged her eye, or if she cannot see clearly after an injury.

Blepharitis

What is it?
Blepharitis is an inflammation of the edges of the eyelids, which usually affects both eyes. Many children with dandruff get blepharitis.

Symptoms
- Red and scaly eyelids
- irritation in the eyes.

What can I do?

1 Use warm, boiled water to wash your child's eyelids, using a fresh cotton ball for each eye. Hold the warm pad over the closed eyelid for about 5–10 minutes, then rub it gently over the closed eyelid to help loosen any crusting. Do this twice a day, using fresh warm water each time.

2 Gently clean the eyelids with a cotton swab, using warm water mixed with a small amount of baby shampoo.

3 If your child has dandruff, wash her hair with an anti-dandruff shampoo. Use an anti-cradle cap shampoo for a baby.

Conjunctivitis (Pink eye)

What is it?
Also known as "pink eye" because the white of the eye turns pink, conjunctivitis is an inflammation of the lining of the eye and eyelids. It can be caused by a virus or by bacteria, although it is milder when caused by a virus. If your child's eyelids are gummed together with pus when she wakes up, she probably has bacterial, rather than viral, conjunctivitis. If your baby develops any of the symptoms in the first day or two of life, see Sticky eye, page 183.

What can I do?

1 Try to find out whether your child's symptoms are caused by something other than conjunctivitis. She might have an allergy such as hay fever, or she may have a speck of dust or an eyelash in her eye. If she has an allergy, her eyes may be itchy and watering, as well as red and sore.

2 If you think she has conjunctivitis, dip a cotton ball into some warm, boiled water and bathe both of her eyes, using a fresh cotton ball for each one. Start with the infected one, and wipe from the inside corner to the outside. Wash your hands before and afterwards.

Symptoms
- Bloodshot eye
- gritty, sore eye
- discharge of pus
- eyelids gummed together after sleep.

☎ Seek medical help
Consult your doctor as soon as possible if you think your child has conjunctivitis or if her eyes are bloodshot and sore.

What might the doctor do?
The doctor may prescribe antibiotic drops or ointment for a bacterial infection, which will cure it. Viral conjunctivitis needs no treatment, but may last a few weeks.

Stye

What is it?
A stye is a painful, pus-filled swelling on the upper or lower eyelid. It is caused by an infection, usually bacterial, at the base of an eyelash.

Some styes simply dry up, but most of these come to a head, and then burst within about a week, relieving the pain. Styes are not serious and you can treat them at home. Try to stop your child from touching the stye to prevent the infection from spreading.

Symptoms
● Red, painful swelling on the eyelid
● pus-filled centre appearing in the swelling.

What can I do?

1 Dip a cotton ball in hot, but not boiling, water, squeeze it out, and press it gently onto your child's stye. This will help to bring the stye to a head more quickly, and encourage the release of pus. Repeat this for two or three minutes, three times a day until the stye bursts.

2 When the stye bursts and releases the pus, the pain is relieved. Wash the pus away very gently with a cotton ball that has been dipped in warm, boiled water. The swelling will go down very soon.

☎ Seek medical help
Consult your doctor as soon as possible if:
● the stye does not improve after about a week
● your child's whole eyelid is swollen
● the skin all around your child's eye turns red
● your child also has blepharitis (see page 209).

Strabismus (Cross-eye)

What is it?
Normally, both eyes look in the same direction at the same time, but in a child with a strabismus one eye focuses on an object while the other does not follow it properly.

A newborn baby's eyes do not always work together correctly, so intermittent cross-eyes is common. This is nothing to worry about. But if your baby's eyes don't move together by the time he is three months old, talk to your doctor. He may have strabismus.

Strabismus may be constant, but in some children, it comes and goes. However, children do not grow out of strabismus, so it is essential to have it treated. The younger the child, the more successful the treatment.

Symptoms
● Eyes looking in different directions.

How can I check for strabismus?
When your baby is about three months old, hold a toy 20cm (8in) from his face, and move it slowly from side to side. Check that his eyes work together to follow the moving object.

☎ Seek medical help
Consult your doctor if you think your child has strabismus.

What might the doctor do?
The doctor will check your child's vision and may give him a patch to wear over his stronger eye for several hours each day, so that he is forced to use his weak eye. A toddler may need to wear glasses. If your child is under two, this treatment will probably cure his strabismus within a few months. If your child has severe strabismus caused by muscle weakness, he may need to have an operation to correct the defect and straighten his eyes.

Ear problems

Most ear problems in small children arise from an infection of the outer or middle ear. Acute middle ear infections may cause severe pain and pus may build up behind the eardrum, causing it to burst. (The hole should heal within a few weeks.) Occasionally, the infection may spread into the bone behind the ear.

Ear canal *is the tube running from the outer ear to the middle ear*

Middle ear cavity *contains three tiny bones that transmit sound signals to the inner ear*

Auditory nerve *takes sound signals to the brain*

Eardrum *vibrates in response to sound waves*

Eustachian tube *leads to the back of the throat. It is much shorter in children than in adults, making it prone to blockage*

Outer ear

Anatomy of the ear
Each ear consists of three parts. From the outer ear (the only visible part), a slightly curved canal leads to the eardrum. Behind this is a cavity, the middle ear, in which lie three small bones that transmit sound vibrations to the inner ear, the part of the ear that contains the structures concerned with hearing and balance.

Outer ear infection

What is it?
The skin lining the outer ear canal becomes inflamed when your child has an outer ear infection. This may happen if he swims a lot in either a lake or pool, or because he has poked or scratched his ear, and it has become infected. Children with eczema are especially prone to such infections if they get water in their ears.

What can I do?

1 Give your child the prescribed dose of acetaminophen syrup to relieve the pain.

2 Make sure that water doesn't get into the affected ear at bathtime, and just sponge his hair clean. Don't let your child go swimming until the infection clears up.

> ☎ Seek medical help
> **Consult your doctor as soon as possible** if you think your child has an outer ear infection.

What might the doctor do?
Your doctor will probably prescribe antibiotic ear drops to clear the infection. Ask your child to lie on his side and keep still while you squeeze out drops into the affected ear. Keep him in this position for about a minute afterwards.

Symptoms
● Pain in the ear that is worse when the child touches his ear or lies on it
● redness in the ear canal
● discharge from the ear
● itchiness inside the ear.

Wax in the ear
Wax sometimes accumulates in the ear, giving a feeling of fullness or partial deafness. If your child has a lot of ear wax, very gently wipe away any visible wax with a cotton ball, but don't poke anything into the ear. If this doesn't help, consult your doctor.

Middle ear infection

What is it?

Earache is commonly caused by an infection of the middle ear. If your child has a middle ear infection, the cavity behind his eardrum becomes infected or inflamed, usually because an infection has spread from the throat. The tube that runs from the throat to the ear is very short and narrow in a child, and so is obstructed easily. Generally, only one ear is infected.

By the time your child is seven or eight years old, the eustachian tube (see page 211) will have increased in width, making your child much less prone to these infections.

Symptoms

- Very painful ear which may stop your child sleeping
- crying and rubbing or tugging at the ear, if your child can't yet talk well enough to complain of earache
- crying, loss of appetite, and general signs of illness in young babies, especially after a cold
- fever
- partial deafness.

What can I do?

1 To relieve your child's earache, fill a hot water bottle with warm, **not hot,** water, and wrap it in a towel. Then let him rest his ear against it. Don't give a hot water bottle to a baby who is too young to push it away if it is too hot – heat a soft cloth, and hold it against your baby's ear instead.

2 If your child's ear is very painful, and is causing him a lot of discomfort, try giving the recommended dose of acetaminophen syrup. This should relieve the pain.

3 If you notice a discharge, don't clear it away or probe his ear – just put a clean handkerchief over his ear. Encourage him to rest his head on the affected side, so that any discharge can drain away.

☎ Seek medical help

Consult your doctor as soon as possible if your child's ear is infected, or has a discharge.

How can I prevent ear infection?

Try to minimize colds by hand washing. Breastfeed your baby and avoid bottle feeding when he is lying down. Immunize your child against flu and pneumococcus (see page 102).

What might the doctor do?

The doctor will examine your child's ears, and may prescribe an antibiotic if he is under two years. If your child is older, the doctor might wait and reassess him to see if the infection resolves without antibiotics.

Glue ear (effusion)

What is it?

Repeated middle ear infections can lead to glue ear, an accumulation of sticky fluid in the middle ear.

☎ Seek medical help

Consult your doctor as soon as possible if you think your child has glue ear.

Symptoms

- Partial deafness after repeated middle ear infections.

What can I do?

Try to minimize the number of ear infections your child has (see above). If you smoke, try to stop. Children of parents who smoke seem to be more prone to ear infections. Do not use over-the-counter cold medications or decongestants as these are not helpful and may be harmful to children under six.

What might the doctor do?

The condition may clear up on its own, so treatment may not be needed. However, a simple operation may be necessary. Under anaesthetic, a hole is made in the eardrum and a tiny tube (a grommet) is inserted. After several months, it will fall out, the hole will heal, and your child's hearing will be back to normal.

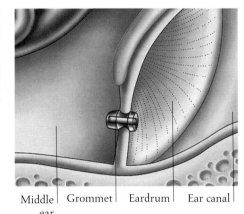

Middle ear | Grommet | Eardrum | Ear canal

The grommet is implanted in the eardrum, to equalize air pressure on either side of it, and to allow the ear to dry out. The grommet is not uncomfortable, and will not affect your child's hearing.

Mouth infections

A baby or child with a mouth infection will have a very sore mouth. Thrush is the most common mouth infection in babies. Children over one are prone to cold sores (see page 230), usually around the lips, but sometimes inside the mouth.

Helping a child with a sore mouth

If your child's mouth is sore, try to make eating and drinking as painless as you can. Allow warm meals to get cool before giving them to your child, since hot food generally hurts more than cold, and offer her plenty of very cold drinks. If she is reluctant to eat or drink, try some of the suggestions given here.

Let your child drink through a straw or use a training cup, because this may be less painful than drinking from a cup.

Soup
This is nourishing and easy to eat, and can be served cold. Alternatively, liquidize food, or chop it very small.

Cold drinks
Serve drinks very cold; avoid fruit juice, since it is very acidic.

Ice cream
Your child may find cold food, such as ice cream, easy to eat.

Water

Cheese
Encourage your child to finish meals with cheese and a drink of water to help keep her teeth clean, if she can't brush properly.

Thrush

What is it?

Thrush is an oral infection caused by a yeast that lives in the mouth and intestines. The yeast is normally kept under control by bacteria, but sometimes it multiplies out of control, producing a sore, irritating rash. Yeast can also cause a rash in the diaper area. Thrush is not a serious infection, and usually clears up with treatment.

Symptoms

● Creamy yellow, slightly raised patches on the inside of the cheeks, tongue, or the roof of the mouth, which do not come away easily if you try to wipe them off
● reluctance to eat due to a sore mouth
● in babies, a red rash in the diaper area that starts in the creases at the top of the legs.

What can I do?

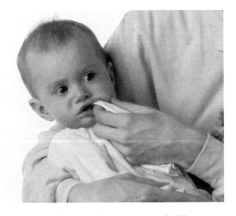

1 Wipe the patches in your child's mouth very gently with a clean handkerchief. If they don't come off easily, she probably has thrush. Don't rub them hard, because if you scrape them off they will leave a sore, bleeding patch underneath.

2 Give your child food that is easy to eat (see above). If you are bottle-feeding, make sure that you sterilize nipples and pacifiers after each feed.

3 If you are breastfeeding, continue to feed as normal, but take extra care with nipple hygiene. Yeast infections may be passed back and forth from mother's nipples to baby's mouth, so you may need treatment as well.

> ☎ **Seek medical help**
> **Consult your doctor as soon as possible** if you think your baby or child has thrush.

What might the doctor do?

Your doctor may prescribe a medicine to be painted on the spots in your baby's mouth just before a feed, or, for a child over about two, lozenges to suck. If you are breastfeeding, the doctor may prescribe an antifungal cream for your nipples. Gentian violet may also be used to treat both baby's mouth and mother's nipples – be prepared for purple staining!

Throat infections

Sore throats are common in children, and often accompany other illnesses, such as colds or flu. Mild sore throats clear up in a few days, but severe infections, particularly if the tonsils are affected, may give your child a fever, and make swallowing painful.

☎ **Seek medical help**

Consult your doctor as soon as possible if your child:
● has such a sore throat that swallowing is painful
● seems generally unwell and has a fever or rash
● has infected tonsils
● has not been immunized against diphtheria.

Sore throat

What is it?
Sore throat is an infection that makes the throat area sore and red. It may be part of a cold or flu (see pages 200–1), a bacterial infection (strep throat), or one of the first signs of other viral illnesses (see pages 203 and 206). Children are prone to earache when they have a throat infection (see pages 211–2).

Symptoms
● Reluctance to eat as it hurts to swallow
● red, raw-looking throat
● earache (see page 211–2)
● slightly raised temperature
● swollen glands.

What can I do?

1 Ask your child to face a strong light and open his mouth. Examine the back of his throat (see page 189). If it is sore, it will look red and raw, and you may see creamy spots.

2 Gently feel down each side of his neck and just below the angle of his jaw-bone, to check whether his glands are swollen (see page 189).

3 Give your child plenty of cold drinks, and purée food if swallowing hurts him. He may find cold food, such as ice cream, less painful to eat than warm food.

4 Take your child's temperature (see page 193), and if necessary give him the recommended dose of acetaminophen to bring his fever down.

What might the doctor do?
Most mild sore throats need no treatment, but it is advisable to get medical advice and diagnosis early, especially if the child has a fever or is generally unwell. If the doctor suspects that the infection is caused by bacteria he may prescribe an antibiotic.

Tonsillitis

What is it?
Tonsillitis is inflammation of tonsils, causing a sore throat and other symptoms. The tonsils are glands at the back of the throat, one on either side, which trap infection, and stop it from spreading.

Symptoms
● Very sore throat
● red and enlarged tonsils, possibly covered with creamy spots
● temperature over 38°C (100.4°F)
● swollen glands on the neck.

What can I do?

1 Examine your child's tonsils and feel his glands (see page 189). If infected, his tonsils will be large and red, and may have creamy spots.

2 Take his temperature (see page 193). Give him acetaminophen or ibuprofen suspension to bring it down, if necessary.

3 Encourage your child to have plenty to drink, especially if he has a fever.

What might the doctor do?
Your doctor will examine your child's throat, and take a throat swab. He may prescribe an antibiotic to clear infection.

If your child has recurrent severe tonsillitis, your doctor may recommend having his tonsils removed. However, this operation is done after a child is four.

Coughs and chest infections

Most coughs in small children are a symptom of a cold or flu (see pages 200–1), which produces a dry, tickly cough. If your child finds breathing difficult and coughs up phlegm, he may have a chest infection (see pages 216–9). However, slightly wheezy breathing is normal for a child with a cold, because his airways are narrow and become narrower if they are swollen. Rarely, a cough may be an early sign of measles (see page 204), and a severe, persistent cough might be whooping cough (see page 207).

Emergency
Call for emergency help immediately if your child:
● has a bluish tinge round his face, mouth, and tongue
● is breathing very rapidly
● is breathing so noisily that it can be heard across the room
● seems to be fighting for breath
● is abnormally drowsy
● is unable to speak or make sounds as usual.

Frequent chest infections
Babies under a year old and children with a long-term chest disorder such as asthma (see page 218) are prone to chest infections. If you smoke, your children are much more likely to develop chest infections than are the children of non-smoking parents.

If your child has frequent chest infections, your doctor may arrange for tests to find the cause.

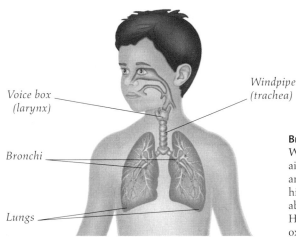

Voice box (larynx)

Bronchi

Lungs

Windpipe (trachea)

Breathing
When your child breathes in, air is sucked down his windpipe and bronchi (the airways) into his lungs, where oxygen is absorbed into his bloodstream. His blood then carries the oxygen all around his body.

Croup

What is it?
Croup is a viral infection of the throat, windpipe, and vocal cords (or larynx). The inflammation of these breathing passages may make it difficult for your child to breathe. Croup can become serious, so you must monitor your child carefully. Attacks of croup tend to occur at night, and if severe, can be frightening for everyone. In older children, this viral infection is called laryngitis.

Symptoms
● Breathing difficulty
● loud crowing sound as breath is drawn in
● barking cough
● hoarse voice.

What can I do?

1 Keep calm, and reassure your child. He is likely to be very frightened, but if he panics, it will be even harder for him to breathe.

2 Create a steamy atmosphere by taking your child into the bathroom and turning on the hot taps. The moist air will soothe his air passages and help him to breathe more easily.

3 Prop your child up on pillows, or hold him on your lap – he will be able to breathe easily in these positions.

☎ Seek medical help
Call your doctor now if your child has difficulty breathing, or if you think he has croup.

4 You can also bundle up your child and take him outside to breathe cold, moist air for five to ten minutes. This often works wonders for croup.

5 Give him acetaminophen for fever and make sure that he drinks plenty of fluids.

6 Do not give him over-the-counter medicine or any medication that might make him drowsy.

What might the doctor do?
The doctor will tell you what to do if the croup recurs and may prescribe a steroid medication. If the attack is severe, the doctor might send your child to the hospital where he will be carefully monitored and may be given a medicated inhalation.

Cough

What is it?

A cough is a protective reflex action that helps to clear any irritants or blockages from the airways. It can be either a reaction to irritation in the throat or windpipe, or the result of an infection of the respiratory tract. It may also be caused by an obstruction in the airways. A cough will generally disappear of its own accord.

A dry, ticklish cough, without sputum, is rarely serious. It probably means that your child's throat or windpipe is irritated, which may be a by-product of a cold, because mucus dribbles down the throat and irritates it. Her throat might also be irritated, if she is with adults who smoke. An ear infection can also cause a dry cough. If your child has a moist-sounding cough, and brings up vomit while she coughs, then she probably has a minor respiratory infection. While most coughs like this are not serious, they can be a symptom of bronchiolitis, bronchitis, or pneumonia (see pages 217–9). Coughing only at night could be a sign of asthma (see page 218).

☎ Seek medical help

Consult your doctor as soon as possible if:
- your baby is under six months
- the cough prevents your child from sleeping
- the cough does not improve in three days
- your child has a recurrent cough.

What might the doctor do?

The doctor will examine your child, and listen to her breathing.

If your child has a dry cough, the doctor may prescribe a cough medicine that will help soothe her throat.

If the cough is particularly chesty, the doctor may carry out some diagnostic tests. He may prescribe antibiotics.

What can I do?

1 If your child has a sudden attack of coughing, check whether she has inhaled a small object, such as a candy or a button (see Choking, page 242), but don't put your fingers down her throat to try to pull it out.

2 If your child has a chesty cough, help her to clear the phlegm from her chest when she is coughing. Support her as she leans forwards. It is okay if she swallows the phlegm.

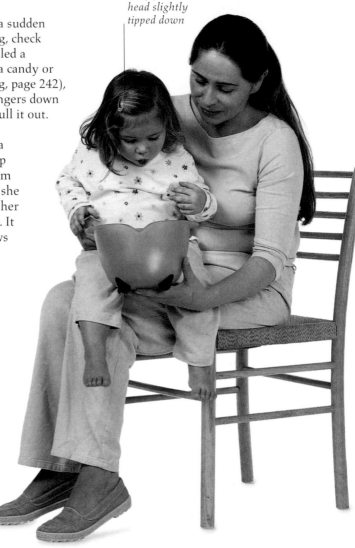

Keep your child's *head slightly tipped down*

3 If your child has a dry cough, a warm drink at bedtime will ease her throat.

4 Make sure that your child's bedroom is not overheated because this will dry out the air. If the air becomes too dry, it will aggravate her cough.

5 Moisten the air in her bedroom at night with a cool-mist humidifier. Remember to disinfect it daily.

6 Keep your child away from cigarette smoke – it can aggravate her cough.

If she is over 18 months *extra pillows will prevent mucus dribbling down her throat at night*

Bronchiolitis

What is it?

Bronchiolitis is a common and usually mild viral illness that causes inflammation of the smallest airways in the lungs, called bronchioles. It occurs in epidemics during the winter. Those most commonly affected are babies under a year old. The risk of a child getting bronchiolitis increases if his parents are smokers, or if he lives in overcrowded accommodation in which viral infections spread more easily.

Your baby may have a runny nose for a day or two, and then suddenly seem much worse, with a fever, dry rasping cough, and rapid or difficult breathing. Mild bronchiolitis usually improves within a week or so.

Symptoms

- Runny nose
- fever
- dry, rasping cough
- rapid or difficult breathing
- wheezing
- feeding difficulties.

What might the doctor do?

For a mild attack, your doctor may prescribe a bronchodilator drug to make breathing easier.

In more severe cases, your baby may be admitted to the hospital where oxygen can be given, and the baby can be fed through a tube inserted through his nose and into the stomach or, sometimes, intravenously. Most children are able to return home in 3–10 days.

The cough may persist for a few weeks longer. Although there are no lasting after effects, for the next few years many children who have had bronchiolitis tend to suffer from wheezing whenever they have a cold.

What can I do?

1 Give your baby plenty of drinks to make sure that he is getting enough fluids.

2 No drug will alter the course of the illness, but acetaminophen suspension will help bring down his temperature.

3 Increase the humidity in your child's bedroom with a cool-mist humidifier. This will help to relieve your child's breathing.

☎ Seek medical help

Consult your doctor as soon as possible if:
- your child is breathing faster than usual, or his breathing is laboured or wheezy
- your child is having difficulty feeding
- your child looks bluish around the lips.

4 Raise the head of your baby's crib or bed slightly by putting a book with a 1.5in (4cm) spine under each leg (see page 201). If your baby is over 18 months, you can give him an extra pillow.

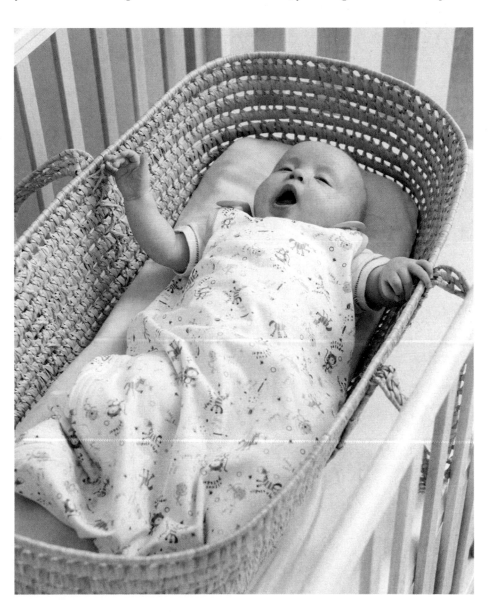

Bronchitis

What is it?

Bronchitis is an inflammation of the lining of the bronchi (the main air passages leading to the lungs). It usually follows a viral infection, such as a cold, flu, or sore throat, because the infection spreads downwards, but the inflammation may also be caused by a bacterial infection.

Your child probably won't feel particularly ill, but he may have difficulty sleeping if his cough tends to be worse at night.

Symptoms

- Rattly cough
- slight wheeziness
- slight temperature
- runny nose.

What can I do?

1 Help to relieve wheezy breathing, and clear your child's lungs, when he has a coughing fit. Support your child as he leans forwards, and pat his back.

2 Take your child's temperature and, if it is raised, give him acetaminophen or ibuprofen suspension. Also give him plenty of water to drink.

3 Raise the head of the baby's crib by placing a book under the legs. When your older child goes to bed, try to prop him up in bed with extra pillows (see page 216).

☎ Seek medical help

Call for emergency help immediately if your child shows any of the emergency signs listed on page 215. **Consult your doctor as soon as possible** if you think your child may have bronchitis, and call him again if he:

- is not improving after two days
- coughs up greenish-yellow coloured phlegm
- develops a high temperature.

What might the doctor do?

If your doctor thinks your child has a bacterial infection he might prescribe an antibiotic to eliminate it.

Asthma

What is it?

Asthma is a series of recurrent episodes of narrowing of the tiny airways leading to the lungs, which makes breathing, especially breathing out, difficult. In young children it is usually triggered by colds and viral infections, not by allergies. Mild asthma is common, and children who develop it at a very young age are more likely to grow out of the condition as they grow older.

Symptoms

- Coughing, particularly at night, or after exercise
- slight wheeziness and breathlessness, especially during a cold
- attacks of severe breathlessness, when breathing is shallow and difficult
- feeling of suffocation during an asthma attack
- pale and sweaty skin during an attack
- blue tinge round the lips during a severe attack.

Put a small cushion *on his lap for him to lean on*

What can I do?

1 Keep calm, and reassure your child. If he has had previous attacks, give him whatever medicine the doctor has prescribed. If this has no effect, **call for emergency help.**

2 Sit your child on your lap, and help him to lean slightly forwards – this makes it easier for him to breathe. Don't hold him tightly – let him settle into the most comfortable position.

3 If your child prefers to sit on his own, give him something to rest his arms on – a table top or pile of pillows, for example – so that he leans forwards.

Pneumonia

What is it?

Pneumonia is an inflammation of the lungs, which causes breathing difficulty. Usually only a portion of the lungs is affected, but in severe cases both lungs may be affected.

In young children, pneumonia is nearly always due to the spread of an upper respiratory tract infection, such as a cold or flu, and is usually caused by a virus, not bacteria.

Occasionally, pneumonia is the result of a tiny amount of food being inhaled into the lungs, causing a small patch of inflammation and infection.

Pneumonia is most common in babies under a year old. Although it is a serious disease, most babies who are otherwise healthy will usually recover completely in about a week, and it will not result in any long-term damage to the lung tissues.

Symptoms

- Deterioration in a sick child
- raised temperature
- dry cough
- rapid breathing
- difficult or noisy breathing.

☎ Seek medical help

Call for emergency help immediately if your child develops any of the emergency signs listed on page 215. **Call your doctor now** if you think your child has pneumonia.

What can I do?

1 Prop your child up with extra pillows in bed, so that he can breathe more easily. Raise the head of your baby's crib with books (see page 201).

2 Take your child's temperature and, if it is raised, try to reduce it by giving him the recommended dose of acetaminophen or ibuprofen suspension.

3 Make sure your child has plenty to drink, especially if his temperature is raised.

What might the doctor do?

The doctor will advise you how to care for your child, and if the infection is bacterial, he may prescribe an antibiotic. If your child is very ill, he might need to be treated in a hospital.

Emergency

Call for emergency help immediately if your child:
- has a bluish tinge on his tongue or around his lips
- is severely breathless
- does not start to breathe more easily 10 minutes after taking his medicine
- becomes unresponsive.

☎ Seek medical help

Call your doctor now if this is your child's first asthma attack. **Consult your doctor as soon as possible** if you think your child may have asthma.

What might the doctor do?

If your child's asthma is mild, the doctor may recommend a bronchodilator drug that he can inhale whenever he has symptoms. If he has the symptoms daily, a drug to prevent attacks every day may be prescribed. During a severe attack, the doctor may send your child to the hospital.

Preventing asthma attacks

Try to find out what causes your child's asthma attacks by keeping a record of when they occur. Vigorous exercise and over-excitement can bring on an attack. Some other common triggers are shown here.

Feather-filled cushions or duvets
Change these for ones with a synthetic filling, and air them regularly.

House dust mites
Reduce house dust by vacuuming and damp mopping, rather than sweeping and dusting. Cover your child's mattress with a plastic sheet. Consider buying special bedding that reduces dust levels.

Pollen, especially from grass and trees
Discourage your child from playing in long grass.

Animal fur
If you have a pet, speak to your doctor, who may recommend allergy testing.

Cigarette smoke
Don't let people smoke near your child.

Stomach pain

Stomach pain can be a symptom of many disorders, including gastroenteritis and urinary tract infections. It may also be caused by vomiting, and can accompany illnesses, such as tonsillitis and measles.

Your child may complain of a stomach ache if he feels generally unwell, knows he is about to be sick, or if he has a pain elsewhere but can't quite describe its precise location.

Dealing with a stomach ache

What causes stomach pain?

Many children have recurrent bouts of stomach pain when something makes them feel anxious or insecure. Provided that your child's pain is not severe and lasts for only an hour or two, you needn't worry; try to find out what is bothering him, and reassure him.

However, if your child is in severe pain for a few hours you should take it seriously. He might have appendicitis, although this is extremely rare in children under three. Typically, appendicitis pain is felt around the navel for a few hours, then moves to the lower right part of the abdomen.

Waves of severe stomach pain at intervals of about 15–20 minutes in a baby or toddler may mean that his bowel has become blocked.

What can I do?

1 Take your child's temperature. If it is slightly raised, he may have appendicitis, especially if the stomach pain is severe, or seems to be located around his navel. Don't give him a pain killer to ease it, or anything to reduce his temperature.

2 If you think your child may have appendicitis, don't give him anything to eat or drink. Give him some water only if he is thirsty. Seek medical help immediately.

3 Comfort your child by giving him cuddles and extra attention.

4 If you don't suspect appendicitis, fill a hot water bottle with warm water and wrap it in a towel. Let your child lie down with this held against his stomach.

> ☎ **Seek medical help**
>
> **Call your doctor now** if your child:
> ● develops any other symptoms
> ● has stomach pains for longer than three hours.
> **Consult your doctor** if your child has frequent stomach pain.

Wrap the hot water bottle *securely in a towel*

Emergency

Call for emergency help immediately if your baby or child:
● screams with pain at intervals of about 15–20 minutes, and goes pale when he screams
● passes dark red stools that resemble redcurrant jelly
● has severe stomach pain for longer than three hours
● has severe stomach pain combined with a raised temperature.

What might the doctor do?

The doctor will examine your child to try to find out the cause of his stomach pain. The treatment will depend on his diagnosis, but stomach pain often needs no treatment. If the doctor suspects appendicitis or a blocked bowel, he will arrange for your child to go to the hospital for an emergency operation.

Constipation, vomiting, and diarrhea

A minor change in your child's diet can cause temporary constipation or diarrhea. Vomiting or diarrhea may accompany almost any illness, and can also be caused by excitement or anxiety.

Frequent vomiting or severe diarrhea can quickly make a baby or a young child dehydrated. This is a serious condition and must be treated promptly (see page 222).

Constipation

What is it?
If your child has constipation he passes stools less frequently than usual, and they are harder than normal. Children's bowel habits vary greatly: some children have a bowel movement twice a day, others go only once every two or three days. Whatever your child's regular pattern is, it is quite normal and nothing to worry about unless it suddenly changes.

☎ Seek medical help
Consult your doctor as soon as possible if your child:
● cries or complains of pain when moving his bowels
● has streaks of blood in his stools, or on his diaper or underwear
● has constipation for more than three days.

What can I do?

1 Don't worry if your child is temporarily constipated, it won't do him any harm. Don't give him a laxative, because this will upset the normal action of his bowels, and don't add sugar to his bottle.

2 Give your child plenty of fluids to drink, especially if the weather is hot – this will help to soften his stools. Prune juice will ease his constipation.

3 Don't hurry your child when he is sitting on the potty, but on the other hand, don't let him remain there for too long.

4 Try to include more fibre in your child's diet (see below). This provides the bulk that facilitates bowel movement.

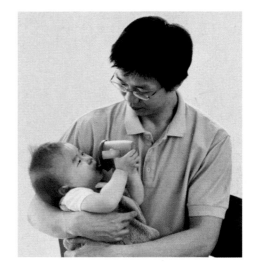

What might the doctor do?
The doctor may prescribe a mild laxative, and give you some advice on your child's diet. If your child has streaks of blood in his stools he could have a small tear in the lining of his anus. This usually heals when the constipation is treated.

Good sources of fibre
Some examples of foods rich in fibre are shown here. Fresh foods are always the best. Wash vegetables and fruit thoroughly, remove stems and seeds, and peel for a child under one year old. Purée the food for a baby under eight months (see pages 110–1).

Fresh fruit
Offer your child a variety of fruit, such as slices of peeled pear, peach, and banana.

Wholegrain bread

Wholegrain breakfast cereal

Dried fruit
Prunes and apricots are ideal for young children.

Vegetables
Mashed potato and lightly cooked broccoli or carrots are high in fibre. Celery can be served raw.

Vomiting

What is it?
When your child vomits, she will bring up most of the contents of her stomach. Most cases clear up within 24 hours, but young children and babies can dehydrate rapidly, so make sure your child drinks plenty of fluids.

Babies under about six months old often regurgitate a small amount of their feeds. This is perfectly normal – your baby is not vomiting.

Identifying and treating dehydration
Your child may be dehydrated if she shows one or more of the symptoms listed below:
- dry mouth and lips
- dark, concentrated urine
- no urine passed for six hours
- sunken eyes and fontanelle
- abnormal drowsiness or lethargy.

To prevent dehydration, use an oral rehydration solution (ORS) to replace regular formula feeds or supplement breast milk. Give a little fluid frequently (every 10 to 15 minutes) by small cup, spoon, or syringe, and increase breastfeeds.

What can I do?

1 Hold your child over a bowl and comfort her while she is vomiting (see page 199). Wipe her face afterwards and give her some sips of water.

2 Make sure that your child has plenty to drink – she needs 1–1½ litres (2–3 pints) a day. Use an oral rehydration solution available from your pharmacist, and offer her a little every hour. If your baby won't take a bottle, try using a teaspoon or a medicine syringe (see page 195).

☎ Seek medical help
Call your doctor now if your child:
- vomits and seems abnormally drowsy
- throws up greenish-yellow vomit
- has vomited repeatedly for more than four to six hours
- shows any signs of dehydration.

What might the doctor do?
The doctor will examine your child to find out what is making her vomit, and will then treat her according to the diagnosis.

If she shows signs of dehydration, the doctor may recommend persevering with oral rehydration fluids or may arrange for her to be admitted to the hospital, where she can be given fluids intravenously.

Gastroenteritis

What is it?
Gastroenteritis is an infection in the stomach and intestines that can be caused by contaminated food. It is serious in babies, because it can dehydrate them very quickly, but it is rare in breastfed babies. A mild attack in a child over two years old is not serious.

Symptoms
- Vomiting and nausea
- diarrhea
- stomach cramps
- loss of appetite
- raised temperature.

What can I do?

1 Make sure that your child drinks about 1–1½ litres (2–3 pints) a day. Give an oral rehydration solution (ORS) available from your pharmacist. Oral rehydration is successful in at least 95 percent of cases.

2 Don't give your child anything to eat until she stops vomiting, then introduce bland foods. Continue your baby's usual milk feeds (see page 185) after vomiting ends.

3 Give her acetaminophen if she has a fever.

4 Let your child wear a diaper again if she has just grown out of them.

5 Make sure that your child washes her hands properly after using her potty and before eating. Wash your own hands after changing her diaper and before preparing food.

Note: Breastfed babies should continue to breastfeed.

Diarrhea

What is it?

If your child has diarrhea, she will pass watery stools more frequently than normal. This may be the result of eating food that is too rich for her or contains more fibre than she is used to. It may also be caused by an infection. Give your child plenty of fluids to prevent dehydration.

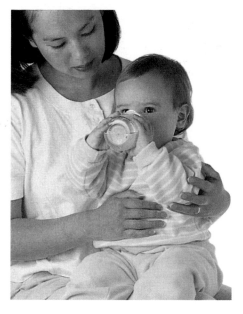

☎ Seek medical help

Call your doctor now if your child:
- has had diarrhea for more than 24 hours
- has blood in her stools
- shows any signs of dehydration (see page 222).

What can I do?

1 Make sure that your child always has plenty of water to drink. An oral rehydration solution is ideal (see Identifying and treating dehydration, page 222). Do not give your child fruit juice or a sugar solution as they can make diarrhea worse.

2 Put your child in a diaper again if she has just grown out of them. This will prevent any unnecessary soiling.

3 Always pay careful attention to hygiene: wash your hands after changing your baby's diaper and before preparing her food, and make sure that your child washes her hands after using the potty and before eating.

Treatment of diarrhea

If your baby is not taking her feeds, replace all feeds (other than breast milk) with an oral rehydration solution (ORS, see page 222).

The quantity required **per hour** depends on her age: from 30 to 90ml (1 to 3oz) for a baby under 6 months, to 125 to 250ml (4 to 8oz) for a child over two. If she is vomiting, give her 15ml (1tbsp) every 10 to 15 minutes. As the diarrhea becomes less frequent, return to your baby's usual feeds of formula or whole milk and food in small, frequent feedings.

What might the doctor do?

The doctor will examine your child to find out the cause of her diarrhea, and will treat her according to the diagnosis. If your child has become dehydrated, the doctor may prescribe oral rehydration fluids. If she is very dehydrated, he might arrange for her to be admitted to the hospital, where she can be given extra fluids intravenously.

☎ Seek medical help

Call your doctor now if your child:
- is under two and you suspect she may have gastroenteritis
- is over two and has had symptoms of gastroenteritis for more than two days.

What might the doctor do?

The doctor will probably treat your child for dehydration and may advise you to give her only liquids for a few days. He may also ask for a sample of your child's stools.

"What steps can I take to prevent gastroenteritis?"

Clean all your baby's feeding equipment thoroughly for as long as she drinks formula or milk from a bottle (see pages 100–1). Wash your baby's bowls and cups in very hot water. Dry them on paper towels rather than with a dish towel, or use a dishwasher.

Pay careful attention to your personal hygiene, especially when preparing food. Put prepared bottles of formula or milk in the refrigerator – never store them warm in an insulated container since bacteria thrive in warm conditions. If you store any cooked food, don't keep it in the refrigerator for longer than two days and make sure it is thoroughly heated when you serve it.

Heat kills the bacteria that can cause gastroenteritis.

If you are travelling, ask your doctor about any precautions you should take, particularly with regard to water, fruit, and salads. Always take an oral rehydration powder with you, in the event your child develops gastroenteritis while you are away.

Rotavirus is the most common cause of acute diarrhea in children under two years of age. A vaccine to prevent rotavirus is available in Canada (see page 202). You may want to discuss this with your doctor.

Q&A

Bladder, kidney, and genital problems

Most urinary system infections are due to bacteria entering the urethra, and spreading up into the bladder. They are quite common in young children, and are usually not serious. Some children are born with minor abnormalities of the urinary system that make them prone to such infections. Minor infections of the genitals are often part of the symptoms of diaper rash (see page 182).

The urinary system
Your child has two kidneys that filter his blood. The clean blood returns to his bloodstream, while the waste product (the urine) drains into his bladder, where it collects until he is ready to urinate.

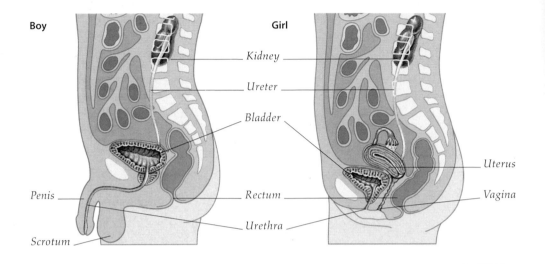

Boy — Penis, Scrotum

Girl — Kidney, Ureter, Bladder, Uterus, Rectum, Vagina, Urethra

Urinary system infections

What are they?
Any part of the urinary system – the kidneys, the bladder, and the connecting tubes – can become infected with bacteria. Infections are more common in girls because the tube from the bladder (the urethra) is shorter than in a boy, and its opening is nearer to the anus, so germs can spread to it more easily.

Symptoms
- Urinating more often than usual
- pain when urinating
- pink, red, or cloudy urine
- change in odour of the urine
- raised temperature
- listlessness
- loss of appetite
- abdominal pain.

What can I do?

1 If your child seems unwell, check to see whether her urine looks pink or cloudy. Note whether she is urinating more frequently than usual, and whether it seems to hurt her to pass urine. If your child is still in diapers, you probably won't be able to tell that urination is frequent or painful, but you may notice a change in odour of the urine.

2 Make sure that your child has plenty to drink, to keep her kidneys flushed out.

3 Take your child's temperature and, if it is raised, give her the prescribed dose of acetaminophen or ibuprofen suspension to reduce it.

> ☎ **Seek medical help**
> **Consult your doctor as soon as possible** if you think your child has a urinary system infection.

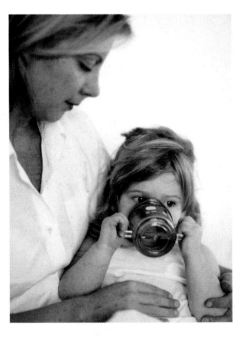

What might the doctor do?
The doctor will examine your child, and if he suspects an infection will ask you to take a sample of her urine. If your child has an infection, the doctor will prescribe an antibiotic. He may also arrange for special tests or investigations to check her kidneys and urinary tract.

Genital problems in girls

What can go wrong?
A little girl's vagina can become sore due to diaper rash (see page 182), a yeast infection, or pinworms (see page 232).

If your daughter has a blood-stained or smelly discharge from her vagina, she may have pushed something into it. Newborn girls often produce a white or blood-stained discharge for a few days, and this is nothing to worry about. After this age until just before puberty, a discharge is abnormal, and should be investigated by a doctor.

What can I do?
1 If your daughter's bottom is sore or red, don't use soap when you wash it as this may irritate it even more – just use water, and dry it thoroughly. Always wipe from the front to back, so that germs can't spread forwards from her anus.

2 Allow your child to go without a diaper for as long as possible each day, and don't put plastic pants over her diapers as they prevent air circulating to her bottom.

3 If your daughter has a discharge from her vagina, check whether she has pushed something into it. If she has, **consult your doctor as soon as possible.**

Symptoms
- Soreness or itching in or around the vagina
- redness around the vagina
- discharge from the vagina.

☎ Seek medical help
Consult your doctor as soon as possible if your daughter:
- has a discharge from her vagina
- still has symptoms after two days of home treatment
- has pushed something into vagina.

What might the doctor do?
The doctor will examine your daughter, and may take a sample of the discharge. If she has something lodged in her vagina, he will remove it gently. If she has an infection, he may prescribe antibiotics to be taken by mouth, or a cream to be applied to the affected area, depending on the cause of her symptoms.

Genital problems in boys

What can go wrong?
The foreskin, which covers the tip of the penis, can become inflamed or infected (balanitis), often as part of diaper rash (see page 182).

If a swelling develops in your son's groin or scrotum, he may have a hernia (a loop of intestines bulging through a weak area in the wall of the abdomen), which will require medical attention.

What can I do?
Wash and dry his foreskin carefully at each diaper change, and let him go without a diaper for as long as possible each day. Use a mild detergent and rinse diapers and underwear well.

How can I prevent inflammation?
Don't try to pull your son's foreskin back – it may not retract until he is at least four. If you try to force it, you may inflame his foreskin.

☎ Seek medical help
Consult your doctor as soon as possible if:
- your son's foreskin looks red or swollen, or if there is any discharge
- you think your son may have a hernia
- your son's hernia becomes painful, the bulge grows or changes in any other way.

Symptoms
Inflamed foreskin
- Red, swollen foreskin
- discharge of pus from the penis.

Hernia
- Soft, painless bulge in the groin or scrotum, which may disappear when your child lies down, and get bigger when he coughs, sneezes, or cries.

Circumcision
This is an operation to remove the foreskin. If you are thinking of having your son circumcised, first discuss it with your doctor. Like any other operation, it carries a small risk, so it is usually done only for religious or specific medical reasons.

What might the doctor do?
If your son's foreskin is inflamed, the doctor may prescribe an antibiotic cream. If your son has a hernia your doctor will recommend that he has an operation to repair it. If the hernia is painful or tender, the doctor may send him to hospital immediately for emergency surgery.

Skin problems

Minor skin problems are common in childhood. Most clear up quickly, but some are very contagious, and must be treated promptly. If your child has a rash combined with other signs of illness, she may have an infectious illness (see pages 203–8). For other problems, see below.

Quick diagnosis guide
One or more red spots, or a rash, see Spots and boils, Hives, Heat rash (below and opposite), Insect stings (page 252), or, if dry and scaly, see Eczema (page 228).
Raw, cracked areas, usually on or around the lips, or on the cheeks and hands, see Chapped skin (page 229).
Small blisters or crusty patches on or around the mouth, see Cold sores and Impetigo (pages 230–1).
Hard lump of skin, usually on the hands or feet, see Warts (page 230).
Itchy head, see Lice and nits (page 232).
Intense itching around the anus, see Pinworms (page 232).

Dealing with itching
Many skin problems cause itching, and since scratching can make the skin infected, it is important to relieve your child's itchiness.
● Dress her in cotton clothes, since cotton is less irritating to the skin than wool or other fabrics.
● Moisturize the skin with gentle, unscented moisturizer.
● Add therapeutic oil to your child's bath.
● Buy cotton scratch mitts for her to wear in bed.

Spots and boils

What are they?
A spot or pimple is a small red swelling, usually on the face. A boil is an infection in the skin that causes a large, painful lump, which then produces a head of pus in the middle. Boils are most likely to occur on the face or on pressure points such as the buttocks, but they can appear anywhere on the body.

Don't worry if your child gets occasional spots, but recurrent boils may be a sign of illness.

Symptoms
Spot
● Small, red, painless lump.

Boil
● Painful, red lump that gradually gets larger
● white or yellow centre of pus appearing after a day or two.

☎ Seek medical help
Consult your doctor as soon as possible if:
● your child has a spot that looks inflamed
● your child has a boil in an awkward or painful place
● the centre of pus does not appear three days after the boil first developed
● red streaks spread out from the boil.
● your child gets boils on a frequent basis.

What can I do?

1 If your child gets occasional spots, simply ignore them. They will clear up in a few days without treatment. If she tends to dribble, and the spots appear around her mouth, smear a small amount of barrier cream over the area.

2 If your child has a boil, or a spot that looks inflamed, gently clean it, and the skin around it, with a cotton ball and water.

3 If it is rubbed by clothing, or is in a painful place such as on the buttocks, cover it with a sterile dry dressing.

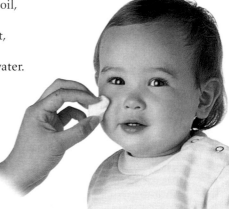

4 The boil will come to a head and burst of its own accord in a few days. Don't squeeze it – this may spread the infection. After it has burst, clean it gently with a cotton ball dipped in antiseptic cream, and keep it covered until it has healed.

What might the doctor do?
The doctor may lance the boil and drain away the pus, and might prescribe a cream. If your child has a lot of boils, or if they keep recurring, the doctor may prescribe a course of antibiotics.

Hives

What is it?

Hives (also known as urticaria) is an intensely itchy rash of red patches. The patches usually fade after a few hours, but new ones may appear. Hives may be caused by an allergy to certain foods (for example, milk or a citrus fruit) or drugs (for example, penicillin), exposure to strong sunshine, or most commonly, a viral infection.

Symptoms

● Itchy rash of raised red patches (welts), sometimes with a pale centre
● welts varying in length from 1mm to 1cm (1/16 to 1/2 in)
● larger welts joining together
● sudden swelling of lips, face, and tongue (angioedema).

What can I do?

1 Antihistamines, available over the counter, will usually help hives. However, they may make your child drowsy.

2 If the rash is caused by an allergy, try to find out what your child is allergic to, so that it can be avoided in future. The rash often develops a few hours after contact with an allergen, so try to remember whether, for example, she has recently eaten a new food.

☎ Seek medical help

Call your doctor now if your child's face, tongue, or throat is swollen. Call 911 if she is having difficulty breathing. If you have an Epipen, use it while you wait for the ambulance.
Consult your doctor as soon as possible if:
● the rash does not disappear within four hours
● your child has frequent attacks.

What might the doctor do?

The doctor may prescribe more antihistamine medications and also recommend allergy testing. If your child's face, tongue, or throat is swollen, she may need an injection to reduce the swelling. You may receive a prescription for an Epipen, which you should administer if she has a severe allergic reaction in the future.

Heat rash

What is it?

Heat rash is a faint rash caused by overheating. It is more common in babies than in children, and usually appears on the upper back, chest, or in skin creases, where sweat can gather. It is not a serious disorder, and you can treat it yourself at home.

Symptoms

● Pink rash on the face or in skin creases
● the site may be itchy.

☎ Seek medical help

Consult your doctor as soon as possible if the rash has not faded 12 hours after your child cools down.

What can I do?

1 Take off any heavy bedding and remove a layer of your baby's clothing. Let him sleep dressed in just an undershirt and diaper.

2 Give him a bath in lukewarm water. Pat his skin dry gently, leaving it slightly damp so that he cools down as his skin dries. When he is dry, dress him in cotton clothing.

3 Take your baby's temperature and, if it is raised, give him the recommended dose of acetaminophen or ibuprofen suspension.

How can I prevent heat rash?

Dress your baby in light clothes when the weather is hot, with cotton next to his skin rather than wool or a man-made fibre. Keep him in the shade, or put a sun canopy over him.

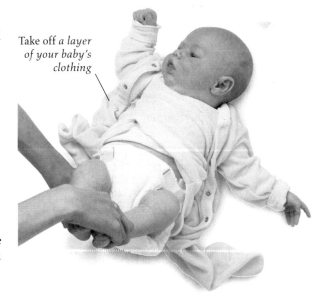

Take off a layer of your baby's clothing

What might the doctor do?

The doctor will check that the rash is just a heat rash. If it is, your baby needs no medical treatment. If the rash has another cause, the doctor will treat that.

Eczema

What is it?

Eczema is an allergic condition or skin inflammation marked by areas of inflamed, itchy, red, scaly skin. It most commonly affects the face and skin creases, such as the inside of the elbows and the back of the knees, although it can appear anywhere on the body.

It usually first appears between the ages of three months and two years, then improves as the child grows older. About half of all children with eczema grow out of it by the age of six, and nearly all of them grow out of it by puberty. Your child is more likely to develop eczema if other members of the family suffer from eczema or from any other allergic condition, such as asthma or hayfever.

Symptoms

- Itchy, red, scaly, dry patches, usually on the face or in skin creases
- clear fluid oozing from the affected areas.

☎ Seek medical help

Consult your doctor as soon as possible if:
- your child's eczema is very widespread or very itchy
- fluid is weeping from the eczema.

What might the doctor do?

The doctor may prescribe a cream, and if the area is infected, an antibiotic. If your child is allergic to a particular food, your doctor can advise you how to give him a balanced diet while avoiding that food.

What can I do?

1 When you give your child a bath, use a mild, hypoallergenic soap or therapeutic bath oils in the water. Rinse well with water.

2 After a bath, apply an unscented moisturizing cream to his skin. Consider applying petroleum jelly to your baby's damp skin to help trap moisture.

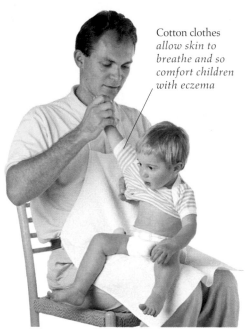

Cotton clothes allow skin to breathe and so comfort children with eczema

3 Dress your child in cotton, rather than wool. In cold weather, put cotton clothing under warmer layers.

4 Try to stop your child scratching the affected areas – put scratch mitts on him at night if this seems to help, and keep his fingernails short.

5 Try to discover a possible cause of the allergy. Common allergens include foods (especially dairy produce and wheat), animal fur, woollen clothes, and laundry detergent and fabric softener. Anxiety can trigger eczema, so find out if anything is worrying your child.

6 When your child's eczema is bad, keep him away from anyone with chickenpox or a cold sore because of greater risk of infection.

Sunburn

What is it?

Sunburn is sore or reddened skin caused by over-exposure to ultra-violet rays from the sun. The skin becomes hot and tender, and may blister if badly burnt. Babies and young children, especially those with fair hair and blue eyes, are particularly vulnerable to it. Sun exposure during childhood is the greatest single cause of skin damage and skin cancer.

Symptoms

- Red, sore areas of skin
- blisters appearing on badly affected areas
- flaking or peeling skin a day or two later.

What can I do?

1 Take your child inside or into the shade as soon as his skin begins to look red. Bear in mind that the worst symptoms of sunburn are likely to be delayed for a few hours.

2 Cool any reddened areas of skin with cold water, then apply a soothing after-sun lotion.

Preventing sunburn

Avoid being in the sun for long periods of time and try to minimize exposure during the hottest time of the day, between 10 a.m. and 2 p.m. Your baby should always be covered up in the sun and your older child should wear a sun hat with a wide brim and back flap, sunglasses with 100 percent UV protection, and loose, protective clothing. Apply a sun block with sun protection factor (SPF) of at least 30 on all areas of exposed skin **before** your child goes outside and reapply regularly, particularly if he has been in the water.

Choose a hat *that protects your child's neck*

☎ Seek medical help

Consult your doctor as soon as possible if:
- your child has a fever and seems unwell
- blisters appear over a large area.

What might the doctor do?

The doctor may recommend a soothing and protective cream.

Chapped skin

What is it?

Chaps are small cracks in the skin that occur when the skin becomes dry after being exposed to cold or hot, dry air. Chapping is not serious, but it can be painful.

What can I do?

1 Moisturize your child's lips with lip balm, and apply moisturizing cream or petroleum jelly to his skin.

2 Use baby oil or lotion to wash the area, and keep his hands warm and dry. If your child habitually licks his lips, encourage him to stop as this can cause chapping.

Symptoms

- Tiny cracks in the skin, usually on or around the lips, or on the cheeks or hands
- bleeding if the cracks are deep.

☎ Seek medical help

Consult your doctor as soon as possible if:
- the cracks do not heal after three days
- the cracks become red, sore, or pus-filled.

What might the doctor do?

The doctor might suggest a moisturizer or, if the area is infected, prescribe an antibiotic.

Cold sores

What are they?

Cold sores are small blisters, usually on or around the lips but they sometimes develop inside the mouth or elsewhere on the face. They may be tender and painful.

They are caused by a strain of the herpes simplex virus that, once it has infected a child, lies dormant in the skin and tends to flare up occasionally. So if your child has had a cold sore, he is liable to get others in the future. Strong sunlight can trigger a recurrence, and so can a minor illness, such as a cold (which is why they are known as cold sores). Anxiety or emotional stress may also reactivate the virus.

Symptoms

- Raised, red area that tingles or itches, usually around the mouth
- small, painful yellow blisters forming about a day later
- blisters crusting over after a day or two
- fever and general illness during the first attack.

What can I do?

1 At the first sign of a cold sore, hold an ice cube against the affected area for 10 minutes. This may prevent the blister developing.

Wrap an ice cube in a cloth and hold it against your child's lip

2 Keep his hands clean, and stop him from touching the sore, as he could spread the infection to his eyes.

3 Since cold sores are very contagious, don't let your child kiss other people and, if he tends to put toys into his mouth, don't let him share them with other children until the sore has gone.

4 If your child has ever had a cold sore, protect his lips from strong sunlight with a sunscreen because sunlight can trigger a recurrence.

☎ Seek medical help

Consult your doctor as soon as possible if:
- your child has a cold sore for the first time
- your child's cold sore starts to ooze or spread
- your child has a cold sore near his eyes.

What might the doctor do?

Cold sores usually resolve on their own. The doctor may prescribe an antiviral cream, which should be applied on the cold sore at the first sign of an attack.

Warts

What are they?

A wart is a lump of hard, dry skin; a plantar wart is a wart on the sole of the foot. They are caused by a virus that invades the skin, and are contagious. Most children get them occasionally. Warts are not painful and disappear spontaneously, usually after a few months, so treatment is not necessary. Plantar warts tend to be painful because of the pressure put on them whenever the child walks or wears shoes, so they should be treated promptly.

Symptoms

Wart
- Hard lump of dry skin.

Plantar wart
- Hard, painful area on the sole of the foot, perhaps with a tiny black centre.

What can I do?

1 If your child has a wart simply ignore it, unless it is on his genitals or by his anus or if it is painful to walk on. It will disappear on its own probably after a few months, although some last for a year or more.

Impetigo

What is it?

Impetigo is a bacterial skin infection that may develop when a rash such as eczema or a cold sore becomes infected, although even healthy skin can sometimes become infected with impetigo. It most often affects young children, especially babies.

It usually affects the skin around the mouth and nose, and the diaper area in babies, but it can occur anywhere on the body. Impetigo isn't a serious disorder in children, but in a young baby it can spread over a large area and make him quite ill. It is very contagious, so it is important to have it treated promptly.

Symptoms

- Rash of small, red spots
- blisters forming over the spots
- the spots burst, then form large brownish-yellow scabs
- fever and general illness in a young baby.

What can I do?

1 Keep your child's washcloth and towel separate from those of the rest of the family, and wash them frequently so the infection doesn't spread.

2 Try to keep him from touching the affected area – don't let him suck his thumb or pick his nose, as this could spread the infection.

3 If your doctor has prescribed a cream, remove the crusts each day before applying it by wiping them with a damp cotton ball. Don't rub hard, but persevere until the crusts loosen.

4 Pat the area dry with a tissue or paper towel and throw it away immediately, so that the infection can't spread.

5 Keep your child away from other children, especially young babies, until he has had 48 hours of treatment.

Wipe the crusts gently *with a cotton ball dipped in warm, soapy water*

☎ Seek medical help

Call your doctor now if your baby is under three months old and suddenly develops widespread impetigo. **Consult your doctor** if you think your child has impetigo.

What might the doctor do?

The doctor may prescribe a cream and tell you to wipe away the crusts (see left) before applying it. If the infection is widespread, he may prescribe an antibiotic.

Cover the plantar wart *with an adhesive bandage.*

☎ Seek medical help

Consult your doctor if:
- your child's warts multiply
- your child has a wart on his genitals or anus
- your child has a plantar wart that doesn't resolve.

2 If your child has a plantar wart, try an over-the-counter remedy from your pharmacist. Remove dead skin from the surface of the wart by rubbing with a pumice stone. Cover a plantar wart with an adhesive bandage and it may disappear spontaneously. Keep your child's washcloth and towel separate.

What might the doctor do?

If home treatment is not successful, your doctor may prescribe a medicated compound to be applied to the wart, or may use liquid nitrogen to "freeze" it. Warts sometimes recur even after they have been treated.

Head lice

What are they?

Lice are tiny insects that infest the hair, and make the child's head itchy. Their minute white eggs (nits) cling to her hair roots. Lice spread very easily from one head to another, so treat the whole family if your child picks up lice. Tell your friends to check their children's heads, and tell the staff at your child's daycare or school. Keep her at home until she is treated.

Symptoms

- Itchy head
- tiny white grains firmly attached to the hairs near the roots
- red bite marks under the hair.

What can I do?

1 Ask your pharmacist for a lotion or shampoo to kill the lice and nits. Also buy a fine comb to remove the lice and nits after treatment.

2 Follow the instructions carefully for the lotion or shampoo. Leave it on her hair for as long as specified and rinse her hair well. Then comb it thoroughly with the special comb, wiping the comb with a tissue between each stroke. Reapply in 7 to 10 days as specified.

3 Wash hats and pillowcases in hot water and dry in a hot dryer for 15 minutes. Seal toys and bedding in plastic bags for 14 days and the nits will die.

Use a cotton ball *to apply the lotion*

4 Do not use products with lindane on children under two as it can be toxic. Other chemical-free methods, such as "smothering" lice with mayonnaise or olive oil, are safe but not as effective as the medicated lotions. There is no evidence that tea tree oil eradicates head lice.

Pinworms

What are they?

Pinworms are tiny, white thread-like worms, about 1cm (½in) long, that infect the gut. They can enter the body in contaminated food, and then live in the bowels, coming out at night to lay eggs around the anus, and causing intense itchiness. They are common in children, and are harmless, although the itching may be very uncomfortable. In little girls, the worms may crawl forwards to the vagina. The eggs are easily transferred, so it is sensible to treat the whole family if your child is infected.

Symptoms

- Intense itching around the anus, which is usually worse at night
- intense itching around the vagina
- tiny white worms in the stools or around the anus.

What can I do?

1 Contact your doctor if you think your child has pinworms. A simple test can confirm this infection.

2 The pinworms can be treated with an oral medication, which may take up to two weeks to work. Your doctor might repeat the treatment after two weeks. He may also suggest treating the whole family.

3 Keep her fingernails short, and discourage nail-biting or thumb-sucking which could re-infect her.

4 Make sure that the whole family washes their hands thoroughly after going to the toilet and changing diapers, and before preparing and eating food.

5 If your child no longer wears diapers, make sure she wears pyjamas or cotton underwear under her nightgown. Wash her clothing and bed linens in hot water, and dry them in a hot dryer.

Hygiene measures

The eggs can survive for two weeks outside the body on underwear and bedding so after taking the medication, clean "risk areas" thoroughly to prevent reinfection:

- Clean beds and bedrooms thoroughly. Wash all bed linens, sleepwear, towels, cuddly toys, and vacuum mattresses. Don't allow eating in the bedroom.
- Make sure the whole family washes their hands thoroughly after going to the toilet and before eating. Use a nail brush to clean the nails properly.
- Don't share towels or washcloths.

6 Give her regular baths or showers, and wash around her anus and vagina first thing every morning to get rid of any eggs laid overnight.

Epilepsy

Epilepsy, which causes recurrent convulsions, affects about 1 in 200 people. Many people with epilepsy experience their first seizure before the age of 20. A seizure is caused by excessive electrical discharges by brain cells. The most common cause of convulsion in children is a high fever (see page 194), but this is not considered a form of epilepsy. A single seizure does not mean your child has epilepsy. However, do seek medical advice to rule out any serious underlying condition.

What is it?

Epilepsy is currently defined as a tendency to have recurrent seizures, caused by bursts of abnormal electrical activity in the brain. In many cases the cause of epilepsy is unknown (see page 194). With treatment, many children grow out of it. There are several different types of epilepsy; two common forms in childhood are absence attacks (partial seizures where only part of the brain is affected) and generalized seizures (where the whole brain is affected) – see symptoms box.

What can I do?

1 During a generalized seizure, stay with your child and protect her from injury by removing any harmful objects nearby. Don't try to restrain her.

2 After the seizure, turn her on her side in the recovery position (see page 241). Don't wake her if she falls asleep, but make sure that she is breathing properly (see page 238).

3 Try to avoid letting your child get into situations that could be dangerous if she has a seizure – for example, put a gate at the top of the stairs, and don't leave her alone in the bath. But don't be over-protective – she shouldn't feel that her epilepsy makes her abnormal.

What might the doctor do?

The doctor may send your child to hospital for tests. He may also prescribe a drug to help control the seizures; if so, tell the doctor if your child's behaviour changes in any way, but don't stop giving her the drug.

The recovery position
If your child has a seizure, place her in the recovery position, and tilt her chin to keep her airway open, and ensure that she is breathing properly. Leave her in this position until she regains consciousness. If she falls asleep, let her wake naturally.

Symptoms

Partial seizures (absence attacks)
- Sudden cessation of movement
- dazed expression
- complete recovery in a few seconds.

Generalized seizures (tonic-clonic seizures)
- Sudden unconsciousness, so your child falls down
- stiff arms and legs
- twitching or jerky movements
- possible loss of bladder or bowel control
- sleeping, or gradual return to consciousness, after the twitching movements have stopped.

☎ Call an ambulance

Call an ambulance now if your child has:
- a major seizure for the first time
- a major seizure lasting more than three minutes
- a series of seizures in rapid succession.

Consult your doctor if you think your child has absence attacks.

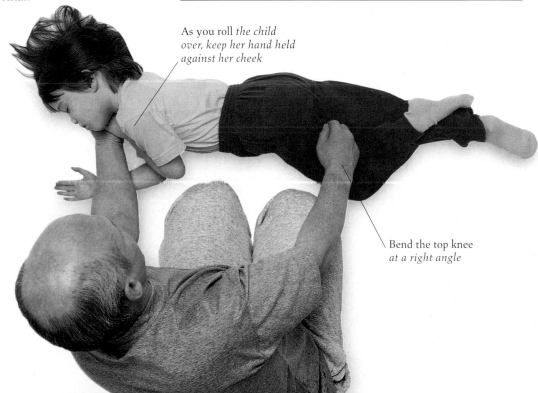

As you roll *the child over, keep her hand held against her cheek*

Bend the top knee *at a right angle*

Your child's safety

About a quarter of all injuries that happen in the home involve children under four, but there are a number of ways you can make your house safer. The best way to keep your child safe is to keep him under your watchful eye. Make sure that the safety equipment you buy for the house conforms to Canadian safety standards, and use it only for the age of child it is designed for. Buy new if possible. Second-hand items may not comply with safety regulations.

Safety in your home

Children are vulnerable to accidents because their desire to explore and experiment far outstrips their common sense and forethought. Many accidents can easily be prevented, and it is your responsibility to make sure that your child can't injure himself and his world is safe for him to play in and explore.

Kitchen

Your kitchen is full of potential hazards for a child, and these dangers are increased if you are busy. Keep him away from the cooking area when you are cooking – an infant seat or a playpen is ideal. Don't forget that stove burners, kettles, and irons stay hot long after you have switched them off. At mealtimes, keep hot dishes near the centre of the table so that your child can't grab them. Don't use a table cloth because he can pull it, and spill hot things over himself.

Store *plastic bags and plastic wraps out of your child's reach*

Fit *a child-resistant lock on your fridge or freezer*

Fit a guard *around your stove, and turn your saucepan handles away from the front. Use the back burners rather than the front ones*

Make sure that *your child can't get to your garbage bin*

Buy *coiled electrical cords, or make sure your cords are short*

Push *hot drinks to the back of kitchen surfaces*

Keep *all household cleaners and bleaches in a cupboard with a child-resistant catch*

Keep *sharp utensils such as kitchen knives in a drawer with a child-resistant catch*

Don't let *your child touch the oven door while it is hot*

Keeping your baby safe

With each new skill he develops, your baby will find ways of running into danger, so you must think ahead to avoid hazards. He will learn to roll over when he is very young, so if you need to lay him down for even a moment, put him on the floor.

He will soon grab things, so make sure that anything he can reach is safe to handle, and too large to swallow or choke on. Don't eat, drink, carry anything hot, or smoke while you are holding your baby. Never leave him alone with a bottle – he could choke. Always use the safety harness on his stroller and high chair. Don't put him in an infant seat on a high surface – it could easily fall off. Don't leave a young child alone with your baby: he might pick him up and drop him, or give him dangerous objects to play with.

Bedroom

Your child will spend a lot of time in his bedroom, so make sure it is safe. Don't put a pillow in his crib until he is at least two, and don't use loose plastic sheeting as a waterproof mattress cover. Never attach his toys to the crib with cords – they might wind around his neck. Keep large toys out of the crib – your child could use them as stepping stones to climb out – and don't string toys across the crib once he can stand. His toys should be non-toxic and non-flammable, and must have no sharp edges or pieces small enough to swallow.

Fix *safety catches on the windows, so that they can be opened only a little way. Open sash windows from the top*

Cover *hot radiators with a towel*

Store *toys in a low cupboard or shelf, so your child can reach them without climbing*

Make *sure that your furniture is sturdy and has rounded edges. You can buy corner pieces to cover sharp edges*

Keep *diaper changing materials in a box with a lid*

Change *your baby's diaper on the floor*

Use flame-resistant *bedding and sleepwear*

Set *the crib mattress to its lowest position before your baby can pull himself to standing*

Bathroom

Never leave a child under four alone in the bath, or in the bathroom if the bathtub is full, even for a few seconds. Use a non-slip bath mat. Set your water heater lower than 55°C (130°F), and run the cold water into your child's bath first. Test the temperature before putting your child in. Other accidents that may occur in the bathroom can easily be prevented:
- Keep all medicines out of your child's reach in a cabinet with a lock or a child-resistant catch.
- Cover any heated towel bars with towels.
- A portable electric heater should not be used anywhere your child might reach it.
- Keep cleaning supplies and the toilet brush in a cupboard with a child-resistant catch.
- Put razors and cosmetics out of your child's reach.
- If you have a shower with a glass screen, replace the screen with a curtain, or install safety glass.

In the yard

Keep an eye on your child when he is playing in the yard. Never let your child play in or near a wading pool without supervision, and empty the pool after use. If you have a pond, cover or fence it securely. Make sure that the plants in your garden aren't poisonous. Teach your child not to eat any berries. Fix child-resistant locks on all gates. Don't let your child play in an area where you have recently used pesticide, weed-killer, or fertilizer.

Keep the whole pond covered with wire netting or surround it with a sturdy fence. Children can drown in a few centimetres of water

Lock away all your gardening and other tools, and any weed killer, fertilizer, and pesticide

The sand in your child's sandbox should be too shallow for him to bury himself. Teach him not to throw sand. Cover the sandbox when not in use, as dogs and cats could foul the sand, which is a hygiene risk

Put your child's play equipment on grass or sand, not on a hard surface

Living room

When you buy upholstered furniture, make sure that it will not give off toxic fumes if you have a fire. Always use a fireplace screen. Keep the television out of your child's reach.

Don't leave cigarettes, matches, alcohol, sewing equipment, or coins lying around. Keep indoor plants out of his reach, as some are poisonous.

If you have low glass panels in doors or windows, use toughened, laminated, or wire-net glass, or apply a transparent safety film, or put coloured stickers on them, so that your child can see where the glass is. Avoid glass-topped tables.

Hall and stairs

Fix safety gates at the top and bottom of the stairs before your child can crawl or climb. Make sure that the hall, stairs, and landings are well lit, and that the railings

aren't so wide apart that your child could fall through. Install door knob covers on the front and back doors, and a smoke detector. Repair loose tiles or tears in rugs. On polished wooden floors don't let your child wear socks without shoes.

Cars

Your child should always travel in a car seat that is officially approved for his age and weight (see pages 158–59). Children should never travel in the front seat of a car with air bags – the middle position of the back seat is the safest for a single car seat. Use child-proof locks on the doors and windows, and don't let your child lean out of the window or put his hand out while you are travelling. Never leave your child alone in the car.

Be extra cautious when your child is playing outside. Check where he is before you close the car door and when backing

out of a driveway. If he is just behind your car, you will not see him in the rearview mirror.

Electricity

Electric shocks from any power source can be very serious, so be extra cautious:
- Switch off electrical appliances when you are not using them.
- Wrap extension cords with electrical tape at the junctions.
- Cover unused sockets with childproof socket covers, or mask them with heavy insulating tape.
- Check all electrical cords regularly, and replace those with exposed wires.
- Don't let your child play with electrically powered toys until he is at least four years old.

First aid

This chapter will help you deal with various injuries yourself and indicate when medical help is necessary. Always treat the most serious injury first. Sometimes it may be faster to take your child to the hospital rather than call an ambulance (911 in most urban areas), but see below for occasions when you must call an ambulance. If your child is badly injured, she will need urgent medical treatment, but you should give first aid while waiting for emergency help to arrive.

Getting your child to a hospital

Call for an ambulance, or better still ask someone else to phone, if:
- your child is unconscious
- you think your child might have a head or spinal injury
- you think she needs special treatment while travelling.

If you take your child to the hospital yourself, there should be one person to drive, while the other sits in the back with your child and continues to give first aid.

If your child is unconscious, don't leave her alone even to call an ambulance. If she is not breathing and you are on your own, give her cardiopulmonary resuscitation (CPR) (see page 239) for two minutes before calling for help.

Warning

If there is a chance that your child has injured her neck or spine – for example, after a fall from a height – don't move her unless her life is in danger. Leave her in the position you found her while you check whether or not she is breathing. If you need to perform cardiopulmonary resuscitation (CPR), turn your child on her back very gently, keeping her head, neck, and back aligned. Ideally, get help so that one person supports her head and neck while you turn her body.

First aid kit

Keep a supply of first aid equipment in a clean, dry container, and replace anything you use as soon as possible. Take some antiseptic wipes with you on outings, to clean cuts and scrapes.

One elastic bandage

Gauze bandage rolls

Hypoallergenic tape
This is useful for sticking on dressings, and drawing together the edges of large cuts.

Calamine lotion
This will soothe sunburn and insect bites and stings.

Non-adherent, absorbent, sterile wound dressings
These peel off a wound easily.

Triangular bandage
This can be used to make a sling or secure a dressing.

Resuscitation mask
This plastic pocket mask protects you and the casualty from cross infection during CPR.

Alcohol-free antiseptic wipes

Tweezers

Scissors

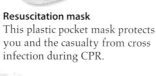

Prepared wound dressings
These consist of a pad attached to a bandage, and are easy to use.

Non-latex disposable gloves

Safety pins

Assorted adhesive bandages
Use these for dressing minor cuts and grazes.

Life-saving techniques

Every second counts! Familiarize yourself with lifesaving skills so that you can act quickly in an emergency. CPR (cardiopulmonary resuscitation) guidelines were just in the process of changing when this book went to press. The sequences shown here reflect these changes, but it is essential that you obtain proper training and up-to-date information about the life-saving combination of cardiac compressions and rescue breathing. This section is not meant to replace a CPR/first aid course. If possible, take a course as it could save your child's life. Contact your local St. John Ambulance office to find out about first aid and CPR classes near you.

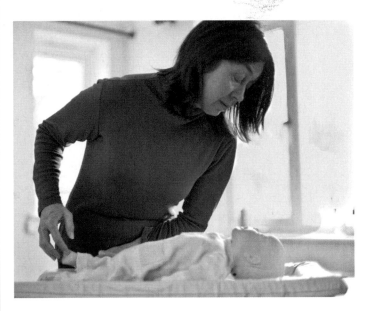

Checking for responsiveness

Unconsciousness is a potentially life-threatening condition that requires immediate medical assistance. To assess whether your baby is unconscious, tap the soles of her feet, for a child, tap her shoulder and call out her name loudly. If there is no response, it is likely that she is unconscious. **Never** shake a baby.

If she responds, she's conscious. Assess and treat any other injuries. Don't move her unless it's absolutely essential, and attend to life-threatening injuries, such as breathing difficulties, severe bleeding, or burns first.

If she doesn't respond, she is unconscious; check to see if she is breathing (see below).

> ## Emergency
> **Call for emergency help immediately** if your baby or child becomes unconscious, even if this is only for a few seconds.

Opening the airway and checking breathing

1 Place your baby on a firm surface. Put one hand on her forehead, and tilt her head back slightly. Place the forefinger of your other hand on the point of her chin and lift it. For a child, put two fingers on the chin. Keep your fingers away from her neck.

2 Check for normal breathing for no more than 5 seconds. If your baby is not breathing normally (for example, if she is gasping), start CPR.

If she is breathing normally, cradle her in your arms with her head lower than her body (see page 241), and call for emergency help.

If she is not breathing normally, ask someone to call an ambulance while you begin CPR immediately. If you are on your own, continue CPR for five cycles (approximately 2 minutes) before stopping to call for help.

Cardiopulmonary resuscitation (CPR) for a baby up to 12 months

1 Make sure your baby is on her back on a firm surface, such as a table. A thin pad under her shoulders helps keep the airway open, but don't waste time looking for one.

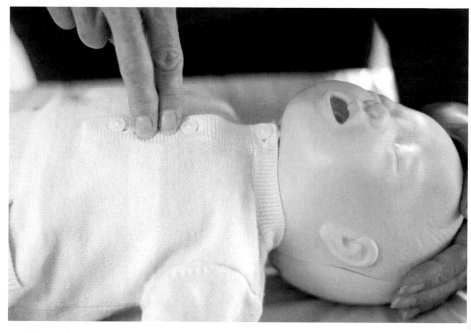

2 Begin chest compressions. Support your baby's head with one hand, and place two fingers of your other hand on the centre of her chest just below the nipple line. Press straight down sharply to compress the chest by at least one third of its depth or 4cm (1½in).

3 Release the pressure, but don't remove your fingers, and allow the chest to come back up. Repeat to give **30** compressions at a rate of at least 100 per minute.

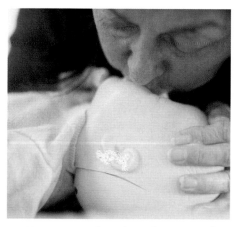

4 Begin rescue breaths. Take a normal breath, then seal your lips around her mouth and nose and blow gently into the mouth for about one second until you see the chest rise.

5 Still supporting her head, remove your lips and watch the chest fall back. Repeat to give **two** rescue breaths.

If the chest does not rise, the airway may not be open correctly; adjust the head position and try again.

6 Give another 30 chest compressions followed by two rescue breaths. Continue to give chest compressions and rescue breaths at a rate of 30:2 until the baby begins to breathe again, the emergency help arrives, or you are too exhausted to keep going

If you are on your own, give CPR for two minutes before stopping to call an ambulance.

If she starts breathing normally, hold her in the recovery position (see page 241).

If you are untrained in CPR or unsure of your skills, provide chest compressions only and await advice from the EMS.

Life-saving techniques *continued*

Cardiopulmonary resuscitation (CPR) for a child over one year

1 Check for responsiveness by asking your child if he is okay. Gently tap his shoulders and call his name. If there is no response, send a bystander for help and an AED (automated external defibrillator), if available. If you are alone, give five cycles of CPR (approximately two minutes) before you go for help.

2 Open his airway and check quickly for normal breathing (for no more than 5 seconds). If he is not breathing or gasping, start CPR immediately.

3 Make sure your child is on his back on a firm surface. Begin chest compressions. Kneel level with your child's chest and place the heel of one hand or both hands on the centre of his chest. Make sure your fingers are raised and off the ribs. If an AED is available, use it as soon as possible.

4 Press straight down sharply to compress the chest by at least one third of its depth or 5cm (2in). Release the pressure, and allow the chest to come back up. Repeat to give **30** compressions at a rate of at least 100 per minute.

5 Begin rescue breaths. Take a normal breath, then pinch his nose, seal your lips around his mouth, and blow gently into the mouth until you see the chest rise (about one second).

6 Still supporting his head, remove your lips , release his nostrils, and watch his chest fall back. Repeat to give **two** rescue breaths.

If the chest does not rise, the airway may not be open correctly; adjust the head position, and try again.

7 Give another 30 chest compressions followed by two rescue breaths. Continue to give chest compressions and rescue breaths at a rate of 30:2 until your child begins to breathe again, the emergency help arrives, or you become too exhausted to keep going.

If you are on your own, give CPR for two minutes before stopping to call an ambulance.

If he starts breathing normally, place him in the recovery position (see opposite).

If you are untrained in CPR or unsure of your skills, provide chest compressions only and await advice from the EMS.

The recovery position

Put your child into this position if she is unconscious but breathing normally. This keeps the airway open as the tongue cannot fall back and block the airway, and it allows any fluid to drain from her mouth. For a baby, see right.

Warning
If you suspect a back or neck injury several people are needed to place the child into the recovery position. One person should support the head while another rolls her over. A third can help keep the back straight. Keep the head and neck in a straight line at all times.

For a child over one year

1 Kneel beside your child. Tilt her head back and lift her chin forwards. This keeps her air passages open while you put her in the recovery position.

Her head *must be tilted well back with the chin jutting forward*

2 If necessary, straighten her legs. Bend the arm nearest to you so that it makes a right angle and lay it on the ground, with the palm of the hand upwards.

3 Bring her other arm across her chest. Hold the back of her hand against her opposite cheek.

Move *her furthest arm across her chest and bend it*

4 Use your free hand to clasp gently under the thigh furthest from you. Leaving the foot flat on the ground, pull the knee up to bend the leg. Keeping your child's hand against her cheek to support her head, pull on the thigh of the bent leg to roll her towards you and onto her side.

5 Adjust her arm and leg so she cannot fall forwards, and tilt her head. Call an ambulance.

Bend *her top leg into a right angle at the hip and knee to prevent her from rolling forwards*

Recovery position for a baby
A baby under the age of one should be cradled in your arms with her head tilted down to avoid obstruction of her airway and prevent her from choking on her tongue.

Choking

This happens when a small object or piece of food blocks the windpipe, causing coughing and breathing difficulty. It is important to dislodge the object quickly, so that the child can breathe normally. Choking is common in young children who tend to put everything they get hold of into their mouths.

Emergency

Call for emergency help immediately if:
- your child stops breathing or you cannot remove the blockage
- your child continues to choke after you think you have removed the blockage
- your child becomes unconscious.

Helping a baby under 12 months

1 Assess your baby's breathing. If he can cough forcefully or breathe, don't interfere and let him try to cough up the object. If he cannot cough forcefully or cannot breathe, proceed to step 2 (back blows).

Keep his head low and give five sharp blows on the back

2 Pick him up and, supporting his head and neck, turn him face down over your knee. Make sure that his head is lower than his body. Give five forceful back blows with the heel of your hand on the upper part of his back.

3 Turn him face up, supporting his head and neck. If he is still choking, give five chest thrusts. Use two fingers just below the nipple line and depress the chest by at least one third of its depth or 4cm (1½in).

4 Repeat steps 2 and 3, alternating back blows and chest thrusts until either the airway is cleared, help arrives, or the baby becomes unconscious. If the baby is unconscious, ask a bystander to call 911 while you start full resuscitation (see pages 238–39). If you are alone, call 911 after five cycles of CPR (approximately two minutes).

Helping a child over one year

1 Stay with your child and encourage him to cough up the obstruction. Do not interfere unless his cough becomes weak, or he emits a high pitched crowing noise when he breathes. If that happens, tell him that you are going to help him.

2 Stand or kneel behind him and wrap your arms around his waist. To find the correct position, find his hip bones with your hands. Place your fist midline above the level of the other hand (it should be just at or above the navel) and, holding the fist with your other hand, press inward and upward with a sudden, forceful thrust.

3 If the obstruction doesn't clear with five abdominal thrusts, proceed to back blows. Make him bend forwards. Give him five sharp blows between the shoulder blades.

4 If the back blows fail, give another five abdominal thrusts followed by five back blows. Repeat the cycle until either help arrives, the child recovers, or he becomes unconscious. If he is unconscious, proceed to CPR and ask a bystander to call 911. If you are alone, call 911 after five cycles.

Warning

- If the baby or child loses consciousness at any point, begin CPR (see page 240). Check for the obstruction in the mouth each time you open the airway to give a rescue breath.
- Any baby or child who has been given thrusts must be checked by a doctor afterwards.

Suffocation

Anything that is lying across your child's face may block his mouth and nose, and prevent him from breathing.

What can I do?

1 Remove whatever is covering your child's face.

2 Check to see if your child is conscious and breathing (see page 238).

Emergency

Call for emergency help immediately if your child:
- becomes unconscious
- stops breathing, even if only for a few seconds
- shows any worrying symptoms.

If he is not breathing, start CPR immediately (see pages 239–40), and ask someone to call for emergency help.

If he is unconscious but breathing, place him in the recovery position (see page 241), then call for emergency help.

If he is conscious, simply comfort and reassure him while you wait for emergency service to arrive.

Drowning

Babies and children can drown even in very shallow water. When a young child's face is submerged, her automatic reaction is to take a deep breath to scream, rather than to lift her face up out of the water.

What can I do?

Get the child out of the water if it is safe to do so. Lift her very gently, and make sure you do not twist her back. Carry her with her head lower than her body, so that water can drain from her mouth. Once she is out of the water, lay her down and check for consciousness and breathing (see page 238).

If she is conscious, take off her wet clothes, replace them with dry clothes, and wrap her up to keep her warm.

If she is breathing normally but is unconscious, place her in the recovery position so that water can drain from her airways. Call for emergency help. If possible lay her on a coat or blanket, and replace any wet clothing with dry clothes. Wrap her in a blanket to keep her warm.

If she is not breathing, ask someone to call for emergency help. Clear any obvious debris, such as seaweed, from her mouth, and begin CPR. If you are on your own shout for help, but give CPR for five cycles (approximately 2 minutes) before stopping to call the emergency services.

Emergency

Call for emergency help immediately if your child has been rescued from drowning, even if she isn't unconscious, as water may have entered her lungs.

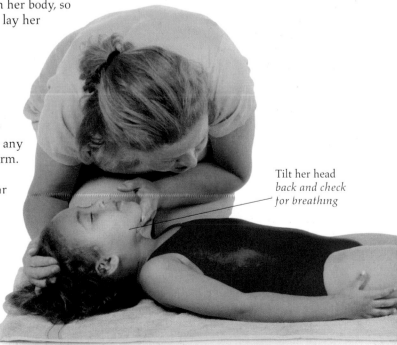

Tilt her head *back and check for breathing*

Warning

It is vital to keep your child warm as children can develop hypothermia after even a short period in cold water.

Shock

Shock is a condition in which blood pressure suddenly drops, depriving the body's vital organs of oxygen. It can occur as a reaction to any severe injury, especially heavy bleeding or severe burns.

Symptoms
- Pale, cold, sweaty skin
- blue or greyish tinge inside the lips or under the fingernails
- rapid and shallow breathing
- restlessness
- drowsiness or confusion
- unconsciousness.

Emergency
Call for emergency help immediately if your child is in shock.

What can I do?

1 Lay your child down, ideally on a blanket to protect him from the cold ground. Raise and support his legs high on a pile of cushions or a chair. If you suspect a broken leg, or a poisonous bite on his leg, do not raise the affected area.

2 Cover him with a blanket or coat, or cuddle him, to keep him warm. **Do not** try to warm him up with a hot water bottle or an electric blanket – this only draws blood away from the vital body organs to the skin.

3 If he complains of thirst, moisten his lips with a damp cloth. **Do not** give him anything to eat or drink.

4 If he becomes unconscious, check his breathing (see page 238).

If the child is not breathing, start CPR immediately (see pages 239–40).

If the child is breathing normally, put him into the recovery position (see page 241).

Poisoning

Post the number of the nearest Poison Control Centre by your phone. Poisoning is one of the most common emergencies in young children.

What can I do?

1 Call for emergency help immediately if you think that she has swallowed something poisonous.

2 If you see signs of burning around your child's mouth, wipe her face and mouth with a wet cloth. Do not give fluids.

3 Do not try to make her vomit. Induce vomiting only on the advice of your doctor or the Poison Control Centre. If she vomits, keep a sample as this can help the emergency services to identify what she took.

4 Save any containers that might have held poison and take them to the emergency department with you.

If she loses consciousness, check breathing, and be prepared to begin CPR if she is not breathing.

If she is unconscious but breathing, place her in the recovery position.

Symptoms
Your child's symptoms will depend on the type of poison she has swallowed. You may notice any of these signs:
- stomach pain
- vomiting
- symptoms of shock (see above)
- seizures
- drowsiness
- unconsciousness
- burns or discolouration around the mouth if your child has swallowed a corrosive poison
- poison or empty container nearby.

Warning
If a child needs CPR and there is poison around her mouth, place a pocket mask over her mouth first.

Burns and scalds

All burns and scalds carry a serious risk of infection. A burn that causes only superficial reddening of the skin and is less than 2–3cm (1in) is a minor burn, and can be treated at home first before you seek medical advice. Any deeper burn or burns that affect a larger area need medical attention as there is also a risk of shock if a lot of fluid is lost from the burn.

> ## Emergency
> **Get your child emergency medical help immediately** if:
> - the burn covers an area of more than about 2–3cm (1in)
> - the burn was caused by an electric shock (see page 251)
> - the casualty is a baby
> - the burn has affected all the layers of skin (deep), however small it is.

Minor burns

What can I do?

1 Cool the burn immediately by holding it under cold running water for 10 minutes or until the pain eases.

2 Cover with a clean non-fluffy dressing. Don't use an adhesive bandage as the burned area may be more extensive than you think. Seek medical advice.

Do not burst any blisters – they protect the damaged area underneath while the new skin is growing.

Do not put any cream, lotion, or adhesive dressing on the burn.

Burning clothes

What can I do?

1 Stop the child from moving since movement will fan the flames. Lay your child on the ground with the burning area up.

2 Put out the fire by throwing water on it or smothering the flames with a rug, blanket, or heavy curtain, keeping this away from your child's head if possible.
Don't throw water over him if he is near an electrical appliance that is turned on.
Don't try to smother the flames with nylon or any other flammable fabric.

3 When the flames are out, treat your child for a major burn (see right).

Major burns

What can I do?

1 To stop the burning and relieve the pain, cool the burn with cold running water for 10 minutes or until pain eases.

Do not immerse a young child in cold water as there is a risk of hypothermia.

2 While cooling the burn, remove clothing from around the burned area before it swells. Cut clothing away if required.

Do not remove anything sticking to the burn. Never touch or burst any blisters.

3 Cover the burn with a clean, non-fluffy material to protect it from infection. If you don't have a sterile dressing, a clean handkerchief or a pillow case will do. The dressing does not need to be secured. Ensure that the child remains warm to prevent the onset of hypothermia. Seek emergency medical help immediately.

4 Check for symptoms of shock. If she complains of thirst, moisten her lips with a damp cloth, but do not give her anything to drink. Take her to the hospital.

Serious bleeding

If blood spurts from a wound or if bleeding continues, try to stem the flow so that the blood has a chance to clot. Use disposable gloves; alternatively wash your hands before and after treatment.

Emergency
Take your child to hospital as soon as you have given first aid if he has been bleeding heavily.

What can I do?

1 Press a sterile dressing or pad of clean non-fluffy material over the wound. If there is a foreign object embedded in the wound, treat as below.

2 Raise the injured part above the level of his heart to reduce the blood flow to the area.

3 Lay your child down, keeping his injury raised and supported if possible. Keep pressing on the injury for at least 10 minutes.

4 Secure the original pad with a bandage. If blood seeps through the first dressing, place another one on top and secure it.

5 If blood seeps through the second dressing, too, do not remove them. Add more dressings and continue to apply pressure. Seek emergency help if you cannot control the bleeding.

6 Check for symptoms of shock (see page 244), and treat your child for this if necessary.

Embedded objects

Small pieces of dirt in a cut will be washed out by bleeding. However, if your child has a foreign object stuck in a wound do not attempt to remove it as you may cause more damage. Try to stop the bleeding, bandage, and take your child to the hospital.

Emergency
● **Take your child to hospital as soon as you have given first aid** if he has something embedded in a wound.
● Treat for shock if necessary (see page 244).

What can I do?

1 Help your child rest. Apply pressure on either side of the object and raise the injured part above the level of your child's heart. **Do not** try to remove any objects that are embedded in a wound as you may cause further damage and bleeding.

Apply pressure *on either side of the wound*

2 Loosely place a piece of clean gauze over the wound and object to minimize the risk of infection.

3 Use spare bandage rolls to build up padding to the same height as the embedded object.

Bandage *over padding*

4 Secure the padding by bandaging over it, being careful not to press on the embedded object. Take your child to hospital.

Cuts and scrapes

Cuts and scrapes are common throughout childhood, and you can treat most of them yourself. Make sure that you keep your child's tetanus injections up to date. Treat an animal bite as a cut, but if your child receives a poisonous bite or sting, see page 252.

Emergency
Take your child to hospital as soon as you have given first aid if:
- the cut is large or deep
- the cut is jagged or gapes open
- your child has cut his face badly
- the cut or scrape is very dirty
- your child has a puncture wound (a deep cut with a small opening in the skin) caused by something dirty.

☎ Seek medical help
Seek medical help as soon as possible if the area around the wound later becomes tender and red – it may be infected.

What can I do?

1 Wash your hands. Clean the cut by holding it under running water for some time, or wiping gently around it with an antiseptic wipe or a cotton ball soaked in warm water. Use a clean cotton ball for each stroke. **Do not** remove anything that is embedded in the cut (see opposite).

If your child has been bitten by an animal, wash the wound with soap and water and contact your doctor.

2 If the cut continues to bleed, press a pad such as a clean handkerchief or a non-fluffy cloth firmly on it for a few minutes.

Place a bandage over the cut

3 Put an adhesive bandage or dressing over the cut to help protect the wound and keep it clean. **Do not** put any antiseptic ointment on your child's cut except on your doctor's advice.

4 Keep the cut covered with an adhesive bandage or a dressing until it has completely healed. This ensures that the area remains moist, and helps the cut heal more quickly. Change the bandage or dressing every day.

Nose bleeds

Nose bleeds are very common in young children and can result from a bump on the nose, nose-picking, or excessive nose-blowing. A few children seem prone to nose bleeds, which can be because they have fragile blood vessels in their noses.

What can I do?

1 Apply direct pressure by pinching the entire fleshy part below the bridge of her nose firmly with your thumb and index finger. Lean her forward to allow the blood to drain from the nose and mouth.

2 After 10 minutes, release the pressure gradually. If the bleeding has stopped, have your child sit quietly. If it has not, pinch her nose for another 10 minutes.

3 Don't let your child blow her nose for about 4 hours after the bleeding has stopped.

☎ Seek medical help
Seek medical help if your child's nose is still bleeding just as badly after half an hour. Consult your doctor if your child has frequent, severe nose bleeds.

Head and face injury

Bumps on the head are common in young children. A cut on the forehead or scalp, even a small one, is likely to bleed profusely. If your child has had a severe blow to her head, she may have a concussion, which results when the brain is shaken within the skull, or compression caused by bleeding inside the skull – this may not be apparent for some hours.

What can I do?

1 If your child's head is bruised, hold a cloth that has been wrung out in very cold water, or an ice pack wrapped in a cloth, over the bruise for 15 minutes. This may stop it from swelling. Check the skin underneath the pack regularly, and remove the pack if a red patch with a white waxy centre develops.

2 If there is a wound, place a clean cloth over the cut and press against the wound, just as you would for bleeding anywhere else on the body (see page 246).

Emergency

Call for emergency help immediately if your child has injured her head and shows any unusual behaviour or has any of these symptoms up to 24 hours later:
- unconsciousness, however brief
- vomiting more than twice
- noisy breathing or snoring if your child doesn't normally snore
- difficulty in waking, or abnormal drowsiness
- discharge of clear or blood-stained fluid from her nose or ear
- unusual crying
- severe headache
- dislike of bright light.

3 Watch your child carefully for the next 24 hours in case she develops any of the emergency signs listed above. If she bumped her head badly, wake her every three hours – **if she won't wake up, call for emergency help immediately.**

If a discharge of clear or blood-stained fluid trickles from your child's nose or ear, lay her down with a pad of clean material placed under her nose or ear. If she deteriorates or loses consciousness, assess her condition (see page 238). Be prepared to begin CPR (see page 239–40). If breathing, place her in the recovery position (see page 241). **Call an ambulance.**

Broken teeth

If your child has broken a tooth, or one has become dislodged, put the broken piece in some milk, and take your child and her tooth to your dentist or to hospital immediately.

Put *your child in the recovery position*

Bruises and swelling

A bruise appears when a fall or blow causes bleeding into the tissues beneath the skin, causing swelling and discolouring.

Crushed fingers and toes

If your child has crushed his fingers in a door or window, or dropped something heavy on his foot, hold the injured area under cold running water for a few minutes. If it is very swollen, or still painful after about half an hour, take your child to the hospital.

What can I do?

1 Hold a pad that has been wrung out in very cold water, or an ice pack wrapped in a cloth, over the bruise for about 15 minutes, repeat if necessary. This should help to reduce pain and swelling.

Apply *a cold compress*

2 If your child seems to be in great pain or if it hurts him to use a bruised limb, especially if the swelling is severe, check for any signs of a sprained joint or a broken bone (see opposite).

Sprained joints

If the ligaments that support a joint are damaged, it is said to be sprained. This can cause symptoms very similar to those of a broken bone: if you are not sure which it is, treat as a broken bone (see below).

What can I do?

1 Taking care not to pull or twist the injured joint, gently take off your child's shoe and sock, or any other items that might constrict swelling around the injury.

2 Raise and support the injured joint in the most comfortable position for your child, then hold a cloth wrung out in ice-cold water, or an ice pack wrapped in a cloth, on the joint for 15 minutes, to reduce swelling and pain.

3 A thick layer of cotton wrapped around the joint may feel comforting. However, if you have any doubt, immobilize the joint as for a fracture (see below). In either case, seek medical attention as soon as you have given first aid.

Emergency
Get medical help as soon as you have given first aid.

Symptoms
- Pain in the injured area
- swelling and, later, bruising
- difficulty moving the joint.

Fractures and dislocated joints

Broken bones are unusual in young children – their bones have not hardened, so they are flexible and tend to bend rather than break. Sometimes there may be a partial break, which mends easily. A joint is dislocated if one or more bones slip out of place.

Symptoms
- Severe pain in the injured area
- swelling and, later, bruising
- difficulty moving the injured part
- misshapen appearance to the injured part – a limb may be bent in an odd way, or may look shorter than the uninjured limb.

Tie the bandages on the uninjured side

For a broken leg or ankle, lay your child down and put padding around the injured area and between his knees and ankles. Bandage the injured leg to the uninjured one, securing it above and below the injury. Put some padding under the knots.

What can I do?

1 Expose the injured area by gently removing any constricting clothing (you may need to cut it off) or loosening his shoe. Do not move him unless it is essential.

2 Support the injured part in the most comfortable position for your child. For a broken wrist, arm, or collar-bone, put padding around the injured area and, if your child will let you, gently fold his arm across his chest, then support it in an arm sling, fastening the bandage with a reef knot tied just below the shoulder. Don't try to force his arm into this position. If he can't bend it, surround it with padding, and put a folded triangular bandage right

Arm sling   **Elevation sling**

around the arm and body. If there is bleeding that needs to be reduced, the arm should be raised in an elevation sling. The fingertips are brought up to the level of the opposite shoulder, the sling is wrapped around the arm, passed from the elbow across the back, and tied at the shoulder.

3 Check for symptoms of shock and treat him for this if necessary (see page 244). If you think he has a broken leg, don't raise his legs.

Emergency
Call for emergency help as soon as you have given first aid.

Foreign object in the eye

Eyelashes or particles of dust can easily get into the eye. If your child's eye seems irritated but you can't see anything in it, it may be an eye infection (see page 209).

Symptoms
- Pain in the eye
- red, watering eye
- your child may rub her eye.

Chemicals in the eye

If your child has splashed any chemicals or corrosive fluids in her eyes, wash her eyes out immediately under cold running water, keeping her eyelids apart with your fingers. If only one eye is affected, tilt her head so that the injured eye is lower, and the chemical cannot wash over into the uninjured one. Then cover the eye with a pad, and take your child to a hospital. If possible, take the chemical bottle with you.

What can I do?

1 Wait a few minutes to see if the natural watering of the eye washes the foreign object away. Try to stop your child from rubbing her eye.

2 Sit your child down, facing the light. Separate the eyelids. Ask her to look right, left, up, and down. Make sure that you examine all of the eye.

3 If you can see the foreign object, wash it out using a jug of clean water. Aim for the inner corner, so that water will wash over the eye. Or, use a damp swab or handkerchief to lift it off.

4 If an object is under the eyelid, you can ask an older child to clear it by lifting the upper eyelid over the lower. You will need to do this for a younger child; wrap her in a towel first to stop her grabbing your arms. If the eye is still red or sore once the object has been removed, take her to the hospital.

A foreign object that cannot be removed

Cover the eye with a sterile dressing. Reassure the child and take her to the hospital.

Foreign object in the ear

Insects may crawl into your child's ear, and children may push small objects into their ears. Don't let your child play with beads or similar small objects until she is old enough to understand that they should not be put into her ears.

Symptoms
- Tickling in the ear
- partial deafness
- your child may rub or tug at her ear.

What can I do?

1 If your child has an insect in her ear, she may be very alarmed. Sit her down and support her head with the affected ear uppermost. Gently flood the ear with tepid water so that the insect floats out. If you can't remove the insect, take your child to hospital.

2 Children often push things into their ears. A hard object may become stuck. This may result in pain and temporary deafness; it may damage the ear drum. Do not attempt to remove the object, even if you can see it. Reassure your child and ask her what she put into her ear. Take your child to the hospital.

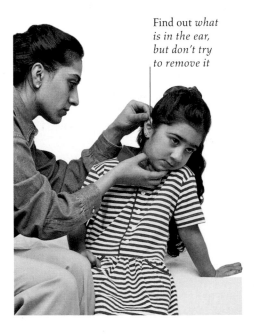

Find out *what is in the ear, but don't try to remove it*

Foreign object in the nose

Children sometimes stuff small pieces of food or other objects, such as beads or marbles, up their noses.

Symptoms
● Smelly, blood-stained discharge from the nose.

What can I do?
If your child can blow her nose, help her to do so, one nostril at a time. If this does not dislodge the object, take her to the hospital immediately.

Electric shock

A mild electrical shock gives only a brief pins-and-needles sensation. A severe one can knock your child down, render her unconscious, and stop both breathing and heartbeat. Electric current can also burn. Factors that affect the severity of the injury are: the voltage, the type of current, and the path of the current. Be aware that a high-voltage jolt may cause the child to fall resulting in spinal injuries and fractures.

Electrical burns
Electricity can burn where the current enters the body and where it leaves, so your child may have burns where she touched the electrical source and anywhere that was in contact with the ground. Although these burns may look small, they are often very deep.

What can I do?

1 Switch off the current, at the source if possible.

If you can't do this, stand on an insulating material – such as a rubber mat, a pile of dry newspapers, or a phone directory. Separate your child from the electrical source by pushing the cable away, using a dry, non-conducting object, such as a wooden chair or broom handle.

If nothing is available, drag your child away, insulating your hand as much as you can by wrapping it in a dry cloth or newspaper. Grasp your child's clothes, and avoid touching her skin.

2 Check to see if your child is conscious (see page 238).

If she is unconscious, check her breathing. If she is not breathing, start CPR (see page 239–40) immediately. If your child is breathing, put her in the recovery position (see page 241).

If she is conscious, comfort and reassure her. Look for symptoms of shock (see page 244).

3 Examine her for any burns: check areas that were in contact with the electrical source or the ground (burns will look red or scorched, and may swell). If you find any, treat them as severe burns (see page 245).

Emergency
Call for emergency help as soon as you have given first aid if:
● your child was unconscious, even if only for a few seconds
● she has any electrical burns.

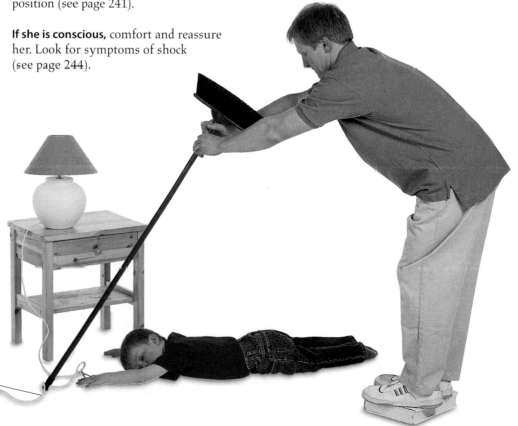

Move *the cable rather than your child's arm*

Minor bites and stings

While they may be painful and uncomfortable, most bites or stings from plants and insects are not usually life threatening for your child. However, a few people develop a serious allergic reaction to stings that can lead to shock, and therefore need urgent medical treatment.

Symptoms
- Sharp pain
- redness
- slight swelling
- itching.

What can I do?

1 If your child has been stung by a bee, check whether the stinger has been left in the skin. Brush or scrape it off with a flat object, such as a credit card. Do not use tweezers or your fingers as you may squeeze more poison out.

2 Hold a cloth that has been wrung out in ice cold water over the sting.

3 Soothe the area around the sting, which will quickly become red, swollen, and itchy, by dabbing it gently with a cotton pad dipped in rubbing alcohol or a paste of baking soda and water.

If your child has been stung in his mouth, the swelling of tissues in the mouth may cause the airway to become blocked. Give him a cold drink or, if your child is over two, let him suck an ice cube. Call for emergency help.

Emergency
Take your child to the emergency department as soon as you have given first aid if he:
- has difficulty breathing
- develops a widespread rash with welts
- feels dizzy, or faints
- develops symptoms of shock (see page 244)
- has a sting inside his mouth.

Snake and spider bites, and scorpion stings

Bites from snakes and poisonous spiders and scorpion stings are always serious for young children. Snake bites carry a risk of tetanus, but your child can be vaccinated against this.

What can I do?

1 Calm your child, and help him lie down. Keep the bitten part still, and position it below the level of his heart.

2 Call for emergency help. Meanwhile, wash the bite with soap and water, but do not suck out any poison.

3 Carefully place a clean, sterile dressing over the affected area.

4 Immobilize the limb with padding. If the hand or foot feels numb or cold, loosen the bandages.

5 Reassure your child. Keep him still to stop the venom from spreading through the body.

6 Check for shock. If he loses consciousness, check his breathing.

Symptoms
Your child's symptoms will depend on what has bitten or stung him; some symptoms may not appear for a few hours:
- severe pain
- one or two puncture marks
- swelling
- nausea or vomiting
- difficulty breathing
- shock (see page 244)
- seizures
- drowsiness
- unconsciousness.

Emergency
Call an ambulance immediately. Give first aid while waiting for help, if your child has been bitten by a snake, spider, or a scorpion.

Clean *and dry the wound*

Raise the heart *above the level of the bite*

Frostbite

Frostbite is damage to tissue due to exposure to cold. It is most likely to happen to body parts that are the furthest away from the heart, such as the fingers, toes, or ears.

Symptoms
- Skin is cold, hard, and white
- fingers, toes, or ears become red and painful when warmed.

What can I do?

1 Put the frozen part of your child's body under your arm.

2 If frostbite is severe, and medical help is not available, immerse the affected area in warm water.

3 If there is tissue damage, take the child to your doctor.

☎ Seek medical help
Get medical advice if:
- there is tissue damage
- your child is lethargic or disoriented.

Thorns and splinters

Thorns or tiny splinters of wood, glass, or metal will often become embedded in a child's hands or feet. They carry a risk of infection because they are rarely clean.

What can I do?

Grasp the end of the splinter with tweezers

1 Clean the area around the splinter with soap and water, and gently pat it dry.

2 Using a pair of tweezers, grasp the end of the splinter as close to the skin as you can. Carefully draw it out at the same angle that it entered the skin.

3 If a small thorn or splinter has gone straight down into the skin, and is not painful, it is best to leave it alone. It will probably work its own way out. Watch for signs of infection.

☎ Seek medical help
Get medical advice if:
- a splinter is embedded
- the embedded splinter is glass or metal
- the area around a splinter becomes red, swollen, or tender 48 hours later.

Blisters

Blisters form when burns, scalds, or repeated friction damage the skin. The fluid-filled blister forms on the top layer of the skin to protect the new skin that is forming underneath.

Cover the blister with a special blister bandage to prevent your child's shoe from rubbing it

What can I do?

1 Don't burst or prick the blister or try to remove the top layer of skin. This will leave the raw skin open to infection. Protect it with a dressing. Dress your child in clothes that will not rub against it.

2 If the blister bursts, cover with an adhesive bandage with a large enough pad to cover the whole blister, or a special blister bandage.

Growth charts: girls

Growth charts are an important way to monitor your child's growth. They provide you with the information to interpret how well your child is growing. The charts below show average growth (the solid line), and the range of normal measurements. Your doctor will check your baby's progress by weighing and measuring her regularly and marking her own growth curve on a similar chart. The shape of her curve should run parallel to the "average" curve: this shows a healthy rate of growth.

Head circumference

Your nurse practitioner or doctor will pass a tape measure around your baby's head (see page 81). During the first year, head circumference is an easy-to-measure yardstick of healthy growth.

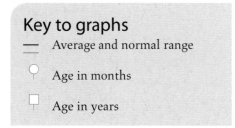

Key to graphs

— Average and normal range

○ Age in months

□ Age in years

Data sources:
World Health Organization (WHO) Child Growth Standards (2006) and WHO Reference (2007), adapted for Canada by Dieticians of Canada, Canadian Paediatric Society, the College of Family Physicians of Canada, and Community Health Nurses of Canada.

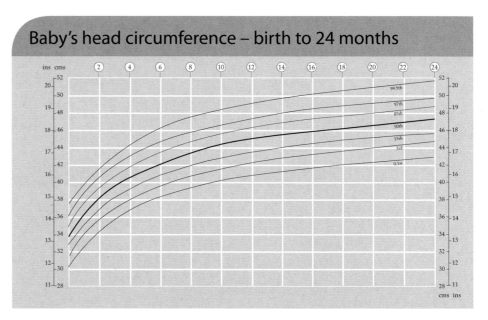

Baby's head circumference – birth to 24 months

Your child's height

Once your child is able to stand unaided, measure her against a wall every six months. She should stand close to it, without shoes and with feet together. Use a ruler at right angles to the wall to mark her height, then measure the distance to the floor. Don't worry if your child has periods of slow growth interspersed with spurts; but if two consecutive measurements seem very low, consult your doctor.

Data sources:
World Health Organization (WHO) Child Growth Standards (2006) and WHO Reference (2007), adapted for Canada by Dieticians of Canada, Canadian Paediatric Society, the College of Family Physicians of Canada, and Community Health Nurses of Canada.

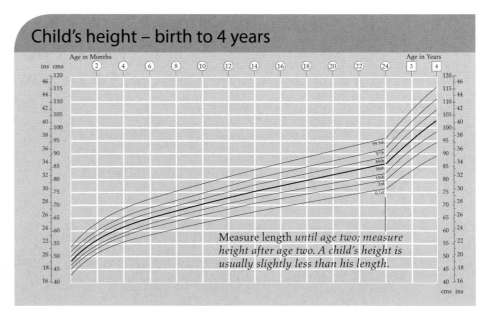

Child's height – birth to 4 years

Measure length until age two; measure height after age two. A child's height is usually slightly less than his length.

Your baby's weight

Your baby's weight gain is a vital indicator of her general health and well-being throughout the first year. Do remember that the range of "normal" weights at a given age is very wide. Ask your nurse practitioner or doctor to weigh your baby once a month, and more often if you are at all worried that she might not be gaining normally.

Data sources:
World Health Organization (WHO) Child Growth Standards (2006) and WHO Reference (2007), adapted for Canada by Dieticians of Canada, Canadian Paediatric Society, the College of Family Physicians of Canada, and Community Health Nurses of Canada.

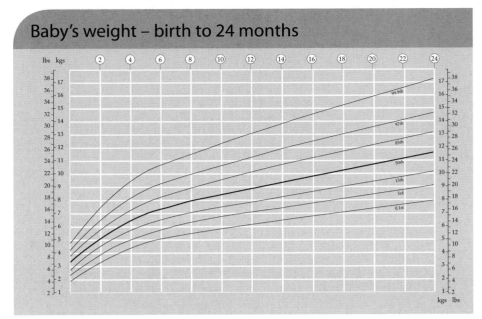

Your child's weight

After her first birthday, weigh your child naked about every six months. She won't put on weight steadily, but the periods of slow and rapid growth should balance out. She shouldn't lose weight. If she seems overweight, she probably only needs to mark time until her height catches up. Ask your doctor's advice if her weight drops, or if two consecutive measurements are less than you would expect. Although it's normal, try to resist comparing her weight to others of her age.

Data sources:
World Health Organization (WHO) Child Growth Standards (2006) and WHO Reference (2007), adapted for Canada by Dieticians of Canada, Canadian Paediatric Society, the College of Family Physicians of Canada, and Community Health Nurses of Canada.

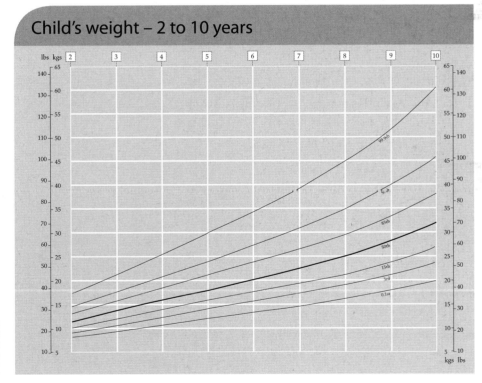

Healthy bodies, healthy weights

With over one third of Canadian children being overweight, it is important to build in healthy nutrition and life habits from a young age. Healthy eating starts with breastfeeding (which has a protective effect against childhood obesity) and continues with Canada's Food Guide. However, it is equally important to build regular activity into your child's routine. We know that regular exercise builds strong bones, strengthens muscles (including the heart), and achieves a healthy weight. Young children are constantly moving. However, as they get older, they start to spend more time watching television and playing computer games. You can have fun helping your child stay active by limiting her time spent in front of the TV or computer screen and encouraging enjoyable physical activity. Set an example and include your child as you take the stairs, go on "adventure walks," or play outside. Rake leaves or shovel snow together. Play sports together. Dance! You will both experience the benefits and fun of healthy activity.

Growth charts: boys

The charts below show average growth (the solid line), and the range of normal measurements. Your doctor will check your baby's progress by weighing and measuring him regularly and marking his own growth curve on a similar chart. The shape of his curve should run parallel to the "average" curve: this shows a healthy rate of growth. However, the growth charts are not diagnostic instruments, but just tools that contribute to forming an overall clinical impression for the child being measured.

Head circumference

Your nurse practitioner or doctor will pass a tape measure around your baby's head (see page 81). During the first year, head circumference is an easy-to-measure yardstick of healthy growth.

Key to graphs

— Average and normal range

○ Age in months

□ Age in years

Data sources:
World Health Organization (WHO) Child Growth Standards (2006) and WHO Reference (2007), adapted for Canada by Dieticians of Canada, Canadian Paediatric Society, the College of Family Physicians of Canada, and Community Health Nurses of Canada.

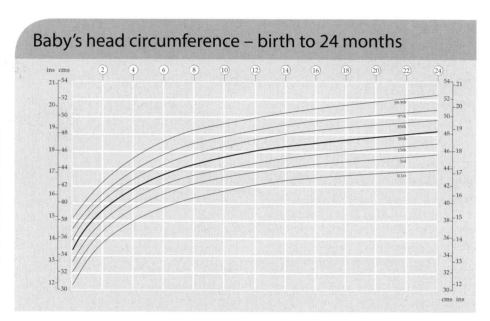

Baby's head circumference – birth to 24 months

Your child's height

Once you child is able to stand unaided, measure him against a wall every six months. He should stand close to it, without shoes and with feet together. Use a ruler at right angles to the wall to mark his height, then measure the distance to the floor. Don't worry if your child has periods of slow growth interspersed with spurts; but if two consecutive measurements seem low, consult your doctor.

Data sources:
World Health Organization (WHO) Child Growth Standards (2006) and WHO Reference (2007), adapted for Canada by Dieticians of Canada, Canadian Paediatric Society, the College of Family Physicians of Canada, and Community Health Nurses of Canada.

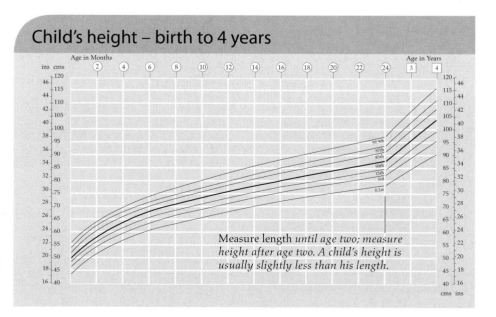

Child's height – birth to 4 years

Measure length until age two; measure height after age two. A child's height is usually slightly less than his length.

Your baby's weight

Your baby's weight gain is a vital indicator of his general health and well-being throughout the first year. Ask your nurse practitioner or doctor to weigh him once a month, and more often if you are at all worried that he might not be gaining normally.

Data sources:
World Health Organization (WHO) Child Growth Standards (2006) and WHO Reference (2007), adapted for Canada by Dieticians of Canada, Canadian Paediatric Society, the College of Family Physicians of Canada, and Community Health Nurses of Canada.

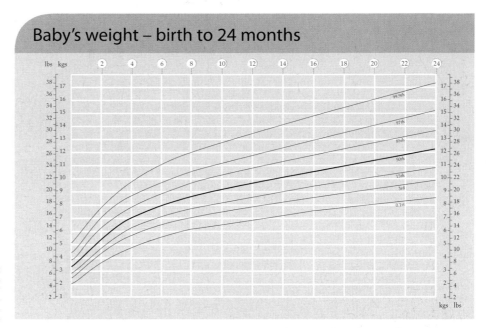

Baby's weight – birth to 24 months

Your child's weight

After his first birthday, weigh your child naked about every six months. He won't put weight on steadily, but the periods of slow and rapid growth should balance out. He shouldn't lose weight: if he seems overweight, he probably only needs to mark time until his height catches up. Ask your doctor for advice if his weight drops, or if two consecutive measurements are less than you would expect. Your doctor will help evaluate your child's weight using tools such as body mass index (BMI) and growth charts.

Data sources:
World Health Organization (WHO) Child Growth Standards (2006) and WHO Reference (2007), adapted for Canada by Dieticians of Canada, Canadian Paediatric Society, the College of Family Physicians of Canada, and Community Health Nurses of Canada.

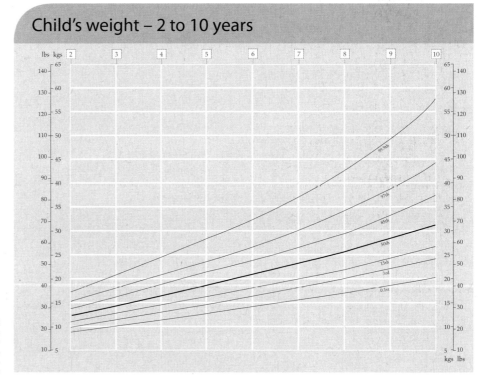

Child's weight – 2 to 10 years

Healthy bodies, healthy weights

With over one third of Canadian children being overweight, it is important to build in healthy nutrition and life habits from a young age. Healthy eating starts with breastfeeding (which has a protective effect against childhood obesity) and continues with Canada's Food Guide. However, it is equally important to build regular activity into your child's routine. We know that regular exercise builds strong bones, strengthens muscles (including the heart), and achieves a healthy weight. Young children are constantly moving. However, as they get older, they start to spend more time watching television and playing computer games. You can have fun helping your child stay active by limiting his time spent in front of the TV or computer screen and encouraging enjoyable physical activity. Set an example and include your child as you take the stairs, go on "adventure walks," or play outside. Rake leaves or shovel snow together. Play sports together. Dance! You will both experience the benefits and fun of healthy activity.

Useful addresses

Prenatal resources

Babycenter Canada
www.babycenter.ca
Information on pregnancy and childbirth

Canadian Association of Midwives
59 Riverview Road
Montréal, QC
H8R 3R9
(514) 807-3668
www.canadianmidwives.org

Doulas of North America
1582 S. Parker Road, Ste 201
Denver, CO 80231
(888) 788-3662
www.dona.org

Healthy Canadians
www.healthycanadians.ca

International Childbirth Education Association
1500 Sunday Drive, Ste 102
Raleigh, NC 27607
(800) 624-4934
www.icea.org
Includes Canadian resources for finding a childbirth class or a doula

Lamaze International
2025 M Street, NW, Ste 800
Washington, D.C. 20036-3309
(202) 367-1128
www.lamaze.org

Motherisk
Main tel: (416) 813-6780
Alcohol and Substance Use helpline:
1-877-327-4636
Morning Sickness helpline:
1-800-436-8477
HIV and HIV Treatment helpline:
1-888-246-5840
www.motherisk.org
Information on the safety of medications, infections, chemicals, personal products, and everyday exposures during pregnancy and breastfeeding

My Fertility
16750 route Transcanadienne
Kirkland, QC
H9H 4M7
(514) 426-7300
www.myfertility.ca

Preeclampsia Foundation
6767 N Wickham Road, Ste 400
Melbourne, FL 32940
(800) 665.9341
www.preeclampsia.org

Society of Obstetricians and Gynaecologists of Canada
780 Echo Drive
Ottawa, ON
K1S 5R7
(613) 730-4192 / (800) 561-2416
www.sogc.org

Women's Health Matters
Women's College Hospital
76 Grenville Street, Room E140
Toronto, ON
M5S 1B2
www.womenshealthmatters.ca

Smoking cessation in pregnancy

Pregnets
(416) 535-8501 xt 6343
www.pregnets.org

Postpartum resources

BC Reproductive Mental Health Program
BC Women's Hospital & Health Centre
4500 Oak Street
Vancouver, BC
V6H 3N1
(604) 875-2424
www.bcwomens.ca

Breastfeeding Committee for Canada
P.O. Box 30071
North Vancouver, BC
V7H 2Y8
www.breastfeedingcanada.ca

Canadian Mental Health Association
Phenix Professional Building
595 Montreal Road, Ste 303
Ottawa, ON
K1K 4L2
(613) 745-7750
www.cmha.ca
Help with depression and postpartum psychosis

La Leche League Canada
P.O. Box 700
Winchester, ON
K0C 2K0
(613) 774-4900
www.lllc.ca

Postpartum Support International
6706 SW 54th Avenue
Portland, OR 97219
(800) 944-4773
www.postpartum.net
Includes resources for Canadians

Nutrition

Health Canada
In pregnancy:
www.hc-sc.gc.ca/fn-an/nutrition/prenatal/index-eng.php
For infants and children:
www.hc-sc.gc.ca/fn-an/nutrition/child-enfant/index-eng.php

Infant and child health

About Kids Health
The Hospital for Sick Children
555 University Avenue
Toronto, ON
M5G 1X8
www.aboutkidshealth.ca

Canadian Institute of Child Health
384 Bank Street, Ste 300
Ottawa, ON
K2P 1Y4
(613) 230-8838
www.cich.ca

Caring for Kids
Canadian Paediatric Society
2305 St. Laurent Boulevard
Ottawa, ON
K1G 4J8
(613) 526-9397
www.caringforkids.cps.ca

Healthy Children
American Academy of Pediatrics
141 Northwest Point Boulevard
Elk Grove Village, IL 60007-1098
(847) 434-4000
www.healthychildren.org

Immunizations

National Advisory Committee on Immunization
www.phac-aspc.gc.ca/naci-ccni

Public Health Agency of Canada
www.phac-aspc.gc.ca/im/iyc-vve/index-eng.php

First aid and safety

Canadian Red Cross
170 Metcalfe Street, Ste 300
Ottawa, ON
K2P 2P2
(613) 740-1900
www.redcross.ca

Child Safe Canada
#102–6449 Crowchild Trail South West
Calgary, AB
T3E 5R7
(403) 202-5900 / (780) 429-5900
www.childsafecanada.com

Children's Safety Association of Canada
385 The West Mall, Ste 250
Etobicoke, ON
M9C 1E7
(416) 620-1584 / (888) 499-4444
www.safekid.org

St. John Ambulance Canada
1900 City Park Drive, Ste 400
Ottawa, ON
K1J 1A3
(613) 236-7461
www.sja.ca

Transport Canada – Car Seat Information
(613) 998-8616 / (800) 333-0371
www.tc.gc.ca/eng/roadsafety/safedrivers-childsafety-index-53.htm

Child care

Canadian Child Care Federation
383 Parkdale Avenue, Ste 201
Ottawa, ON
K1Y 4R4
(613) 729-5289 / (800) 858-1412
www.cccf-fcsge.ca

Parents' groups

Bereaved Parents of Canada
(519) 927-3387
www.bereavedparentsofcanada.ca

Canadian Equal Parenting Groups
www.canadianequalparentinggroups.ca
Directory of groups to support children's relationships with both parents after divorce or separation

Canadian Foundation for the Study of Sudden Infant Death
60 James Street, Ste 403
St. Catharines, ON
L2R 7E7
(905) 688-8884 / (800) 363-7437
www.sidscanada.org

Multiple Births Canada
P.O. Box 432
Wasaga Beach, ON
L9Z 1A4
(705) 429-0901 / (866) 228-8824
www.multiplebirthscanada.org

Special needs

Asthma Society of Canada
4950 Yonge Street, Ste 2306
Toronto, ON
M2N 6K1
(416) 787-4050 / (866) 787-4050
www.asthma.ca

Autism Society Canada
Box 22017, 1670 Heron Road
Ottawa, ON
K1V 0C2
(613) 789-8943 / (866) 476-8440
www.autismsocietycanada.ca

Canadian Diabetes Association
1400-522 University Avenue
Toronto, ON
M5G 2R5
(800) 226-8464
www.diabetes.ca

Canadian Down Syndrome Society
#283–5005 Dalhousie Drive NW
Calgary, AB
T3A 5R8
(800) 883-5608
www.cdss.ca

Cerebral Palsy Support Foundation of Canada
10 Bassett Boulevard, Unit 35
Whitby, ON
L1N 9C3
(905) 259-3421
www.cpsc.ca

Spina Bifida and Hydrocephalus Association of Canada
167 Lombard Avenue, Ste 647
Winnipeg, MB
R3B 0V3
(204) 925-3650 / (800) 565-9488
www.sbhac.ca

Index

A

abbreviations, maternity records 33
abdomen
    signs of illness 190
    stomach pain 220
abdominal examinations
    baby 69, 81
    in pregnancy 35
abnormalities, congenital 19, 35, 36, 37
abscesses, breast 96
absence attacks 233
accidents
    first aid 237–53
    home safety 234–6
acetaminophen, bringing down a
    fever 194
activity games 172
AFP test 36
after pains 71
age of mother 10, 37
aggressive children 176
air travel 25
airway
    choking 242
    opening 238
alcohol 11, 13, 53, 93
allergies
    asthma 218–19
    and breastfeeding 87
    cow's milk 102
    eczema 228
    hives 227
ambulance, when to call 180, 188, 237
amniocentesis 36–7
amniotic fluid 23
amniotomy 66
anaesthesia
    Caesarean section 67
    epidural 64
    surgery on children 191
anatomy scans 36
anemia 34, 38
anencephaly 11
anger, and crying 119
animal bites 247
ankles, swollen 35, 42
anti-colic nipples 99
antibiotics 195
antibodies 21, 92
anxiety
    and crying 119
    separation anxiety 127, 160
    sleep problems 127
Apgar score 63
appendicitis 220
appetite, loss of 180, 186
aprons, waterproof 134
ARA-supplemented formula milk 103
areola 22, 91, 93
aspirin, safety 196, 203
assisted delivery 66
asthma 218–19
au pairs 161

B

babies
    bathing and washing 134–43
    breastfeeding 87–97
    clothes 128–33
    crying 117–19
    diapers 146–55
    giving medicine to 195
    growth and learning 162–77
    handling 82–6
    newborn screening 69
    play 86
    safety 235
    sex of 15
    sleep 120–27
    small for dates 38–9, 70
    travel 156–9
    see also newborn babies; premature
        babies; toddlers
"baby flat head" 120
baby lotion 148
baby monitors 121
baby oil 148
baby wipes 148
babysitters 160
babywalkers 167
back
    avoiding problems 44
    back injuries 237, 241
back labour 59
bacteria
    bottle-feeding and 101, 104
    food safety 53
    Group B streptococcus 57
bad behaviour and consequences 176
bad dreams 177
balanitis 225
balls 167, 173
barrier cream 148, 150, 151
bassinets 126, 156
bath mats 134
bath seats 140
bathing babies 134–43
bathrooms, safety 235
baths 134
bedding 121, 123
bedrooms
    equipment 120–21
    safety 235
beds
    caring for a sick child 199
    co-sleeping 87, 126
    home birth 55
bedtime routines 120, 122, 124–5, 127
bedwetting 155
bee stings 252
behaviour
    dealing with bad behaviour 176
    rewarding good behaviour 176
    symptoms of illness 186, 189
bibs 108
bilirubin 70
biophysical profile scan 36
birth 32–3, 61–3
birth centres 32
birth partners 58, 61
birthing balls 59
birthmarks 69
bisphenol A (BPA) 98
bites, first aid 252
biting, aggressive children 176
bladder
    after birth 71
    problems in children 224
blankets 121
    security 161, 177
bleeding
    after birth 63, 71
    gums 20, 40
    hemorrhage 63
    miscarriage 39

nose bleeds 247
    serious injuries 246
    vaginal 39
blepharitis 209
blisters 253
blocked ducts 96
blood
    disorders 37
    in stools 180
    tests 34, 36, 37, 69
    see also bleeding
blood pressure 35, 38, 40
body temperature 192–3
    babies 123
    chilling 184
    and crib death 123
    fever 180, 193–4
    overheating 184
    taking 189, 190, 193
    thermometers 189, 192–3
boiling method, sterilizing equipment 101
boils 226
bonding 87, 97
bones
    diagnosis guide 187
    fractures 249
books, reading to children 173
booster seats 109
booties 129
boots 133
bottle brushes 100
bottle-feeding 98–107
    away from home 105
    burping babies 99, 107
    demand feeding 88
    diaper contents 146
    equipment 98–101
    formula milk 99
    giving a bottle 106–7
    hygiene 100–101, 104
    making up feeds 102–6
    problems 106
    quantities 102
bottles 98
bouncing chairs 162
bowel movements
    abnormal-looking stools 223
    after birth 71
    blood in stools 180
    constipation 16, 17, 40, 221
    diaper contents 146
    diarrhea 101, 146, 185, 223
    meconium 31, 69, 146
    potty-training 154–5
bowls 108
boys
    cleaning bottom 135, 137, 151
    diapers 149
    genital problems 225
    newborn babies 69
brain
    concussion 248
    development of 25
    diagnosis guide 187
    epilepsy 233
    meningitis 208
bras 23, 29, 96
Braxton Hicks contractions 24, 30, 31, 56
breast pads 96
breast pumps 95
breast shells 96
breastfeeding 87–97
    after birth 62

changing to bottle-feeding 106
    demand feeding 88, 92
    diaper contents 146
    duration of 97
    latching on 90, 91
    milk coming in 93
    older babies 97
    and periods 73
    positions 90–91
    problems 96
    sick babies 198
    twins 88
    and vitamin D 92
    weaning 97
breasts
    after breastfeeding 93
    blocked ducts 96
    bras 23, 29
    engorged 93
    expressing milk 94–5
    leaking 96
    mastitis 96
    milk production 92
    newborn baby 69
    in pregnancy 16, 18, 20, 24
    signs of pregnancy 12
breath holding attacks 177
breathing
    cardiopulmonary resuscitation
        (CPR) 239–40
    checking 238
    in labour 49, 59, 60
    suffocation 243
breathlessness 40
breech birth 67
bronchiolitis 217
bronchitis 218
bruises 248
burns 245, 251
burping babies 88, 107
"butterfly mask" 21

C

Caesarean section 67, 72
caffeine 53, 93
calcium 40, 50
candida 42
car travel
    car seats 158–9
    potty-training and 155
    in pregnancy 21
    safety 158, 236
    soothing babies 125
cardiopulmonary resuscitation
    (CPR) 239–40
caregivers, childminding 161
carriages 122, 156–7
cat arching exercise 72
catching balls 173
cats, safety 13
celiac disease 223
cervix 14
    dilation 57, 60
    immunization against cancer 202
    incompetent 38
chairs, for babies 109
changing mats 147, 148
chapped skin 229
check-up, six-week 73
cheese 53
chemicals, in eye 250
chest compressions 239–40
chest infections 215, 217–19

Acknowledgments

Dorling Kindersley would like to thank the author, **Elizabeth Fenwick,**, for writing the original English edition of the book.

This revised edition
Out thanks to:
Medical consultants: **Dr Elizabeth Owen** and **Dr Su Laurent**
Healthcare consultant: **Ann Peters R.N H.V**
First-aid consultants: **Jemima Dunne** and **Dr. Viv Armstrong**

Child Growth Charts provided and approved by **WHO Multicentre Growth Reference Study Group**

Editorial assistance: **David Isaacs** and **Kate Meeker**
Design Styling: **Sara Kimmins**
Artworks: **Debbie Maizels and Philip Wilson**
Picture credits
Picture Researcher **Jenny Baskaya**
Picture Librarian **Romaine Werblow**

The publisher would like to thank the following for their kind permission to reproduce their photographs:
(Abbreviations key: t=top, b=bottom, r=right, l=left, c=center)

Alamy: Boccabella Debbie 21tl; Janine Wiedel 64bl; Martin Bobrovsky 117tl; Peter Griffin 140bc; Sabine Koldeweyh 119tr; Ulrich Niehoff 234tl ;
Corbis: Andrew Brookes 195tl; Aurelie and Morgan David de Lossy 159tc; Centers for Disease Control 203br; Corbis Yellow 117cc; Fabrice Lerouge 158tr; Image Source 97br; Kevin Dodge 156tl; Laura Dwight 146b; Left Lane Productions 159br; Marina Dempster 68tl; Nico Hermann 54tl; Tammy Hanratty 174tl; **Genesis Film Productions Limited:** Neil Bromhall 23crb; **Getty Images:** American Images Inc 117cl; Andersen Ross 12tl; Ariel Skelley 204br, 237tl; ColorBlind Images 168cl; Dennis O'Clair 1c; Elyse Lewin 125bl, 204bc; Jamie Grill 104br, 192tl; JGI/Jamie Grill 32 tl; Jose Luis Pelaez Inc 17tr; Jupiterimages 175tr; Keith Brofsky 43tl; LWA 70cr; Michael Krasowitz 87tl; PNC 158cl; Steve Wisbauer 148cc; Stockbyte 237cc; Studio Tec/ailead 173bl; Thinkstock 159cc; Vanessa Gavalya 71br; VCL/Justin Pumfrey 166-7c; Victoria Blackie 134tl; **Meningitis Research Foundation:** 208br; **Mother & Baby Picture Library:** Eddie Lawrence 67cr; Ian Hooton 17bl, 32, 33tr, 35tl, 36br, 59tr, 74-75, 80cc, 83r, 89, 178-179, 181c, 198cr, 199cr, 200tl, 202, 224cr, 244cr, 248tc; Moose Azim

96bl; Paul Mitchell 2-3, 8-9, 57tr, 160tl; Ruth Jenkinson, 81br; ©**Mothercare:** 156, 157b; **Science Photo Library:** AJ Photo 70bl; Dr H.C.Robinson 206br; Laurent Bsip 65br; **St John's Institute of Dermatology:** 228cl, 231tr; **St Mary's Hospital:** 183tl; **Sue Ford, Western Ophthalmic Hospital:** 183bl, 209r; **The Wellcome Insitute Library, London:** 209cl, 213bl, 226l, 227cla, 232l; **Dr Ian Williams/ msl:** 182tl, 203r, 210l 214cr, 227bl, 229br, 230tr

Jacket images
Front, Spine: **Getty Images:** LWA
Back: **Mother & Baby Picture Library:** Ian Hooton tr; Paul Mitchell tl

All other images © **Dorling Kindersley**
For further information see:
www.dkimages.com

Original edition
Senior Art Editor **Carole Ash**
Project Editors **Sarah Pearce**
Pregnancy and Birth **Tanya Hines**
Health Care **Claire Le Bas**

Art Editors
Pregnancy and Birth **Rowena Alsey**
Health Care **Tina Hill**
Production Manager **Michel Blake**
Editorial Direction **Daphne Razazan**

Picture credits
Picture Researcher **Anna Grapes**
Picture Librarians **Melanie Simmonds, Marcus Scott**

Illustrators
Coral Mula: all line artwork except 14t;
Nick Hall: 14t; **Kevin Jones Associates:** 234, 235, 236; **Richard Tibbitts:** 14, 16, 18, 20, 22, 24, 28, 30

Photography
Andy Crawford assisted by Gary Ombler, **Antonia Deutsch** assisted by Pamela Cowan, **Trish Gant, Steve Gorton, Dave King, Ray Moller, Stephen Oliver, Susannah Price, Steve Shott**

Loan or supply of props
Avent (baby feeding equipment); Mothercare; Baby B's, Fulham, London, England; Diana Dolls Fashions Inc., Stoney Creek, Ontario; The Nursery Collection, Watford, England; Porter Nash Medical, London, England; Seward Ltd., London, England. **Special thanks to:** Mary Snyder at Snugli, Inc.; Gerry Baby Products Company, Denver, Colorado; Judi's Originals, Scottsdale, Arizona.

Consultants
Dorling Kindersley acknowledges the contribution of the following consultants to the original edition:
Professor R. W. Taylor MD, FRCOG, Head of Department of Gynaecology, The United Medical Schools of Guy's and St. Thomas's Hospitals, London; **Professor Jon Scopes** MB, PhD, FRCP, Department of Paediatrics, St. Thomas's Hospital, London; **Christine Williams** RGN, HV, FWT, Health Visitor and Family Planning Nurse; **Janice Leighton** RGN, RM, Community Midwife; **Alan McLaughlin** RGN, Department of Clinical Neurology, St Thomas's Hospital, London.